Diagnosis and Nonsurgical Management of Osteoarthritis

Third Edition

Kenneth D. Brandt, MD

Professor of Medicine and
Professor of Orthopedic Surgery
Indiana University School of Medicine;
Director, Indiana University
Multipurpose Arthritis and
Musculoskeletal Diseases Center
Indianapolis, Indiana

D1115539

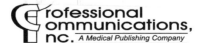

**rofessional
ommunications,
nc.** *A Medical Publishing Company*

Published by
Professional Communications, Inc.

Marketing Office:
400 Center Bay Drive
West Islip, NY 11795
(t) 631/661-2852
(f) 631/661-2167

Editorial Office:
PO Box 10
Caddo, OK 74729-0010
(t) 580/367-9838
(f) 580/367-9989

For orders only, please call
1-800-337-9838

or visit our website at
www.pcibooks.com

ISBN: 1-884735-87-8

Printed in the United States of America

DISCLAIMER
The opinions expressed in this publication reflect those of the author. However, the author makes no warranty regarding the contents of the publication. The protocols described herein are general and may not apply to a specific patient. Any product mentioned in this publication should be taken in accordance with the prescribing information provided by the manufacturer.

This text is printed on recycled paper.

DEDICATION

To Jill, David, Susan, and Paul

ACKNOWLEDGMENT

I remain grateful to my colleagues and friends involved in basic research, clinical research, and health services research in osteoarthritis (OA). I have cited their work extensively. It serves as the basis of our knowledge about OA, which has expanded strikingly in the past few years. Because of their efforts, management of OA today is better and safer than it has been previously.

I am grateful also to my patients, who have taught me much about OA and the burdens it imposes on people, and to my students and Fellows, whose questions repeatedly lead us to reconsider staid ideas and approaches and remind us that we do not have all the answers.

My appreciation goes to Deborah Jenkins, whose clerical assistance was extremely helpful in the preparation of this edition and, as was the case with the first two editions, my special thanks go to Kathie Lane for her help in assembling this extensively revised new edition. Finally, my thanks go to Phyllis Freeny and Malcolm Beasley for their help in publication of the monograph.

TABLE OF CONTENTS

TABLES

FIGURES

ix

COLOR PLATES

Foreword

The third edition of this monograph, like its predecessors, was written chiefly for primary care physicians. It is my hope that in it they will find practical information concerning the diagnosis and management of osteoarthritis (OA). Although the discussion is directed toward the general internist and specialist in family medicine, rheumatologists, orthopedic surgeons, arthritis health professionals, and researchers in academia or the pharmaceutical industry may also find it informative.

The interval between publication of the first and second editions of this book was 4 years; the span between the second and third editions is about 1 year shorter and changes between the second edition and this one are considerable. Chapters on drug therapy and nonpharmacologic therapy have been extensively revised. However, there are still gaps in our understanding of OA and its treatment, and many questions remain to be answered.

In the past few years, physicians, patients, and the lay public have been the recipients of a vast amount of information relating, for example, to the efficacy and safety of acetaminophen (ACET) and coxibs; nutracenticals, such as glucosamine; nonpharmacologic measures for treatment of OA, such as tidal irrigation of the knee and arthroscopic lavage and débridement; disease-modifying OA drugs (DMOADs); intra-articular hyaluronan therapy; and opioids for management of OA pain.

In the past 5 to 10 years, great strides have been made in understanding the pathogenetic mechanisms underlying the breakdown of joint tissues in OA. This new information is being used to develop drugs that we hope will modify the progression of joint damage in OA and, perhaps, even prevent or reverse such damage. The rate at which we are acquiring knowledge about pathogenetic mechanisms in OA, however, has outpaced the rate at which methodology suitable for evaluation of the effects of potential DMOADs has been developed. To date, none of the imaging modalities (a variety of radiographic protocols, magnetic resonance imaging, ultrasonography) or biochemical/immunochemical "markers" proposed for this use have been validated.

In the foreword to the second edition, we expressed concern that drugs that might slow the rate of progression of articular cartilage damage might not be accompanied by decreases in joint pain or mobility or improvement in other outcomes that are clinically important to the patient; that concern remains. Research priorities are sometimes not congruous with those of patients with OA.

Many physicians and patients still consider that OA is the inevitable result of aging or "wear-and-tear." This is reflected by continued usage of the inaccurate, depressing term, "degenerative joint disease." Consider the sense of inevitability and futility that label generates. OA is often viewed (incorrectly) as a condition that, once it becomes symptomatic, follows an inexorably progressive and downhill course, much like Alzheimer's disease. Physicians who convey this view to their patients do them a disservice. Many patients with OA can be made better; many will do well—perhaps, even better—without our intrusion.

It is important for both the patient and physician to understand that even though there is no cure for OA today, *much* can be done to relieve joint pain, improve mobility, and enhance quality of life. It is the objective of this monograph to assist the physician and, thereby, the patient, by providing information that may be useful in management of this disease.

1
Definition of Osteoarthritis

In 1994, at a workshop, "New Horizons in Osteoarthritis," sponsored by the American Academy of Orthopaedic Surgeons, the National Institute of Arthritis, Musculoskeletal, and Skin Diseases; the National Institute on Aging; the Arthritis Foundation; and the Orthopaedic Research and Education Foundation, osteoarthritis (OA) was defined more succinctly:[1]

"Osteoarthritis is a group of overlapping distinct diseases which may have different etiologies, but with similar biologic, morphologic, and clinical outcomes. The disease processes not only affect the articular cartilage, but involve the entire joint, including the subchondral bone, ligaments, capsule, synovial membrane, and periarticular muscles. Ultimately, the articular cartilage degenerates with fibrillation, fissures, ulceration, and full thickness of the joint surface."

Depending on the absence or presence of an identifiable local or systemic etiologic factor, OA has been classified into idiopathic (or primary) and secondary forms. **Table 1.1** depicts the classification scheme developed in the 1986 international conference on OA.[2]

Idiopathic OA is divided into localized and generalized forms. In the latter, OA involves three or more joint groups. For example, a patient with OA localized to the hands but involving one or more distal interphalangeal joints, one or more proximal interphalangeal joints, and the thumb base would be classified as having idiopathic generalized OA. As long as it conforms to the above definition, generalized OA may occur with or without hand involvement.

It is difficult to apply definitions such as that cited above to the diagnosis of OA in an individual subject in the community or a patient in a clinic setting. Criteria for case definition *in community populations* have traditionally relied on the presence of radiographic features of OA. However, the use of radiographic criteria alone to define cases for *clinical studies* of OA has limitations: Although a statistically significant association exists between radiographic changes of OA and reported pain in both the hip and the knee, in the *individual patient* the correlation between the severity of radiographic changes and severity of symptoms is often poor.

Over the past decade, the Subcommittee on OA of the American College of Rheumatology's Diagnostic and Therapeutic Criteria Committee has published classification criteria for OA of the knee,[3] hand,[4] and hip (**Tables 1.2, 1.3, and 1.4**).[5-7] In each case, the classification schemes are based on combinations of symptoms, physical findings, and laboratory and radiographic features. The sensitivity, specificity, and accuracy of the classification criteria of OA of the knee, hand, and hip approach or exceed 90%.

Because the major inclusion parameter in each case is "joint pain for most days of the prior month," the American College of Rheumatology criteria identify patients with *clinical* OA. This contrasts with the identification of OA based on radiographic features alone. Because most subjects with radiographic evidence of OA do not report joint pain, estimates of the prevalence of OA will be lower when based on the college's criteria than when based on traditional radiographic criteria.

REFERENCES

1. Keutttner K, Goldberg VM. Introduction. In: Keuttner K, Goldberg VM, eds. *Osteoarthritic Disorders*. Rosemont, Ill: American Academy of Orthopaedic Surgeons; 1955:xxi-xxv.

2. Brandt KD, Mankin HJ, Shulman LE. Workshop on etiopathogenesis of osteoarthritis. *J Rheumatol.* 1986;13:1126-1160.

3. Altman R, Asch E, Bloch D, et al. Development of criteria for the classification and reporting of osteoarthritis. Classification of osteoarthritis of the knee. Diagnostic and Therapeutic Criteria Committee of the American Rheumatism Association. *Arthritis Rheum.* 1986;29:1039-1049.

4. Altman R, Alarcon G, Appelrouth D, et al. The American College of Rheumatology criteria for the classification and reporting of osteoarthritis of the hand. *Arthritis Rheum.* 1990;33:1601-1610.

5. Altman R, Alarcon G, Appelrouth D, et al. The American College of Rheumatology criteria for the classification and reporting of osteoarthritis of the hip. *Arthritis Rheum.* 1991;34:505-514.

6. Altman RD. Classification of disease: osteoarthritis. *Semin Arthritis Rheum.* 1991;20(suppl 2):40-47.

7. Silman AJ, Hochberg MC. *Epidemiology of the Rheumatic Diseases*. Oxford, UK: Oxford University Press; 1994.

TABLE 1.1 — CLASSIFICATION OF OA

IDIOPATHIC

Localized

• Hands	– Heberden's and Bouchard's nodes (nodal)
	– Erosive interphalangeal arthritis (non-nodal)
	– First carpometacarpal joint
• Feet	– Hallux valgus
	– Hallux rigidus
	– Contracted toes (hammer/cock-up toes)
	– Talonavicular
• Hip	– Eccentric (superior)
	– Concentric (axial, medial)
	– Diffuse (Coxae senilis)
• Spine	– Apophyseal joints
	– Intervertebral joints (disc)
	– Spondylosis (osteophytes)
	– Ligamentous (hyperostosis, Forestier disease, diffuse idiopathic skeletal hyperostosis [DISH])
• Other single sites	– Glenohumeral
	– Acromioclavicular
	– Tibiotalar
	– Sacroiliac
	– Temporomandibular

Generalized

• Includes ≥3 areas listed above (Kellgren-Moore)

SECONDARY

Trauma
• Acute
• Chronic (occupational, sports)

Congenital or Developmental

• Localized diseases	– Legg-Calvé-Perthes disease
	– Congenital hip dislocation
	– Slipped epiphysis
• Mechanical factors	– Unequal lower extremity length
	– Valgus/varus deformity
	– Hypermobility syndromes

18

Metabolic

- Ochronosis (alkaptonuria)
- Hemochromatosis
- Wilson's disease
- Gaucher's disease

Endocrine

- Acromegaly
- Hyperparathyroidism
- Diabetes mellitus
- Obesity
- Hypothyroidism

Calcium Deposition Diseases

- Calcium pyrophosphate dihydrate deposition
- Apatite arthropathy

Other Bone and Joint Diseases

- Localized — Fracture
  - Avascular necrosis
  - Infection
  - Gout
- Diffuse — Rheumatoid (inflammatory) arthritis
  - Paget's disease
  - Osteopetrosis
  - Osteochondritis

Neuropathis (Charcot's joint)

Endemic

- Kashin-Beck disease
- Mseleni disease

Miscellaneous

- Frostbite
- Caisson disease
- Hemoglobinopathies

Brandt KD, et al. *J Rheumatol.* 1986;13:1126-1160.

TABLE 1.2 — ALGORITHM FOR CLASSIFICATION OF OA OF THE KNEE

Clinical

1. Knee pain for most days of prior month
2. Crepitus on active joint motion
3. Morning stiffness ≤30 minutes in duration
4. Age ≥38 years
5. Bony enlargement of the knee on examination

Osteoarthritis is present if items 1, 2, 3, and 4 *or* items 1, 2, and 5 *or* items 1 and 5 are present. Sensitivity is 89%; specificity is 88%.

Clinical, Laboratory, and Radiographic

1. Knee pain for most days of prior month
2. Osteophytes at joint margins
3. Synovial fluid analysis typical of OA
4. Age ≥40 years
5. Morning stiffness ≤30 minutes in duration
6. Crepitus on active joint motion

Osteoarthritis is present if items 1 and 2 *or* items 1, 3, 5, and 6 *or* items 1, 4, 5, and 6 are present. Sensitivity is 94%; specificity is 88%.

Altman R, et al. *Arthritis Rheum.* 1986;29:1039-1049; and Altman R. *Semin Arthritis Rheum.* 1991;20(suppl 2):40-47. Reproduced from: Silman AJ, Hochberg MC. In: *Epidemiology of the Rheumatic Diseases.* Oxford, UK: Oxford University Press; 1993.

TABLE 1.3 — ALGORITHM FOR CLASSIFICATION OF OA OF THE HAND

Clinical

1. Hand pain, aching, or stiffness for most days of prior month
2. Hard tissue enlargement of ≥2 of 10 selected hand joints*
3. <3 swollen MCP joints
4. Hard tissue enlargement of ≥2 DIP joints
5. Deformity of ≥2 of 10 selected hand joints

Osteoarthritis is present if items 1, 2, 3, and 4 *or* items 1, 2, 3, and 5 are present. Sensitivity is 92%; specificity is 98%.

Abbreviations: DIP, distal interphalangeal; PIP, proximal interphalangeal; MCP, metacarpophalangeal; CMC, carpometacarpal.

---

* Ten selected hand joints include the second and third DIP joints, second and third PIP joints, and first CMC joint of each hand.

Altman R, et al. *Arthritis Rheum.* 1990;33:1601-1610; and Altman RD. *Semin Arthritis Rheum.* 1991;20(suppl 2):40-47. Reproduced from: Silman AJ, Hochberg MC. In: *Epidemiology of the Rheumatic Diseases.* Oxford, UK: Oxford University Press; 1993.

TABLE 1.4 — ALGORITHM FOR CLASSIFICATION OF OA OF THE HIP

Clinical, Laboratory, and Radiographic

1. Hip pain for most days of the prior month
2. Femoral and/or acetabular osteophytes on radiograph
3. Erythrocyte sedimentation rate ≤20 mm/h

Osteoarthritis is present if items 1 and 2 *or* items 1, 3, and 4 are present. Sensitivity is 91%; specificity is 89%.

Altman R, et al. *Arthritis Rheum.* 1991;34:505-514; and Altman RD. *Semin Arthritis Rheum.* 1991;20(suppl 2):40-47. Reproduced from: Silman AJ, Hochberg MC. In: *Epidemiology of the Rheumatic Diseases.* Oxford, UK: Oxford University Press; 1993.

2   Epidemiology

Prevalence

Among all of the specific joint diseases, osteoarthritis (OA) is the most frequent cause of rheumatic complaints (**Table 2.1**).[1] More than 80% of everyone over the age of 55 has x-ray evidence of OA. Not all of these individuals are symptomatic, but 10% to 20% of those affected may report limitation of activity due to their OA (**Figure 2.1**).[2,3] Knee OA is the leading cause of chronic disability among the elderly in the United States.[4] However, because of the difficulties associated with diagnosis, estimates of the true prevalence of OA are imprecise. Because of the lack of longitudinal data and difficulty in defining the onset of OA, estimates of incidence are unavailable.

Because age is the most powerful risk factor for OA and the eldest of the "baby boomers" (in the United States, 76 million individuals born between 1946 and 1964) have just recently begun to pass their 50th birthday, we are on the brink of an epidemic of OA. **Figure 2.2** depicts the anticipated growth of the segment of the population over the age of 65 in the United States, with projections to the middle of the next century. It emphasizes the increasing proportion of the elderly in the population.[5,6] It is projected that both the prevalence of arthritis and the proportion of those in whom the disease causes significant limitation of activity will increase.[7]

Risk Factors for OA

Felson has recently provided an up-to-date view of the epidemiology of OA.[8] Epidemiologic studies have defined several risk factors for OA.[9] In view of the growing frequency of this disease, it is particularly important to recognize those that are remediable (**Table 2.2**).

TABLE 2.1— PREVALENCE OF OA IN VARIOUS POPULATIONS

Population	Age (years)	Female (%)	Male (%)
English	≥35	70	69
US whites	≥40	44	43
Alaskan Eskimos	≥40	24	22
Jamaican (rural)	35 to 64	62	54
Pima Indians	≥30	74	56
Blackfoot Indians	≥30	74	61
South African blacks	≥35	53	60
Mean of 17 populations	≥35	60	60

Peyron JG, Altman RD. In: *Osteoarthritis: Diagnosis and Medical/Surgical Management.* 2nd ed. Philadelphia, Pa: WB Saunders Company; 1992:15-37.

■ Age, Gender, Race

Age is the most powerful risk factor for OA. The prevalence of OA at all joint sites increases progressively with age. Radiographic evidence of OA has been found in >80% of people age 70 and older (**Figure 2.1**).[10,11] The National Health and Nutrition Examination Survey found that the prevalence of knee OA increased from <0.1% in people 25 to 34 years old to 10% to 20% in those 65 to 74 years old.[12] Women were about twice as likely as men to be affected and black women twice as likely as white women. Others have found an even higher prevalence of knee OA; in the Framingham Study, the prevalence was 30% between age 65 to 74 years[13] and virtually every study that has examined people >75 years old has found a prevalence >30% and more disease among women than men. OA of the hip is somewhat less common than OA of the knee and does not exhibit this female preponderance, suggesting a difference in the etiology of OA at these two sites.

Although the incidence of hand, hip, and knee OA increases with age, a recent study of subjects with knee OA in a health maintenance organization showed that the inci-

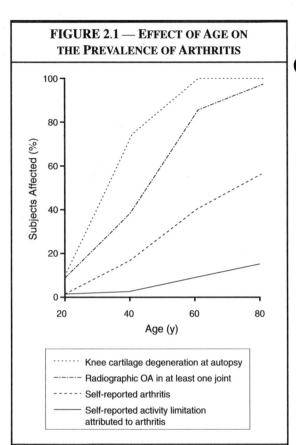

FIGURE 2.1 — EFFECT OF AGE ON THE PREVALENCE OF ARTHRITIS

······· Knee cartilage degeneration at autopsy

─·─·─ Radiographic OA in at least one joint

─ ─ ─ Self-reported arthritis

——— Self-reported activity limitation attributed to arthritis

Loeser RF Jr. *Rheum Dis Clin North Am*. 2000;26:547-567.

dence in women peaked at a rate of 1% per year between ages 70 and 89.[14] Similarly, in other studies, the incidence of symptomatic OA in both sexes appears to level off, or even decline, around the age of 80.[15,16]

■ **Trauma and Repetitive Stress**

Major trauma and repetitive stress have both been implicated as causes of OA. The patient with a trimalleolar fracture will almost certainly develop ankle OA. Studies of humans and animal models demonstrate that loss of ante-

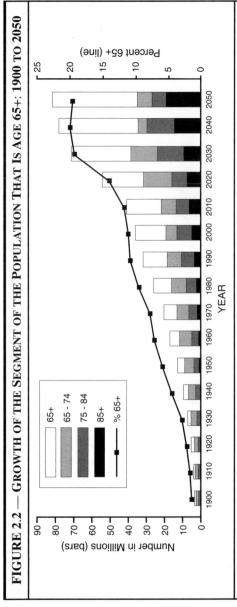

FIGURE 2.2 — GROWTH OF THE SEGMENT OF THE POPULATION THAT IS AGE 65+: 1900 TO 2050

US Bureau of the Census: *Sixty-Five Plus in America.* Pub. P23-178RV; *Population Projections of the United States by Age, Sex, Race, and Hispanic Origin: 1993 to 2050.* Pub. P25-1104. Census data (1900-1990) are as of April 1; projections (2000-2050) are as of July 1.

TABLE 2.2 — RISK FACTORS FOR OA

- Age
- Major joint trauma*
- Repetitive stress and joint overload*
- Obesity*
- Race
- Genetic factors*
- Female gender
- Congenital/developmental defects*
- Quadriceps weakness (knee OA)
- Prior inflammatory joint disease
- Metabolic/endocrine disorders
- Proprioceptive defect* (?)

Abbreviations: OA, osteoarthritis.

* Potentially modifiable.

Hochberg M. *J Rheumatol*. 1991;18:1438-1440.

rior cruciate ligament integrity, damage to the meniscus, and meniscectomy lead to knee OA. Even if the cartilage is not involved at the time of injury, it will degenerate rapidly if the joint is unstable. It has been suggested that prevention of knee injury would decrease the incidence of knee OA in men by some 25% and in women by nearly 14% (**Table 2.3**).[17]

The pattern of joint involvement in OA is influenced by prior vocational or avocational overload. Case-control studies have shown that activities performed by jackhammer operators, shipyard workers, coal miners, and others involved in similar activities lead to OA in the joint(s) exposed to repetitive occupational use.[18] Occupational overuse of the knee joint in jobs that require repeated kneeling, squatting or bending, and lifting of heavy loads is a risk factor for knee OA.[19] It has been calculated that elimination of such jobs would decrease the incidence of knee OA in men by 15% to 30% (**Table 2.3**).[17] Farming carries an especially high risk of hip OA, although the basis for this association has not been elucidated.[20] The effect of physical activity as a determinant of knee OA may be stronger among obese individuals.[21]

TABLE 2.3 — PREVENTIVE STRATEGIES AND POTENTIAL REDUCTION OF KNEE AND HIP OA

Preventive Strategy	↓ Incidence of Knee OA (%)		↓ Incidence of Hip OA (%)	
	Men	Women	Men	Women
Elimination of obesity	27 to 52	28 to 53	26	27
Prevention of knee injury	25	14	—	—
Elimination of jobs requiring knee bending and carrying heavy loads	15 to 30	—	—	—

Abbreviation: OA, osteoarthritis.

Felson DT. *Bull Rheum Dis*. 1998;47:1-4.

If major trauma is excluded, the association between specific athletic activities, especially leisure time rather than professional activities, and OA is somewhat tenuous. In the absence of knee injury, long-distance running and jogging do not appear to increase the risk for knee OA.[22,23] Thus repetitive joint usage of the type associated with athletics—even long-distance running[24]—does not appear to cause the joint damage seen with repetitive occupational use. This may be due, however, to the lack of good long-term studies and the difficulties associated with retrospective assessment of activities.[25] Selection bias (ie, early discontinuation of the athletic activity by those with damaged joints) may account for the discrepancy, although it may also be due to the intensity and duration of the activity. Occupational use commonly involves repeated exposure over many hours of the day, while exposure of the joint to injury by athletes occurs much less frequently.

On the other hand, elite athletes (eg, soccer players, runners, football players) who participate in sports at a highly competitive level or athletes who have incurred joint injuries appear to be at increased risk for developing OA, in comparison with people who participate in low-impact sports.[26,27] A study of former elite long-distance runners and tennis players found a 2- to 3-fold increase in the risk of radiographic knee and hip OA.[28] In another study, the prevalence of x-ray evidence of knee OA was 4.2% in nonelite former soccer players and 15.5% in elite former players but only 1.6% in controls.[29] Furthermore, the effects of high-impact loading of the knee and injury as risk factors for knee OA may be independent; in a study of soccer players 20 to 30 years after knee injuries and partial meniscectomy, 25% of those with an intact anterior cruciate ligament but 71% of those who had ruptured the ligament had knee OA.[30]

■ Obesity

Increased body mass is associated with a marked increase in prevalence of knee OA. This striking association is much less apparent for hip OA. The Framingham data show that being overweight as a young adult—long before any symptoms of OA had developed—strongly predicted the appearance of knee OA in a 36-year period to follow-up.[31] For those in the highest quintile for body mass index at the

29

baseline examination, the relative risk for developing knee OA during this interval was 1.5 for men and 2.1 for women. For severe OA, the relative risk rose to 1.9 for men and 3.2 for women, suggesting that obesity plays an even greater role in the etiology of the most serious cases of knee OA. It has been estimated that elimination of obesity would decrease the incidence of knee OA by about 25% to 50%, and hip OA, by 25% or more (**Table 2.3**).[17] Obese human subjects who have not yet developed OA can reduce their risk by losing weight. In women of average height, a weight loss of only 5 kg was associated with a 50% reduction in the odds of developing symptomatic knee OA.[32]

■ Periarticular Muscle Weakness

Quadriceps weakness is common in patients with knee OA, in whom it has generally been ascribed to disuse atrophy, which is presumed to develop because the patient minimizes usage of the painful limb. However, quadriceps weakness may exist also in subjects with knee OA who have no history of joint pain and in whom quadriceps muscle mass is not diminished but is normal or even increased (as a result of obesity).[33] Longitudinal studies suggest that quadriceps weakness may not only result from painful knee OA but may itself be a risk factor for structural damage.[34,35] Among women with no radiographic evidence of knee OA at the initial examination but who had definite OA changes some 30 months later, baseline knee extensor strength was significantly lower (P <0.04) than that in women who did not develop x-ray changes of OA.[33,34]

When the presence of knee OA (based on x-ray changes, with or without knee pain) as a function of sex, body weight, age, and lower extremity strength was modeled, it was found that each 10-lb/ft increase in knee extensor strength was associated with a 20% reduction in the odds of developing radiographic OA and a 29% reduction in the odds of developing symptomatic knee OA. A relatively small increase in strength (approximately 20% of the mean for men and 25% for women) was predicted to result in a 20% to 30% decrease in the odds of having knee OA.[33]

The importance of the quadriceps muscle in protecting against mechanical damage to the knee lies in the fact that it is the major antigravity muscle of the lower extremity and serves as a brake on the pendular action of the lower limb during ambulation, minimizing the forces generated with heel strike. In addition, the quadriceps is important in stabilizing the knee joint. Hence weakness may generate abnormal stresses on the joint. A placebo-controlled exercise trial is currently in progress to determine whether strengthening the quadriceps muscle can prevent development of knee pain and joint damage in elderly individuals.

■ Genetic Factors

The mother of a woman with distal interphalangeal joint OA is twice as likely to exhibit nodal OA—and the proband's sister three times as likely—as the mother and sister of a nonaffected woman. The mechanism appears to involve autosomal-dominant transmission in females and recessive inheritance in men. The overall prevalence of Heberden's nodes is 10 times greater in women than in men. In 1990, a point mutation was identified in the cDNA coding for type II collagen, resulting in a switch from arginine to cysteine at position 519 in the fibrillar α (II) chain. This abnormality was shown to be associated with familial chondrodysplasia and polyarticular secondary OA in several generations of a kindred (**Figure 2.3**). This provided a clear example of OA developing in association with a generalized genetic defect in the matrix of articular cartilage.[36,37] Transcription defects resulting in single amino acid substitutions at other sites on the type II collagen molecule have subsequently been detected in individuals from additional kindreds with a heritable form of OA, although phenotypically similar kindreds have not revealed any evidence of a mutation. It is possible, however, that defects also exist (eg, in the proteoglycan core protein, minor collagens or noncollagenous protein, or enzymes responsible for the biosynthesis of key matrix macromolecules) that have not yet been identified.

For example, defects in type IX and type XI collagen are associated with OA changes in animal models. Transgenic mice that expressed a1(IX) collagen chains with a central deletion developed OA in association with mild chondrodysplasia.[38] Other investigators have shown that mice deficient in a1(IX) collagen develop severe OA.[39] Genetic abnormalities in type XI collagen, another minor collagen of articular

FIGURE 2.3 — PEDIGREE OF KINDRED WITH GENERALIZED OA AND MILD CHONDRODYSPLASIA

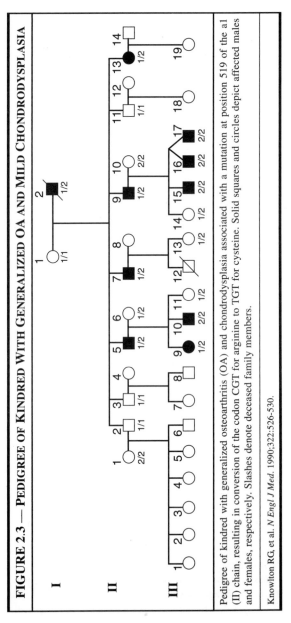

Pedigree of kindred with generalized osteoarthritis (OA) and chondrodysplasia associated with a mutation at position 519 of the α1 (II) chain, resulting in conversion of the codon CGT for arginine to TGT for cysteine. Solid squares and circles depict affected males and females, respectively. Slashes denote deceased family members.

Knowlton RG, et al. *N Engl J Med.* 1990;322:526-530.

cartilage, have also been associated with OA and underlying spondyloepiphyseal dysplasia in humans.[40,41]

Pseudoachondroplasia and multiple epiphyseal dysplasia (both of which are chondrodysplasias) are characterized by short stature and early-onset OA. Genes for both of these disorders have been localized to the short arm of chromosome 19, to which the gene for cartilage oligomeric matrix protein (COMP), a noncollagenous protein synthesized by the chondrocyte, has also been localized. Mutations in COMP have been identified in patients with these disorders.[42]

Local stresses related to joint use and the degree of deformity due to the chondrodysplasia presumably influence the appearance of OA in specific joints in affected members of the described kindreds. It should be emphasized, however, that in those cases of OA in which a genetic defect has been identified, the clinical picture is highly atypical—with OA affecting joints not generally involved in primary OA (eg, the elbow), the disease often becoming apparent as early as adolescence, and, generally, with clear evidence of underlying dysplastic changes. The prevalence of occult genetic abnormalities in cartilage collagen or other matrix macromolecules in individuals with what appears to be typical idiopathic OA remains to be determined. To date, genetic abnormalities have not been identified in patients presenting with a typical clinical picture of idiopathic OA of hip or knee.

■ **Bone Density**

An inverse relationship appears to exist between OA and osteoporosis.[43] Bone density in patients with OA is greater than that in age-matched controls, even at sites remote from the OA joint.[44,45] To some extent, the increase in bone mass may be explained by the association of OA with obesity. It has been suggested that the less-dense subchondral bone absorbs load better than normal bone, so that less stress is transferred to the overlying articular cartilage. Indirect evidence to support this general hypothesis includes the finding of a higher than expected prevalence of OA in subjects with osteopetrosis[46] and in those with greater than average bone mineral density (bone mass).

■ Estrogen Deficiency

Not only is the incidence of OA greater in older women than in older men, both hip and knee OA seem to occur at an accelerated rate in women after the age of 50, ie, roughly the time of menopause. Furthermore, some women develop rapidly progressive hand OA at this time of life.[47] These relationships suggest that postmenopausal estrogen deficiency increases the risk of OA. Cross-sectional studies have consistently suggested that women who have used hormonal replacement therapy are at lower risk for developing knee or hip OA than women who have not used estrogen.[48-52] The reduction in risk of hip OA among estrogen users has been reported to be as great as 40%. Longitudinal studies have also indicated that current estrogen users are at lower risk for knee OA than nonusers, although data from randomized controlled trials are needed before a recommendation can be made that estrogen should be used for prevention or treatment of OA.

While estrogen replacement therapy may prevent structural changes of OA, clinical trial data suggest it does not have a significant impact on symptoms of knee OA.[53]

■ Nutritional Deficiencies

Data suggest that men and women with moderately low serum levels of 25-hydroxy vitamin D are at greater risk for progression (but not initiation) of knee OA than those who have a higher vitamin D level.[54] Similar results were obtained in a prospective radiographic study of hip OA, although the effect of vitamin D on symptomatic OA is unknown.

Data have suggested that reactive oxygen species may contribute to articular cartilage damage in OA.[55] Because vitamin C is a major dietary antioxidant, it is notable that vitamin C deficiency has been suggested to be a risk factor for OA. Subjects in the lowest third of the population with respect to vitamin C intake had three times the risk of progression of knee OA and a greater risk of knee pain than those with a higher vitamin C intake.[56] As was the case for vitamin D deficiency, lower vitamin C intake did not affect the incidence of knee OA.

Risk Factors for Progression of OA

A variety of evidence suggests that the risk factors associated with progression of OA are different from those associated with initiation of joint damage. Several risk factors for knee OA progression are listed in **Table 2.4**. As indicated, once tissue damage is established, low levels of vitamin C or vitamin D may increase the rate of progression of OA, although prospective studies are needed to confirm this possibility. If the individual is obese, weight reduction may have the opposite effect.

TABLE 2.4 — FACTORS ASSOCIATED WITH PROGRESSION OF KNEE OA

- Older age
- Female sex
- Obesity
- Heberden's nodes
- Low dietary intake of vitamin C (?)
- Low dietary intake of vitamin D (?)

Risk Factors for Pain and Disability in Subjects With OA

Most individuals with x-ray evidence of OA do not have joint symptoms. On the other hand, symptoms of OA may be present even in patients with normal joint radiographs. Indeed, in all age groups, the prevalence of knee pain exceeds the prevalence of radiographic evidence of knee arthritis[57] (**Table 2.5**). Risk factors for pain and disability in OA must be differentiated from those related to the pathologic changes. Anxiety, depression, and muscle weakness may all be more important determinants of disability in patients with knee OA than the severity of the pathologic changes.[58] In any given joint, OA may result from a combination of local etiologic factors (eg, trauma) and a diathesis for generalized OA due to genetic predisposition,[59] chondrocalcinosis, generalized hypermobility,[60] or other factors.

Given comparable degrees of pathologic severity, women with OA are more likely to be disabled than men,

TABLE 2.5 — PERCENT OF THE US POPULATION THAT RECALLED HAVING AT LEAST 1 MONTH OF DAILY KNEE PAIN IN THE PAST YEAR COMPARED WITH PREVALENCE OF RADIOGRAPHIC ARTHRITIS*

Age (years)	Knee Pain (%)		Radiographic Arthritis (%)	
	Men	*Women*	*Men*	*Women*
23 to 34	5.7	5.2	NA	NA
35 to 44	7.4	8.1	NA	NA
45 to 54	12.0	11.5	2.3	3.6
55 to 64	11.5	15.0	4	7.2
65 to 74	14.9	19.7	8.4	17.9
25 to 74	9.5	10.9	NA	NA

Abbreviations: NA, not available; US, United States.

* Data are from the National Center for Health Statistics.

Hadler N. In: *Textbook of Osteoarthritis*. Oxford, UK: Oxford University Press; 1998:255-261.

those on welfare more likely than those who are working, and divorced subjects more likely than those who are married. The factors that determine why and when a person with radiographic OA decides to seek medical attention are poorly understood but may be related to the individual's framework of social support and coping skills.[57]

Without minimizing the importance of the above psychosocial factors, it should be noted that in a recent study, magnetic resonance imaging (MRI) differentiated subjects with symptomatic knee OA from asymptomatic subjects of similar age and with comparable radiographic severity. Symptomatic individuals frequently exhibited bone marrow "edema"[61]; large bone marrow lesions were present almost exclusively in those with knee pain and were absent in those with no pain, even in the presence of radiographic disease. The nature of the bone marrow lesions seen on MRI is unclear, but it is unlikely that they represent only extracellular fluid. Severity of symptoms has recently been reported to correlate strongly with MRI evidence of synovitis in subjects with knee OA.[62] In any event, these data raise the possibility that MRI abnormalities could be predictors of symptomatic disease.

REFERENCES

1. Peyron JG, Altman RD. The epidemiology of osteoarthritis. In: Moskowitz RW, Howell DS, Goldberg M, Mankin HJ, eds. *Osteoarthritis: Diagnosis and Medical/Surgical Management.* 2nd ed. Philadelphia, Pa: WB Saunders Company; 1992:15-37.

2. Brandt KD. Osteoarthritis. In: Stein J, ed. *Internal Medicine.* 4th ed. St. Louis, Mo: Mosby Year Book, Inc; 1994:2489-2493.

3. Loeser RF Jr. Aging and the etiopathogenesis and treatment of osteoarthritis. *Rheum Dis Clin North Am.* 2000;26:547-567.

4. Guccione AA, Felson DT, Anderson JJ, et al. The effects of specific medical conditions on the functional limitations of elders in the Framingham Study. *Am J Public Health.* 1994;84:351-358.

5. US Bureau of the Census: *Sixty-Five Plus in America.* Pub. P23-178RV.

6. US Bureau of the Census: *Population Projections of the United States by Age, Sex, Race, and Hispanic Origin: 1993 to 2050.* Pub. P25-1104.

7. Arthritis prevalence and activity limitations—United States, 1990. *Morb Mortal Wkly Rep.* 1994;43:433-438.

8. Felson DT. Epidemiology of osteoarthritis. In: Brandt KD, Doherty M, Lohmander SL, eds. *Osteoarthritis.* 2nd ed. Oxford, UK; Oxford University Press. In press.

9. Hochberg MC. Epidemiologic considerations in the primary prevention of osteoarthritis. *J Rheumatol.* 1991;18:1438-1440.

10. Lawrence RC, Hochberg MD, Kelsey JL, et al. Estimates of the prevalence of selected arthritic and musculoskeletal diseases in the United States. *J Rheumatol.* 1989;16:427-441.

11. Lawrence JS, Bremner JM, Bier F. Osteoarthrosis: prevalence in the population and relationship between symptoms and x-ray changes. *Ann Rheum Dis.* 1966;25:1-24.

12. Davis MA, Ettinger WH, Neuhaus JM, Mallon KP. Knee osteoarthritis and physical functioning: evidence from the NHANES I Epidemiologic Follow-up Study. *J Rheumatol.* 1991;18:591-598.

13. Felson DT, Naimark A, Anderson J, Kazis L, Castelli W, Meenan RF. The prevalence of knee osteoarthritis in the elderly. The Framingham Osteoarthritis Study. *Arthritis Rheum.* 1987;30:914-918.

14. Oliveria SA, Felson DT, Reed JI, Cirillo PA, Walker AM. Incidence of symptomatic hand, hip, and knee osteoarthritis among patients in a health maintenance organization. *Arthritis Rheum.* 1995;38:1134-1141.

15. Felson DT, Zhang Y, Hannan MT, Naimark A, Weissman BN, Aliabadi Levy D. The incidence and natural history of knee osteoarthritis in the elderly. The Framingham Osteoarthritis Study. *Arthritis Rheum*. 1995;38:1500-1505.

16. Hart DJ, Doyle DV, Spector TD. Incidence and risk factors for radiographic knee osteoarthritis in middle-age women: the Chingford Study. *Arthritis Rheum*. 1999;42:17-24.

17. Felson DT. Preventing knee and hip osteoarthritis. *Bull Rheum Dis*. 1998;47:1-4.

18. Cooper C. Occupational activity and the risk of osteoarthritis. *J Rheumatol*. 1995;43(suppl):10-12.

19. Maetzel A, Mäkelä M, Hawker G, Bombardier C. Osteoarthritis of the hip and knee and mechanical occupational exposure —a systematic overview of the evidence. *J Rheumatol*. 1997;24:1599-1607.

20. Croft P, Coggon D, Cruddas M, Cooper C. Osteoarthritis of the hip: an occupational disease in farmers. *BMJ*. 1992;304:1269-1272.

21. McAlindon TE, Wilson PWF, Aliabadi P, Weissman B, Felson DT. Level of physical activity and the risk of radiographic and symptomatic knee osteoarthritis in the elderly: the Framingham Study. *Am J Med*. 1999;106:151-157.

22. Lane NE, Bloch DA, Jones HH, Marshall WH Jr, Wood PD, Fries JF. Long distance running, bone density and osteoarthritis. *JAMA*. 1986;255:1147-1151.

23. Lane NE, Michel B, Bjorkengren A, et al. The risk of osteoarthritis with running and aging: a 5-year longitudinal study. *J Rheumatol*. 1993;20:461-468.

24. Panush RS, Schmidt C, Caldwell JR, et al. Is running associated with degenerative joint disease? *JAMA*. 1986;255:1152-1154.

25. Lindberg H, Montgomery F. Heavy labor and the occurrence of gonarthrosis. *Clin Orthop*. 1987;214:235-236.

26. Panush RS, Lane NE. Exercise and the musculoskeletal system. *Baillieres Clin Rheumatol*. 1994;8:79-102.

27. Lane NE, Buckwalter JA. Exercise: a cause of osteoarthritis? *Rheum Dis Clin North Am*. 1993;19:617-633.

28. Spector TD, Harris PA, Hart DJ, et al. Risk of osteoarthritis associated with long-term weight-bearing sports: a radiological survey of the hips and knees in female ex-athletes and population controls. *Arthritis Rheum*. 1996;39:988-995.

29. Roos H, Lindberg H, Gardsell P, Lohmander LS, Wingstrand H. The prevalence of gonarthrosis and its relation to meniscectomy in former soccer players. *Am J Sports Med*. 1994;22:219-222.

30. Negret P, Donnell ST, Dejour H. Osteoarthritis of the knee following meniscectomy. *Br J Rheumatol.* 1994;33:367-368.

31. Felson DT, Anderson JJ, Naimark A, Walker AM, Meenan RF. Obesity and knee osteoarthritis. The Framingham Study. *Ann Intern Med.* 1988;109:18-24.

32. Felson DT, Zhang Y, Anthony JM, Naimark A, Anderson JJ. Weight loss reduces the risk for symptomatic knee osteoarthritis in women. *Ann Intern Med.* 1992;116:535-539.

33. Slemenda C, Brandt KD, Heilman D, et al. Quadriceps weakness and osteoarthritis of the knee. *Ann Intern Med.* 1997;127:97-104.

34. Slemenda C, Heilman DK, Brandt KD, et al. Reduced quadriceps strength relative to body weight: a risk factor for knee osteoarthritis in women? *Arthritis Rheum.* 1998;41:1951-1959.

35. Brandt KD, Heilman DK, Slemenda C, et al. Quadriceps strength in women with radiographically progressive osteoarthritis of the knee and those with stable radiographic changes. *J Rheumatol.* 1999; 26:2431-2437.

36. Knowlton RG, Katzenstein PL, Moskowitz RW, et al. Genetic linkage of a polymorphism in the type II procollagen gene (COL2A1) to primary osteoarthritis associated with mild chondrodysplasia. *N Engl J Med.* 1990;322:526-530.

37. Ala-Kokko L, Baldwin CT, Moskowitz RW, Prockop DJ. Single base mutation in the type II procollagen gene (COL2A1) as a cause of primary osteoarthritis associated with a mild chondrodysplasia. *Proc Natl Acad Sci USA.* 1990;87:6565-6568.

38. Nakata K, Ono K, Olsen BR, et al. Osteoarthritis associated with mild chondrodysplasia in transgenic mice expressing alpha1(IX) collagen chains with a central deletion. *Proc Natl Acad Sci USA.* 1993; 90:2870-2874.

39. Fässler R, Schnegelsberg PNI, Dausman J, et al. Mice lacking alpha1(IX) collagen develop noninflammatory degenerative joint disease. *Proc Natl Acad Sci USA.* 1994;91:5070-5074.

40. Spranger J. The type XI collagenopathies. *Pediatr Radiol.* 1998; 28:745-750.

41. Sirko-Osadsa DA, Murray MA, Scott JA, Lavery MA, Warman ML, Robin NH. Stickler syndrome involvement is caused by mutations in COL11A2, the gene encoding the alpha2 (XI) chain of type XI collagen. *J Pediatr.* 1998;132:368-371.

42. Briggs MD, Hoffman SM, King LM, et al. Pseudoachondroplasia and multiple epiphyseal dysplasia due to mutations in the cartilage oligomeric matrix protein gene. *Nat Genet.* 1995;10:330-336.

43. Knight SM, Ring EF, Bhalla AK. Bone mineral density and osteoarthritis. *Ann Rheum Dis*. 1992;51:1025-1026.

44. Gevers G, Dequeker J, Martens M, Van Audekercke R, Nyssen-Behets C, Dhem A. Biomechanical characteristics of iliac crest bone in elderly women according to osteoarthritis grade at the hand joints. *J Rheumatol*. 1989;16:660-663.

45. Dequeker J, Goris P, Uytterhoeven R. Osteoporosis and osteoarthritis (osteoarthrosis). Anthropometric distinctions. *JAMA*. 1983;249:1448-1451.

46. Cameron HU, Dewar FP. Degenerative osteoarthritis associated with osteopetrosis. *Clin Orthop*. 1977;127:148-149.

47. Kellgren JH, Moore R. Generalized osteoarthritis in Heberden's nodes. *BMJ*. 1952;1:181-187.

48. Felson DT, Nevitt MC. The effects of estrogen on osteoarthritis. *Curr Opin Rheumatol*. 1998;10:269-272.

49. Nevitt MC, Cummings SR, Lane NE, Genant HK, Pressman AR. Current use of oral estrogen is associated with a decreased prevalence of radiographic hip OA in elderly white women. *Arthritis Rheum*. 1997;37:S212.

50. Hannan MT, Felson DT, Anderson JJ, Naimark A, Kannel WB. Estrogen use and radiographic osteoarthritis of the knee in women. The Framingham Osteoarthritis Study. *Arthritis Rheum*. 1990;33:525-532.

51. Wolfe F, Altman R, Hochberg M, Lane N, Luggan M, Sharp J. Postmenopausal estrogen therapy is associated with improved radiographic score in OA and RA. *Arthritis Rheum*. 1994;37:S231.

52. Samanta A, Jones A, Regan M, Wilson S, Doherty M. Is osteoarthritis in women affected by hormonal changes or smoking? *Br J Rheumatol*. 1993;32:366-370.

53. Nevitt MC, Felson DT, Williams EN, Grady D. The effect of estrogen plus progestin on knee symptoms and related disability in postmenopausal women: The Heart and Estrogen/Progestin Replacement Study, a randomized, double-blind, placebo-controlled trial. *Arthritis Rheum*. 2001;44:811-818.

54. McAlindon TE, Felson DT, Zhang Y, et al. Relation of dietary intake and serum levels of vitamin D to progression of osteoarthritis of the knee among participants in the Framingham Study. *Ann Intern Med*. 1996;125:353-359.

55. Tiku ML, Liesch JB, Robertson FM. Production of hydrogen peroxide by rabbit articular chondrocytes. Enhancement by cytokines. *J Immunol*. 1990;145:690-696.

56. McAlindon TE, Jacques P, Zhang Y, et al. Do antioxidant micronutrients protect against the development and progression of knee osteoarthritis? *Arthritis Rheum.* 1996;39:648-656.

57. Hadler N. Why does the patient with osteoarthritis hurt? In: Brandt KD, Doherty M, Lohmander SL, eds. *Osteoarthritis.* 2nd ed. Oxford, UK: Oxford University Press. In press.

58. Summers MN, Haley WE, Reveille JD, Alarcon GS. Radiographic assessment and psychologic variables as predictors of pain and functional impairment in osteoarthritis of the knee or hip. *Arthritis Rheum.* 1988;31:204-209.

59. Kellgren JH, Lawrence JS, Bier F. Genetic factors in generalized osteoarthrosis. *Ann Rheum Dis.* 1963;22:237-255.

60. Bird HA, Tribe CR, Bacon PA. Joint hypermobility leading to osteoarthrosis and chondrocalcinosis. *Ann Rheum Dis.* 1978; 37:203-211.

61. Felson DT, Chaisson CE, Hill CL, et al. The association of bone marrow lesions with pain in knee osteoarthritis. *Ann Intern Med.* 2001;134:541-549.

62. Hill CL, Gale DG, Chaisson CE, et al. Knee effusions, popliteal cysts and synovial thickening: association with knee pain in osteoarthritis. *J Rheumatol.* 2001;28:1330-1337.

3 Pathology

The pathology of osteoarthritis (OA) reflects both damage to the joint and reaction to that damage.[1-3] Although the most striking gross changes are usually seen in the load-bearing areas of the articular cartilage (**Color Plates 1 and 2**), OA is not a disease of a single tissue (ie, articular cartilage) but a disease of an organ (the synovial joint) in which all of the tissues—subchondral bone, synovium, capsule, ligaments, periarticular muscle, sensory nerves, as well as the cartilage—are involved (**Table 3.1**). OA represents *failure of the joint*. Just as the heart can fail because of a primary disorder of the endocardium, the myocardium, or epicardium, in each case producing a syndrome of congestive heart failure, the joint can fail because of a primary abnormality in the articular cartilage, underlying bone, synovium, or periarticular muscle, in each case producing a syndrome which we recognize as OA.

Most descriptions of the pathology of OA emphasize the progressive loss of articular cartilage that occurs in this disease. Indeed, the integrity of the articular cartilage is essential to normal joint function. Normal joint cartilage (**Color Plate 3**) subserves two essential functions: First, it provides a smooth bearing surface, so that one bone glides effortlessly over the other with joint movement. (The coefficient of friction of cartilage passing over cartilage in a normal joint is some 15 times lower than that of two ice cubes passed across each other.) Second, articular cartilage transmits load so that, eg, during ambulation, as the femur impinges on the tibia, the bones do not shatter.

In the earlier stages of OA, however, the articular cartilage is not attenuated but *thicker* than normal (**Figure 3.1**).[3,4] An increase in water content, reflecting damage to the collagen network, leads to swelling of the cartilage and is associated with an increase in the net rate of synthesis of proteoglycans, the matrix macromolecules that contribute elasticity to the cartilage and endow it with its ability to resist compression. The increase in proteoglycan

TABLE 3.1 — GROSS PATHOLOGIC FEATURES OF OA

- Softening, fibrillation, and, eventually, loss of articular cartilage (although the cartilage may be thicker than normal in the earlier stages of osteoarthritis)
- Eburnation of exposed bone
- Bony remodeling
- Osteophytes
- Subchondral cysts
- Synovitis
- Thickening of joint capsule
- Meniscus degeneration
- Periarticular muscle atrophy

FIGURE 3.1 — HISTOLOGIC SECTIONS FROM THE CENTRAL PORTION OF THE MEDIAL FEMORAL CONDYLES

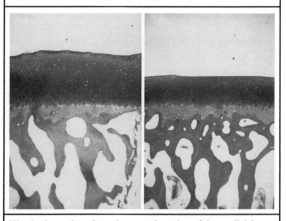

Histologic sections from the central portion of the medial femoral condyles of two knees. The sample from the osteoarthritis (OA) knee (*left*) is thicker than that from the essentially normal contralateral knee (*right*).

synthesis, which represents a repair effort by the chondrocytes, may result in an increase in the total proteoglycan concentration of the tissue. Thus the earlier stages of OA, which in humans may last decades, are characterized by *hypertrophic repair* of the articular cartilage (**Figure 3.2**).

FIGURE 3.2 — MAGNETIC RESONANCE IMAGING SHOWING HYPERTROPHIC REPAIR OF ARTICULAR CARTILAGE IN THE OA KNEE AFTER ANTERIOR CRUCIATE LIGAMENT TRANSECTION

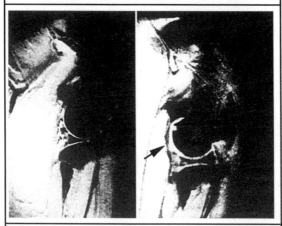

Magnetic resonance image (MRI) of the right (*right*) and left (*left*) knees of a dog *3 years* after transection of the left anterior cruciate ligament, resulting in osteoarthritis (OA). Note the persistence of cartilage thickening on the femoral condyle of the OA knee (*arrow*), in comparison with cartilage of the unoperated contralateral knee, whose thickness is normal.

With progression of OA, the joint surface undergoes thinning and the proteoglycan concentration diminishes, leading to softening of the cartilage. Surface integrity is lost and vertical clefts develop (fibrillation) (**Color Plate 4**). With motion, the fibrillated cartilage is worn away, exposing underlying bone. Areas of fibrocartilaginous repair may appear, but these are inferior to pristine hyaline articular cartilage in their ability to withstand mechanical stress. The

45

chondrocytes, which in normal adult articular cartilage do not undergo cell division, replicate, forming clusters (clones) (**Color Plate 4**). Later, however, the remaining cartilage becomes hypocellular.

In the deep zone of normal articular cartilage, a zone of increased calcification is separated from the uncalcified hyaline articular cartilage by a histologic landmark, the tidemark. In OA, reduplication of the tidemark is common. As many as eight or more tidemarks may be counted, each reflecting a discrete event that altered the mechanical stresses on the cartilage (**Color Plate 5**). In addition, although normal adult articular cartilage is avascular, capillaries from the underlying bone penetrate into the zone of calcified cartilage and beyond into the hyaline cartilage in OA. This vascularization contributes to the remodeling of the cartilage in OA by providing a route for direct penetration of hormones and paracrine factors (cytokines, growth factors). In addition, the penetration of blood vessels through the bone and calcified cartilage weakens the structure, providing a focus for microfractures extending into the cartilage. Fibrocytes grow into these areas and then undergo cartilage metaplasia and form a fibrocartilaginous matrix.

While the loss of cartilage represents the pathologic hallmark of OA, remodeling and hypertrophy of bone are major features. Appositional bone growth occurs in the subchondral region (**Color Plate 6**), leading to the sclerosis that may be seen on x-ray. The abraded bone in the floor of the ulcerated cartilage may take on the gross appearance of polished ivory (eburnation) (**Color Plate 2**). In addition to microfractures of the subchondral trabeculae, bone cysts may be seen (**Color Plate 2** and **Figure 3**.3). These cysts, which reflect localized osteonecrosis, form beneath the surface and weaken the osseous support for the overlying cartilage. The cysts may arise by insudation of synovial fluid through microfractures of the surface into subjacent areas of osteoporotic bone, where they may then become surrounded by new bone. Younger cysts contain loose connective tissue that eventually becomes more fibrotic. In some cases, communication with the joint surface is obvious; in others, no communication is apparent.

Growth of cartilage and bone at the joint margins leads to osteophytes (spurs) (**Figure 3**.3), which alter the contour

FIGURE 3.3 — RADIOGRAPH OF FEMORAL HEAD SURGICALLY REMOVED DUE TO OA

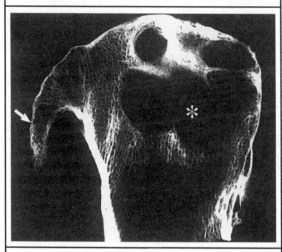

Note the extreme cyst formation in the subchondral bone (*asterisk*) and extreme osteophytosis (*arrow*).

Pritzker KPH. In: *Osteoarthritis*. 2nd ed. Oxford, UK: Oxford University Press. In press.

of the joint and may restrict movement. However, in the absence of other bony changes, eg, subchondral cysts or sclerosis, osteophytes may be a manifestation of aging rather than of OA.[5]

Soft tissue changes include a patchy chronic synovitis[6] (**Color Plate 7**), with lining cell hyperplasia, lymphocytic infiltration, and perivascular lymphoid aggregates. Villus formation may be prominent, suggestive of rheumatoid arthritis. However, in contrast to rheumatoid arthritis, the synovial lining cells do not erode the cartilage at the joint margins or form a pannus infiltrating the cartilage surface. Fragments of articular cartilage and necrotic bone that are lost from the joint surface may become incorporated into the synovial membrane, where they may become surrounded by macrophages, including foreign-body giant cells, and an inflammatory cell infiltrate. The presence of numerous fragments of cartilage and bone within the synovium of an OA joint may reflect a rapidly destructive neurogenic arthritis (ie, Charcot's joint). Thickening of the joint capsule may further restrict movement. In the presence of synovial effusions, loss of compliance of the capsule will lead to expansion of bursal structures that communicate with the joint space. This accounts, for example, for Baker's cysts, which are common in patients with knee OA.

Changes in the ligaments are similar to those in the capsule: dilatation of blood vessels, edema, and increased synthesis of proteoglycans and collagen fibers. Fibrosis may extend to the perineurium and endoneurium and may provide a structural basis for the chronic joint pain of patients with OA. On the other hand, by stretching the collateral ligaments, chronic effusions may lead to joint laxity. The mechanical instability may result in abnormal stresses on the articular surfaces, causing additional joint damage.

Periarticular muscle wasting is common. It may be due to disuse atrophy, as the patient avoids usage of the painful extremity. Alternatively, it may be due to arthrogenous muscle inhibition,[7] with nerve endings in the arthritic joint transmitting impulses to the central nervous system, which reflexly limits the patient's ability to effect a maximal voluntary contraction of the muscle. In any case, because of the importance of periarticular muscle in stabilizing the joint, weakness may be a risk factor for joint damage.

All of the above changes play a role in the clinical signs and symptoms of OA.

REFERENCES

1. Sokoloff L. *The Biology of Degenerative Joint Disease*. Chicago, Ill: The University of Chicago Press; 1969:1-162.

2. Pritzker KPH. Pathology of osteoarthritis. In: Brandt KD, Doherty M, Lohmander LS, eds. *Osteoarthritis*. 2nd ed. Oxford, UK: Oxford University Press. In press.

3. Adams ME, Brandt KD. Hypertrophic repair of the canine articular cartilage in osteoarthritis after anterior cruciate ligament transection. *J Rheumatol*. 1991;18:428-435.

4. Braunstein EM, Brandt KD, Albrecht M. MRI demonstration of hypertrophic articular cartilage repair in osteoarthritis. *Skeletal Radiol*. 1990;19:335-339.

5. Hernborg J, Nilsson BE. The relationship between osteophytes in the knee joints, osteoarthritis and aging. *Acta Orthop Scand*. 1973;44:69-74.

6. Myers SL, Brandt KD, Ehlich JW, et al. Synovial inflammation in patients with early osteoarthritis of the knee. *J Rheumatol*. 1990;17:1662-1669.

7. Hurley MV, Newham DJ. The influence of arthrogenous muscle inhibition on quadriceps rehabilitation of patients with early, unilateral osteoarthritic knees. *Br J Rheumatol*. 1993;32:127-131.

4

Pathogenesis

Although the most obvious changes in the osteoarthritis (OA) joint reside in the cartilage, OA should not be viewed simply as a disease of cartilage. It does not represent the failure of a single tissue but of an *organ*—the diarthrodial joint. Just as congestive heart failure may be due to primary disease of the myocardium, pericardium, or endocardium, the primary abnormality in OA may reside in the articular cartilage, synovium, subchondral bone, ligaments, or neuromuscular apparatus. Nonetheless, given the marked changes that occur in the cartilage in OA, it is essential to appreciate the importance of this tissue in normal joint physiology. Normal joint cartilage (**Color Plate 3**) plays two essential roles:

- First, it provides a remarkably smooth bearing surface, permitting virtually frictionless movement of one bone over the other within the joint (**Figure 4.1**).
- Second, it spreads and transmits load, preventing concentration of stress within the joint (**Table 4.1**).

Essentially, OA develops in either of two settings:

- When the material properties of the articular cartilage and underlying subchondral bone are normal but excessive loads on the joint cause the tissues to fail
- When the applied load is reasonable but the material properties of the cartilage tissue (eg, bone, ligaments, periarticular muscle) are inferior (**Table 4.2**).

Although articular cartilage is highly resistant to wear under conditions of repeated oscillation, repetitive impact loading leads to joint failure.[1] This accounts for the high prevalence of OA in specific joints related to vocational or avocational overload. In general, the earliest progressive degenerative changes in OA occur at sites within the joint that are subject to the greatest compressive loads. It has been suggested that a high proportion of all cases of idiopathic

FIGURE 4.1 — PATHOGENESIS: ARTICULAR CARTILAGE

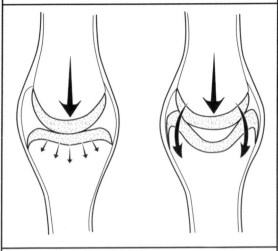

During load-bearing, deformation of the articular cartilage and, especially, the subchondral bone occurs within a joint (*left*). This serves to maximize the contact area and thereby reduce the stress (force per unit area). If this deformity does not occur (*right*), stress will be concentrated, leading to breakdown of the joint.

Brandt KD, Radin E. *Hosp Pract (Off Ed)*. 1987;22:103-107, 110-112, 117-119.

TABLE 4.1 — PHYSIOLOGIC ROLES OF ARTICULAR CARTILAGE

> Provides a smooth bearing surface
> Transmits load

TABLE 4.2 — PATHOGENESIS OF OA

Normal loads
+
Inferior biomaterials
(eg, cartilage, bone, muscle, ligaments)

Excessive loads
+
Normal biomaterials

OA of the hip reflect subtle developmental defects, such as acetabular dysplasia or slipped femoral epiphysis, which increase joint congruity and concentrate loads.

Even if the stresses within the joint are normal, conditions that reduce the ability of the articular cartilage or subchondral bone to deform may lead to OA. For example, in ochronosis, the accumulation of homogentisic acid polymers leads to stiffening of the cartilage; in osteopetrosis, stiffening of the subchondral trabeculae, rather than of the cartilage, occurs. In both conditions, severe generalized OA is common.[2] Development of OA in subjects with familial chondrodysplasia due to a mutation in the cDNA coding for type II collagen[3] (**Figure 2.3**) illustrates the etiologic role that a generalized defect in the articular cartilage matrix may play in this disease.

Mechanisms Protecting the Joint From Stress

The major load on articular cartilage results from the contraction of the muscles that stabilize or move the joint.[4] In normal walking, three to four times the weight of the body is transmitted through the knee joint; during a deep knee bend, the patellofemoral joint is subjected to a load nine to ten times body weight. Adaptive mechanisms must protect the joint from these physiologic loads. Although articular cartilage is an excellent shock absorber in terms of its bulk properties, at most sites it is only 1 to 2 mm thick—too thin to serve as the sole shock-absorbing structure in joints. The additional protective mechanisms that are needed are provided by the subchondral bone and periarticular muscles.

■ Passive Protection: The Subchondral Bone

Normally, in the unloaded state, the opposing surfaces of joints are incongruent. Under load, deformation occurs, maximizing the contact area and hence minimizing the stress (ie, force per unit area).[5] Deformation of the cartilage provides the self-pressurized hydrostatic weeping lubrication needed for effortless motion. However, with increasing load, cartilage deformation alone is insufficient; deformation of the underlying bone must also occur and, under high loads, is more important than deformation of cartilage in reducing stress (**Figure 4.2**).

The highly elastic cancellous subchondral bone, although 10 times stiffer than cartilage, is much softer than cortical bone and serves as a major shock absorber. By providing it with a pliable bed that absorbs energy, cancellous bone protects the overlying cartilage (**Figure 4.2**).[5] If the load is excessive, however, the subchondral trabeculae will fracture. These microfractures then heal with callus formation and remodeling. It has been suggested that because the remodeled trabeculae may be stiffer than normal, a significant increase in the number of microfractures in subchondral bone may be detrimental to normal joint function.[6] If under such circumstances, the bone cannot deform normally with load, the increase in congruity of joint surfaces that occurs with loading is diminished, stresses are concentrated at contact sites on the articular cartilage, and the cartilage fails.

The hypothesis that stiffened subchondral bone drives the destruction of the overlying articular cartilage, however, is not been supported by finite element models. As reviewed by Burr,[7] mathematical modeling studies have shown that even a marked increase in the density of subchondral bone would cause only a modest increase in mechanical stress in the overlying cartilage.[8] The amount of stiffening of the bone required to significantly increase stresses in the cartilage is far beyond that which is likely to occur *in vivo*. Although stiffening of subchondral bone may be an impor-

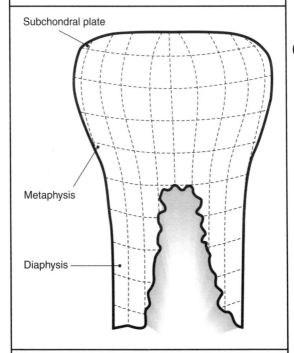

FIGURE 4.2 — PATHOGENESIS: SUBCHONDRAL CANCELLOUS BONE

Subchondral plate

Metaphysis

Diaphysis

The subchondral cancellous bone is arranged in a series of interconnecting longitudinal struts that transmit load stress down to the diaphyseal shaft. Because this bone is pliable, it absorbs energy and protects the overlying articular cartilage from stress during loading of the joint.

Brandt KD, Radin E. *Hosp Pract (Off Ed)*. 1987;22:103-107, 110-112, 117-119.

tant feature of OA, these data suggest that it is not sufficient on a mechanical basis alone to account for the destruction of articular cartilage.

On the other hand, microcracks in the subchondral bone or calcified cartilage can stimulate focal remodeling and account for increased vascularity in OA joints. Microcracks are found routinely in calcified cartilage from femoral heads of middle-aged nonarthritic humans and are associated with foci of vascular remodeling in OA cartilage.[7] Single or repetitive high-impact loads have been shown to cause microcracks,[9] which are followed by focal remodeling of the subchondral bone and degeneration of the overlying articular cartilage. Thus, in contrast to microfractures, microdamage in calcified cartilage, secondary to trauma, may play a role in the pathogenesis of OA.

The subchondral bone in OA may have not only a mechanical effect on the cartilage but also metabolic effects. For example, it has been shown recently that conditioned medium from primary cultures of osteoblasts from OA joints can significantly affect the release of glycosaminoglycans from normal chondrocytes in comparison with the medium of osteoblast cultures from subjects without arthritis.[10] Furthermore, the activity of the plasminogen activator (urokinase)/plasmin system has been shown to be increased in primary cultures of osteoblasts from subchondral bone of humans with OA. In such individuals, levels of insulinlike growth factor 1 are elevated,[11] providing a possible mechanism for the above effect.

Bone mineral density is greater in subjects with OA than in age- and sex-matched controls.[12-14] Bone formation and resorption are both increased in the OA joint, resulting in a decrease in the material stiffness of the bone (*per unit of mass*). However, an increase in the number of subchondral trabeculae, reduction in trabecular separation,[15] and increase in thickness of the subchondral plate result in an increase in *overall* stiffness of the intra-articular bone in OA.[16]

Whether changes in the subchondral bone precede or follow those in the overlying cartilage in OA is unclear. However, even if they are not involved in the initiation of cartilage damage, bony changes may be important in the *progression* of cartilage breakdown in OA. Evidence that changes in bone may precede those in the cartilage is provided by the results of a study in a rabbit model of OA, in which subfracture loads were applied to the patellofemoral joint.[17] Significant reduction in cartilage stiffness was not seen until 12 months after the injury, whereas a progressive increase in the thickness of the subchondral plate was apparent by 6 months. In animal models of OA, thickening of the subchondral plate did not seem to be an early event, but was associated with subsequent progression of cartilage damage.[18,19] In dogs in which knee OA had been induced by transection of the anterior cruciate ligament, treatment with an antiresorptive drug (bisphosphonate) reduced turnover in the subchondral bone but did not affect biochemical, metabolic, or morphologic changes in the overlying cartilage.[20] Furthermore, although the drug inhibited formation of subchondral bone (because this is coupled to bone resorption), it had no effect on osteophytes, in which bone formation is not coupled to resorption but occurs by endochondral ossification.

A placebo-controlled clinical trial examining the possibility that treatment with the antiresorptive drug risedronate can prevent progression of structural damage in humans with OA is currently in progress.

■ Active Protection: The Muscles

Active shock-absorbing mechanisms involve the use of muscles and joint motion in "negative work." While muscle contraction can move a joint, muscles can also act as large rubber bands. When a slightly stretched muscle is subjected to greater stretch as a result of joint motion, it can absorb a large amount of energy. Most of the muscle activity generated during ambulation is not used to propel the body forward but to absorb energy to decelerate the body.

When we negotiate the jump off a ledge or table, we normally land on our toes, come down on our heels, and straighten our flexed knees and hips. During this smooth action, our muscles perform negative work, ie, they absorb energy. As we dorsiflex our ankles, we stretch our gastrocnemius-soleus complex; as we straighten our knees, we stretch our quadriceps; as we straighten our hips, we stretch our hamstrings. The amount of energy absorbed by this mechanism is enormous.[21] Indeed, the energy produced by normal walking is great enough to tear all the ligaments of the knee. That this does not occur routinely attests to the importance and effectiveness of an active energy absorption mechanism.

Small unexpected loads for which we are unprepared are much more damaging to joints than large ones that have been anticipated. Consider what happens when we come down stairs, misjudge a step, and abruptly slip a couple of

steps because our muscles are not prepared to accommo-
date the load—we feel a sharp jolt. To prepare the neuromuscular apparatus to reflexly handle an impact load requires approximately 75 milliseconds. Thus falls of very
brief duration (eg, of only about 1 inch) do not afford sufficient time to bring protective muscular reflexes into play.
Under such conditions, the load is transmitted to the cartilage and bone. In contrast, during a fall from a greater
height, sufficient time is available for activation of the appropriate reflexes, the energy of impact is absorbed by the
lengthening of the muscles surrounding the joint and movement of the joint, and the articular cartilage is thereby pro-
tected.[22] Both muscle atrophy (which may occur in association with OA) and an increase in the latent period of the
reflex (which may occur with peripheral neuropathy due to
aging or other causes) will reduce the effectiveness of this
shock-absorbing mechanism.

After a femoral nerve block, the load rate in normal
subjects who have no force-transient profile during gait increases more than 2-fold (to approximately $150 \times$ body
weight/second).[23] This suggests that a force transient can
be caused by failure to decelerate the lower extremity prior
to heel strike. In normal individuals, minor incoordination
in muscle recruitment, resulting in failure to decelerate the
leg, may generate rapidly applied impulsive forces as high
as $65 \times$ body weight/second at heel strike. Whether this
microincoordination of neuromuscular control, which Radin
and associates have called "microklutziness,"[23] is a risk factor for OA remains to be established, but the possibility is
intriguing.

While the periarticular muscles serve a primary motor
function, Hurley[24] has emphasized the importance of the
sensory function of muscle and of the proprioceptive impulses that originate in muscle and are transmitted to the
central nervous system. Data suggest that muscle weakness,
due either to disuse atrophy or reflex inhibition of muscle
contraction because of intra-articular pathology, may result
in joint degeneration (**Figure 4.3**). Chapter 2, *Epidemiology,* discusses quadriceps muscle weakness as a risk factor
for knee OA in humans.

Sharma[25] has reviewed the evidence of a proprioceptive defect in patients with knee OA. While impaired pro-

FIGURE 4.3 — ROLE OF PERIARTICULAR MUSCLE IN THE PATHOGENESIS OF OA

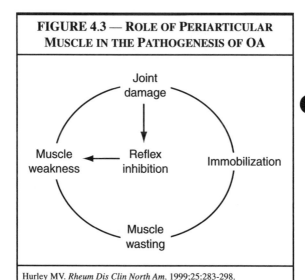

Hurley MV. *Rheum Dis Clin North Am.* 1999;25:283-298.

prioception may be the result of intra-articular damage, proprioceptive defects have been found bilaterally in patients with unilateral knee OA, raising the possibility that an underlying neurologic defect is important in the etiopathogenesis of primary OA.[25] Furthermore, we have shown that interruption of sensory input from the ipsilateral limb rapidly accelerates breakdown of the canine knee after transection of the anterior cruciate ligament.[26]

Cartilage Loss in Osteoarthritis

Cartilage loss is central to OA. The cartilage is slowly degraded, with a progressive decrease in the content of proteoglycans. Because the rates of synthesis of proteoglycans, collagen, hyaluronan (HA), and DNA all are increased in OA, catabolic activity of the tissue is extraordinarily high. Although "wear" may be a factor in the loss of cartilage, it is generally believed that lysosomal proteases (cathepsins) and neutral metalloproteinases (eg, stromelysin, collagenase, gelatinase) account for much of the loss of cartilage in this disease. The proteolytic degradation of cartilage in OA has been reviewed recently by Sandy and Plaas[27] and by Poole and Howell.[28]

The concentration of collagenase in the cartilage increases with severity of the disease and presumably accounts for the destruction of matrix collagen. Despite an increase in HA synthesis,[29] a reduction in cartilage HA content develops,[30] indicating accelerated degradation of the backbone of the proteoglycan aggregate. A specific hyaluronidase has not been isolated from cartilage, but several lysosomal enzymes can cleave HA and chondroitin-6 sulfate.

The slowly progressive loss of cartilage is associated with a loss of aggrecan,[31] resulting in a loss of compressive stiffness and elasticity and an increase in hydraulic permeability of the tissue. The cartilage water content is increased and a change occurs in the arrangement and size of the collagen fibers within the matrix. The biochemical data are consistent with a defect in the collagen network of the cartilage, perhaps due to disruption of the "glue" that binds adjacent collagen fibers together in the matrix.[32] This is perhaps the earliest matrix change to occur in OA and appears to be irreversible. The aggregation defect may be due to an alteration in the HA-binding region of the proteoglycan monomer, a quantitative deficiency in HA, or a deficiency in link protein, a noncollagenous protein that stabilizes the interaction between the proteoglycan and HA. Whatever its basis, it is of considerable importance because the proteoglycans are less constrained within the collagen network than normal.

While the cells in normal adult articular cartilage do not divide, the chondrocytes undergo active cell division in OA cartilage. The new cells are very active metabolically and produce increased quantities of collagen, proteoglycan, and HA. However, the new products do not aggregate well and are not adequately stabilized in the extracellular matrix, so that the mechanical properties of the matrix are inferior to those of normal cartilage. Prior to the loss of cartilage thickness and proteoglycan depletion, the marked biosynthetic (repair) activity of the chondrocytes may lead to an *increase* in proteoglycan concentration, associated with thickening of the cartilage (**Figures 3.1 and 3.2**).[33] Hypertrophic repair is common in the earlier stages of OA in both humans and animal models.[34-37] It is obviously inaccurate to call OA a "degenerative" joint disease.

Many investigators consider that interleukin-1 (IL-1) drives the progression of cartilage breakdown in OA. IL-1 is a cytokine produced by mononuclear cells (including synovial lining cells) and synthesized by chondrocytes, which stimulates the synthesis and secretion of latent collagenase, latent stromelysin, latent gelatinase, and tissue plasminogen activator.[38] The activity of the matrix metalloproteinases (MMPs) is controlled by specific inhibitors (tissue inhibitors of matrix metalloproteinases [TIMPs]) and by activation of the latent enzymes. Serine- and cysteine-proteases, such as the plasminogen activator/plasmin system and cathepsin B, respectively, serve as activators.[39] Other enzymes may also serve to activate the MMPs. For example, collagenase-1, collagenase-3, and 92kD gelatinase may all be activated by stromelysin-1, and 92kD gelatinase by collagenase-3. Membrane-metalloproteinases localized on the surface of the chondrocyte may activate collagenase-3 and 72kD gelatinase.[40]

Intra-articular injection of IL-1 leads rapidly to loss of proteoglycans from articular cartilage of normal rabbits.[41] A similar effect is seen after incubation of normal cartilage from young animals with IL-1 *in vitro*. These observations must be viewed with caution, however, because IL-1 has little effect on proteoglycan release from adult canine, porcine, or human articular cartilage. Furthermore, while proteoglycan synthesis in young porcine cartilage is *inhibited* by concentrations of IL-1 that are lower than those needed to cause matrix degradation in OA, the net rate of proteoglycan synthesis in OA cartilage is greater than that in normal cartilage. Although it can be argued that the effects of IL-1 are focal rather than diffuse, *all* chondrocytes in the OA joint appear to exhibit enhanced biosynthetic activity.

Results of gene therapy experiments offer further indirect evidence of the importance of IL-1 in pathogenesis of OA. In a relatively short-term experiment, in which structural joint damage was relatively mild, transfer of the gene for IL-1 receptor antagonist to the synovial lining of the unstable knee of dogs that had undergone cruciate ligament transection reduced the severity of cartilage degeneration in the OA knee.[42] In the same model, treatment with a selective inhibitor of inducible nitric oxide synthase appeared also to reduce the severity of joint damage.[55] However, synovitis appears to be a less important cause of cartilage breakdown in this canine model than mechanical factors.[56] For example, treatment with prednisone in a dose high enough to inhibit IL-1 production had no effect on the development of OA.[57] More work is needed in this area. Transfer of the gene for IL-1 receptor antagonist to the synovial lining of dogs in which OA had been induced by anterior cruciate ligament transection resulted in a reduction in the severity of cartilage degeneration[42] in comparison with OA joints into which the LacZ gene had been transferred as a control.

Whether their synthesis and release are stimulated by cytokines, such as IL-1, or by other factors (eg, altered mechanical stresses), the neutral metalloproteinases, cathepsins, and plasmin (which can activate latent forms of the metalloproteinases) all appear to be involved in failure of the cartilage in OA. Plasminogen, the substrate for plasmin, may be synthesized by the chondrocytes or may enter the cartilage by diffusion from the synovial fluid. Tissue inhibitors of matrix metalloproteinases and plasminogen activator inhibitor (PAI-1), both of which are synthesized by the chondrocyte, limit the degradative activity of the neutral metalloproteinases and plasminogen activator, respectively. A stoichiometric imbalance exists in OA cartilage between levels of active enzyme, which may be several fold higher than those in normal cartilage, and the level of TIMPs, which may be only modestly increased.[43]

Growth factors (eg, insulinlike growth factor [IGF-1], transforming growth factor-β, basic fibroblast growth factor) drive repair processes that may heal the cartilage lesion or at least stabilize the process.[44] These growth factors modulate catabolic as well as anabolic pathways of chondrocyte metabolism. Not only do they increase proteoglycan synthesis but, by down-regulating chondrocyte receptors for IL-1, they decrease proteoglycan degradation. Although the expression and synthesis of IGF-1 are increased in OA cartilage, the tissue exhibits decreased responsiveness to IGF-1,[45] which may be explained by an increase in local production of IGF-binding proteins.[46]

As discussed in Chapter 7, *Synovial Fluid Analysis*, crystals of calcium pyrophosphate dihydrate (CPPD) or basic calcium phosphate (calcium hydroxyapatite) are often present in synovial fluid of patients with OA.[47] The presence of apatite crystals correlates strongly with x-ray evidence of cartilage degeneration and may be associated with the presence of larger effusions than those in OA joints in which such crystals are not present.[48,49]

Whether the presence of apatite crystals is a cause or result of OA cartilage damage in OA remains unclear. However, apatite crystals have been shown to induce mitogenesis and prostaglandin synthesis in synovial fibroblasts and chondrocytes *in vitro*,[50] and can induce the synthesis and secretion of MMPs capable of causing tissue damage. Apatite crystals are as potent as IL-1 and tumor necrosis factor [TNF] α in inducing secretion of collagenase by human OA fibroblasts[51] and they act synergistically with IL-1 and TNF-α to increase MMP production, suggesting that they may play a role in the pathogenesis of cartilage damage. Their absence from synovial fluid of patients with other joint diseases associated with cartilage breakdown and synovitis, such as rheumatoid arthritis, suggests they have particular importance in OA and are not merely an epiphenomenon.

The "Milwaukee shoulder syndrome" represents a form of destructive OA with some evidence of inflammation in the synovial membrane but minimal synovial fluid leukocytosis.[52] Degeneration of the rotator cuff and severe glenohumeral joint OA are present, with deposition of apatite crystals in the synovial membrane. Crystals released from the degenerating tendons presumably trigger the release of collagenase from mononuclear cells in the synovial membrane, leading to breakdown of the articular cartilage, which perpetuates the release of enzymes from the synovium.

In some cases, CPPD crystal-deposition disease may result in rapidly progressive joint destruction, with a pseudo-Charcot's arthropathy. The relationship between crystals and OA has been reviewed recently by Concoff and Kalunian[53] and by Ryan.[54]

Is Synovitis a Cause of Articular Cartilage Breakdown in OA?

If synovial inflammation were detrimental to articular cartilage in the OA joint, treatment with an NSAID might be indicated even if the effect of the drug on symptoms did not depend on an anti-inflammatory action. However, the relationship of synovitis to cartilage damage in OA is ambiguous. While many consider that IL-1 and perhaps other cytokines released from inflamed synovium drive the breakdown of articular cartilage in OA, there is no direct evidence to support this contention.

Whatever the pathogenetic mechanisms underlying cartilage damage in OA, homeostatic mechanisms may maintain the joint in a reasonably functional state for years. The repair tissue, however, often does not hold up as well as normal hyaline cartilage under mechanical stress. Eventually, at least in some cases, the rate of proteoglycan synthesis falls off, the cells are no longer able to maintain the matrix, and end-stage OA develops, with full-thickness loss of cartilage (**Figure 4.4**).

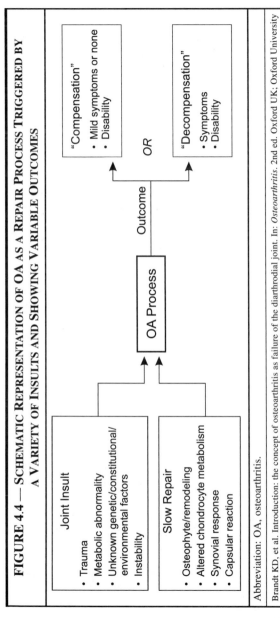

FIGURE 4.4 — SCHEMATIC REPRESENTATION OF OA AS A REPAIR PROCESS TRIGGERED BY A VARIETY OF INSULTS AND SHOWING VARIABLE OUTCOMES

Joint Insult
- Trauma
- Metabolic abnormality
- Unknown genetic/constitutional/environmental factors
- Instability

Slow Repair
- Osteophyte/remodeling
- Altered chondrocyte metabolism
- Synovial response
- Capsular reaction

OA Process

Outcome

"Compensation"
- Mild symptoms or none
- Disability

OR

"Decompensation"
- Symptoms
- Disability

Abbreviation: OA, osteoarthritis.

Brandt KD, et al. Introduction: the concept of osteoarthritis as failure of the diarthrodial joint. In: *Osteoarthritis.* 2nd ed. Oxford UK; Oxford University Press. In press.

REFERENCES

1. Radin EL, Paul IL. The response of joints to impact loading. I. *In vitro* wear. *Arthritis Rheum.* 1971;14:356-362.

2. Schumacher JR Jr. Secondary osteoarthritis. In: Moskowitz RW, Howell DS, Goldberg VM, Mankin JL, eds. *Osteoarthritis: Diagnosis and Medical/Surgical Management.* 2nd ed. Philadelphia, Pa: WB Saunders Company; 1992:367-398.

3. Ala-Kokko L, Baldwin CT, Moskowitz RW, et al. Single base mutation in the type II procollagen gene (COL2A1) as a cause of primary osteoarthritis associated with a mild chondrodysplasia. *Proc Natl Acad Sci USA.* 1990;87:6565-6568.

4. Reilly DT, Mertens M. Experimental analysis of the quadriceps muscle force and patello-femoral joint reaction force for various activities. *Acta Orthop Scand.* 1972;43:126-137.

5. Radin EL, Paul IL. Does cartilage compliance reduce skeletal impact loads? The relative force-attenuating properties of articular cartilage, synovial fluid, periarticular soft tissues and bone. *Arthritis Rheum.* 1970;13:139-144.

6. Radin EL, Parker HG, Pugh JW, Steinberg RS, Paul IL, Rose RM. Response of joints to impact loading. III. Relationship between trabecular microfractures and cartilage degeneration. *J Biomech.* 1973;6:51-57.

7. Burr DB. Bone. Subchondral bone in the pathogenesis of osteoarthritis. Mechanical aspects. In: Brandt KD, Doherty M, Lohmander SL. *Osteoarthritis.* 2nd ed. Oxford, UK: Oxford University Press. In press.

8. Brown TD, Radin EL, Martin RB, Burr DB. Finite element studies of some juxtarticular stress changes due to localized subchondral stiffening. *J Biomech.* 1984;17:11-24.

9. Vener MJ, Thompson RC Jr, Lewis JL, Oegema TR Jr. Subchondral damage after acute transarticular loading: an in vitro model of joint injury. *J Orthop Res.* 1992;10:759-765.

10. Westacott CI, Webb GR, Warnock MG, Sims JV, Elson CJ. Alteration of cartilage metabolism by cells from osteoarthritic bone. *Arthritis Rheum.* 1997;40:1282-1291.

11. Hilal G, Martel-Pelletier J, Pelletier JP, Ranger P, Lajeunesse D. Osteoblast-like cells from human subchondral osteoarthritis bone demonstrate an altered phenotype *in vitro*: possible role in subchondral bone sclerosis. *Arthritis Rheum.* 1998;41:891-899.

12. Nevitt MC, Scott JC, Lane NE, Genant HK, Hochberg MC, Cummings SR. Hip osteoarthritis and bone mineral density in older white women. *Arthritis Rheum.* 1992;35(suppl 9):S42.

13. Hart DJ, Mootoosamy I, Doyle DV, Spector TD. The relationship between osteoarthritis and osteoporosis in the general population: the Chingford study. *Ann Rheum Dis*. 1994;53:158-162.

14. Dequeker J. Inverse relationship of interface between osteoporosis and osteoarthritis. *J Rheumatol*. 1997;24:795-798.

15. Fazzalari NL, Parkinson IH. Fractal properties of subchondral cancellous bone in severe osteoarthritis of the hip. *J Bone Miner Res*. 1997;12:632-640.

16. Burr DB. The importance of subchondral bone in osteoarthrosis. *Curr Opin Rheumatol*. 1998;10:256-262.

17. Newberry WN, Zukosky DK, Haut RC. Subfracture insult to a knee joint causes alterations in the bone and in the functional stiffness of overlying cartilage. *J Orthop Res*. 1997;15:450-455.

18. Dedrick DK, Goulet R, Huston L, Goldstein SA, Bole GG. Early bone changes in experimental osteoarthritis using microscopic computer tomography. *J Rheumatol*. 1991;18(suppl 27):44-45.

19. Dedrick DK, Goldstein SA, Brandt KD, O'Connor BL, Goulet RW, Albrecht M. A longitudinal study of subchondral plate and trabecular bone in cruciate-deficient dogs with osteoarthritis followed for up to 54 months. *Arthritis Rheum*. 1993;36:1460-1467.

20. Myers SL. Effects of a bisphosphonate on bone histomorphometry and dynamics in the canine cruciate-deficiency model of osteoarthritis. *J Rheumatol*. 1999;26:2546-2653.

21. Hill AV. Production and absorption of work by muscle. *Science*. 1960;131:897-903.

22. Jones CM, Watt DG. Muscular control of landing from unexpected falls in man. *J Physiol*. 1971;219:729-737.

23. Radin EL, Yang KH, Riegger C, Kish VL, O'Connor JJ. Relationship between lower limb dynamics and knee joint pain. *J Orthop Res*. 1991;9:398-405.

24. Hurley MV. The role of muscle weakness in the pathogenesis of osteoarthritis. *Rheum Dis Clin North Am*. 1999;25:283-298.

25. Sharma L. Proprioceptive impairment in knee osteoarthritis. *Rheum Dis Clin North Am*. 1999;25:299-314.

26. O'Connor BL, Palmoski MJ, Brandt KD. Neurogenic acceleration of degenerative joint lesions. *J Bone Joint Surg Am*. 1985;67:562-572.

27. Sandy J, Plaas AH. Articular cartilage. Proteolytic degradation of normal and osteoarthritis cartilage matrix. In: Brandt KD, Doherty M, Lohmander SL, eds. *Osteoarthritis*. 2nd ed. Oxford, UK: Oxford University Press. In press.

28. Poole R, Howell DS. Etiopathogenesis of osteoarthritis. In: Moskowitz RW, Howell DS, Altman RD, Buckwalter JA, Goldberg VM, eds. *Osteoarthritis. Diagnosis and Medical/Surgical Management*. 3rd ed. Philadelphia: WB Saunders Company; 2001:29-47.

29. Ryu J, Treadwell BV, Mankin HJ. Biochemical and metabolic abnormalities in normal and osteoarthritic human articular cartilage. *Arthritis Rheum*. 1984;27:49-57.

30. Sweet MBE, Thonar EJ, Immelman AR, Solomon L. Biochemical changes in progressive osteoarthrosis. *Ann Rheum Dis*. 1977;36:387-398.

31. Mankin HJ, Dorfman H, Lippiello L, Zarins A. Biochemical and metabolic abnormalities in articular cartilage from osteoarthritic human hips. II. Correlation of morphology with biochemical and metabolic data. *J Bone Joint Surg*. 1971;53:523-537.

32. Smith GN Jr, Brandt KD. Hypothesis: Can type IX collagen "glue" together intersecting type II fibers in articular cartilage matrix? A proposed mechanism. *J Rheumatol*. 1992;19:14-17.

33. Vikkula M, Palotie A, Ritvaniemi P, et al. Early-onset osteoarthritis linked to the type II procollagen gene. Detailed clinical phenotype and further analyses of the gene. *Arthritis Rheum*. 1993;36:401-409.

34. Bywaters EGL. The metabolism of joint tissues. *J Pathol Bacteriol*. 1937;44:247-268.

35. Châteauvert JM, Grynpas MD, Kessler MJ, Pritzker KP. Spontaneous osteoarthritis in rhesus macaques. II. Characterization of disease and morphometric studies. *J Rheumatol*. 1990;17:73-83.

36. Vignon E, Arlot M, Hartmann D, Moyen B, Ville G. Hypertrophic repair of articular cartilage in experimental osteoarthrosis. *Ann Rheum Dis*. 1983;42:82-88.

37. McDevitt CA, Muir H, Pond MJ. Canine articular cartilage in natural and experimentally induced osteoarthritis. *Biochem Soc Trans*. 1973;1:287-289.

38. Dodge GR, Poole AR. Immunohistochemical detection and immunochemical analysis of type II collagen degradation in human normal, rheumatoid, and osteoarthritic articular cartilages and in explants of bovine articular cartilage cultured with interleukin 1. *J Clin Invest*. 1989;83:647-661.

39. Martel-Pelletier J, Faure MP, McCollum R, Mineau F, Cloutier JM, Pelletier JP. Plasmin, plasminogen activators and inhibitor in human osteoarthritic cartilage. *J Rheumatol*. 1991;18:1863-1871.

40. Martel-Pelletier J. Pathophysiology of osteoarthritis. *Osteoarthritis Cartilage*. 1999;7:371-373.

41. Pettipher ER, Higgs GA, Henderson B. Interleukin 1 induces leukocyte infiltration and cartilage proteoglycan degradation in the synovial joint. *Proc Natl Acad Sci USA*. 1986;83:8749-8753.

42. Pelletier JP, Caron JP, Evans C, et al. In vivo suppression of early experimental osteoarthritis by interleukin-1 receptor antagonist using gene therapy. *Arthritis Rheum*. 1997;40:1012-1019.

43. Dean DD, Martel-Pelletier J, Pelletier JP, Howell D, Woessner JF Jr. Evidence for metalloproteinase and metalloproteinase inhibitor imbalance in human osteoarthritic cartilage. *J Clin Invest*. 1989;84:678-685.

44. Morales TI. Cartilage proteoglycan homeostasis: role of growth factors. In: Brandt KD, ed. *Cartilage Changes in Osteoarthritis*. Indianapolis, Ind: Indiana University School of Medicine; 1990:17-21.

45. Doré S, Pelletier JP, Di Battista JS, Tardif G, Brazeau P, Martel-Pelletier J. Human osteoarthritic chondrocytes possess an increased number of insulin-like growth factor 1 binding sites but are unresponsive to its stimulation. Possible role of IGF-1 binding proteins. *Arthritis Rheum*. 1994;37:253-263.

46. Martel-Pelletier J, Di Battista J, Lajeunesse D, Pelletier JP. IGF/IGFBP axis in cartilage and bone in osteoarthritis pathogenesis. *Inflamm Res*. 1998;47:90-100.

47. Swan A, Chapman B, Heap P, Seward H, Dieppe P. Submicroscopic crystals in osteoarthritic synovial fluids. *Ann Rheum Dis*. 1994;53:467-470.

48. Halverson PB, McCarty DJ. Patterns of radiographic abnormalities associated with basic calcium phosphate and calcium pyrophosphate crystal deposition in the knee. *Ann Rheum Dis*. 1986;45:603-605.

49. Carroll GJ, Stuart RA, Armstrong JA, Breidahl PD, Laing BA. Hydroxyapatite crystals are a frequent finding in osteoarthritic synovial fluid, but are not related to increased concentrations of keratan sulfate or interleukin 1 beta. *J Rheumatol*. 1991;18:861-866.

50. McCarthy GM. Crystal-related tissue damage. In: Smyth CJ, Holer VM, eds. *Gout, Hyperuricemia and Other Crystal-Associated Arthropathies*. New York, NY: Marcel Dekker; 1999:39-57.

51. McCarthy GM, Kurup IV, Westfall PR. Basic calcium phosphate crystals induce mitogenesis and metalloprotease production in human synovial fibroblasts. *Arthritis Rheum*. 1998;41(suppl 9):S300.

52. McCarty DJ, Halverson PB, Carresa GF, Brewer BJ, Kozin F. "Milwaukee shoulder"—association of microspheroids containing hydroxyapatite crystals, active collagenase and neutral protease with rotator cuff defects. I. Clinical aspects. *Arthritis Rheum*. 1981;24:464-473.

53. Concoff AL, Kalunian KC. What is the relation between crystals and osteoarthritis? *Curr Opin Rheumatol.* 1999;11:436-440.

54. Ryan L. Articular cartilage. Crystals and osteoarthritis. In: Brandt KB, Doherty M, Lohmander SL. *Osteoarthritis.* 2nd ed. Oxford, UK: Oxford University Press. In press.

55. Pelletier JP, Jovanovic D, Fernandes JC, et al. Reduced progression of experimental osteoarthritis in vivo by selective inhibition of inducible nitric oxide synthase. *Arthritis Rheum.* 1998;41:1275-1286.

56. Myers SL, Brandt KD, O'Connor BL, Visco DM, Albrecht ME. Synovitis and osteoarthritic changes in canine articular cartilage after anterior cruciate ligament transection. Effect of surgical hemostasis. *Arthritis Rheum.* 1990;33:1406-1415.

57. Myers SL, Brandt KD, O'Connor BL. Low dose prednisone treatment does not reduce the severity of osteoarthritis in dogs after anterior cruciate ligament transection. *J Rheumatol.* 1991;18:1856-1862.

5 Clinical Features

Joints Affected

The joints most frequently affected by osteoarthritis (OA) are (**Figure 5.1**):
- Interphalangeal joints of the hands
- Spine
- Knees
- Hips
- First metatarsophalangeal joint.

In most people with symptomatic OA of peripheral joints, more than one joint is affected. Among 500 subjects with symptomatic OA in peripheral joints, only 6% had symptoms confined to a single joint.[1] The most commonly involved joints were:
- Knees (41%)
- Hands (30%)
- Hips (19%).

In patients with hip OA, congenital or developmental abnormality of that joint (eg, Legg-Calvé-Perthes disease [avascular necrosis of the secondary center of ossification in the femoral head], slipped femoral capital epiphysis, congenital dysplasia)[2-4] may be present. In contrast, congenital or developmental abnormalities are seldom a basis for knee OA, in which a history of prior trauma, meniscectomy, obesity, and certain repetitive vocational activities are dominant risk factors.[2] OA of the spine, which most often affects the lumbar and cervical regions, also is not usually associated with a history of trauma. While secondary OA may involve any diarthrodial joint in the body, in the absence of trauma or of a developmental or congenital abnormality, primary OA is uncommon in the elbow, glenohumeral joint, ankle, and wrist.

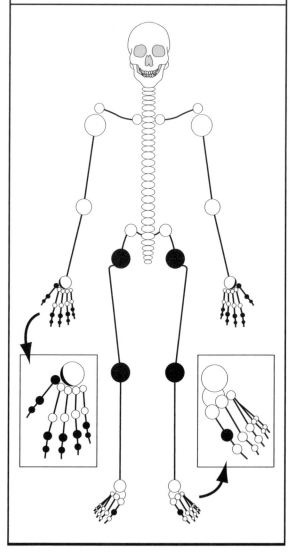

FIGURE 5.1 — HOMUNCULUS SHOWING
JOINTS COMMONLY INVOLVED IN
IDIOPATHIC (PRIMARY) OA

In the vast majority of cases, the clinical feature that leads the patient with OA to seek medical attention is joint pain (**Table 5.1**). Systemic manifestations (eg, fever, anemia, weight loss) are not features of primary OA (**Table 5.2**).[5] Typically, the discomfort has been present for months or years and has been only slowly progressive. The pain is often described as a deep, dull ache, localized to the involved joint, aggravated by use of that joint—especially by weight-bearing in the case of knee or hip OA—and relieved by rest.[5] Although the pain is initially intermittent, with progression of the disease it may become constant, increasingly severe, and disabling. Nocturnal pain interfering with sleep is seen particularly in advanced OA of the hip, in which it is often associated with an effusion of the joint. The presence of night pain in patients with

TABLE 5.1 — COMMON SYMPTOMS AND SIGNS OF OA

Symptoms
- Joint pain
- Joint stiffness
- Crepitus
- Alteration in joint shape
- Functional impairment

Signs
- Crepitus
- Restricted movement
- Tenderness
  - Joint line
  - Periarticular
- Bony swelling
- Soft tissue swelling
- Limp
- Deformity
- Muscle atrophy/weakness
- Increased warmth (±) effusion
- Instability

TABLE 5.2 — CLINICAL FEATURES OF OA

- No primary extra-articular manifestations
- Usually only one or a few joints are symptomatic
- Slow evolution of symptoms and structural damage
- Strong association with age—uncommon before middle age
- Poor correlation between severity of symptoms, disability, and structural change
- Symptoms and signs predominantly relate to joint damage rather than to inflammation

O'Reilly S, Doherty M. In: *Osteoarthritis*. 2nd ed. Oxford, UK: Oxford University Press. In press.

hip OA was found to predict hip joint effusion in over 90% of patients, whereas ultrasonography was much less reliable, predicting effusion in only 70% to 85% of cases.[6]

In patients with OA of the hip, movements requiring internal rotation, in particular, are likely to evoke pain. In those with OA of the knee, extremes of flexion (eg, squatting) or of extension may be painful. In those with OA of the thumb base (**Figure 5.2**) or other joints of the hand, pinch movements and tight grasp, as required for opening a jar, may lead to discomfort.

In some patients with OA, the pain may be referred. For example, pain due to OA of the hip may be referred to the knee. In those with OA of the cervical spine, it may be localized to the shoulder, arm, forearm, or hand; in some cases, pain at these sites may occur in the absence of neck pain. Pain from OA of the cervical or lumbar spine may have a radicular component (ie, it may be sharp and shooting, and aggravated by the increase in intrathecal pressure generated by coughing, sneezing, or straining with a bowel movement). Physical examination may reveal neurologic signs, such as altered sensation, reduced strength, or diminution of a deep tendon reflex, consistent with involvement of a single nerve root.

In addition to joint pain, the patient with OA may complain of joint stiffness. Although morning stiffness is a classic feature of rheumatoid arthritis, it is less well recognized as a feature of OA. While the morning stiffness of rheuma-

**FIGURE 5.2 — CLINICAL FEATURES:
OA OF THE THUMB BASE**

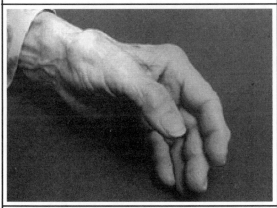

Bony enlargement and squaring of the thumb base caused by bony hypertrophy (osteophytosis) in a patient with osteoarthritis (OA) of the metacarpotrapezial joint.

toid arthritis may persist for hours after the patient awakens, in OA, morning stiffness it usually lasts no more than 20 to 30 minutes. This "gelling" sensation in patients with OA may be prominent not only on arising but after any period of inactivity, such as an automobile ride or an evening in a theater seat. The stiffness induced by inactivity during the day, like morning stiffness, usually subsides rapidly. In those with knee involvement, it typically abates after only a few steps. With progression of the disease, however, the stiffness becomes more prolonged.

Patients with OA often complain of crepitus, the sensation of "cracking" or "popping" of tissues of the involved joint rubbing against each other with movement. Often, crepitus is audible. It is most common in those with OA of the knee.

In other patients with OA, deformity is a complaint. They may note, for example, that one knee has become larger than the other or that the base of the big toe (**Color Plate 8**) or a distal interphalangeal joint (**Figure 5.3**) has become enlarged. In addition, they may complain of angu-

**FIGURE 5.3 — CLINICAL
FEATURES: NODAL OA**

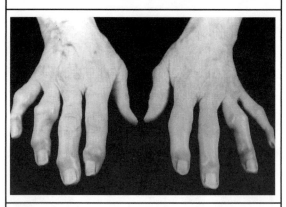

Nodal osteoarthritis (OA) involving both the distal and proximal interphalangeal joints. Note the bony enlargement of the distal interphalangeal joints (Heberden's nodes) and several proximal interphalangeal joints (Bouchard's nodes). Gross deformity is obvious in some joints.

lar deformities, such as bowing of the knees (varus) due to OA of the medial tibiofemoral compartment or squaring of the thumb base due to involvement of the first carpometacarpal joint or metacarpotrapezial joint (**Figure 5.2**). At times, the deformity may be striking (**Color Plate 9**).

In patients with OA of the hip or knee, development of a limp may be a major source of concern, especially when the disturbance is noticeable to others watching the patient walk. Walking on an uneven surface or on a ramp tends to exaggerate the limp.

Origins of Joint Pain in OA

Because articular cartilage is aneural, the joint pain in OA must arise from other structures (**Table 5.3**). In some cases, it may be due to stretching of nerve endings in the periosteum covering osteophytes. In others, it may arise from

TABLE 5.3 — ORIGINS OF JOINT PAIN IN PATIENTS WITH OSTEOARTHRITIS

Tissue	Mechanism of Pain
Subchondral bone	Medullary hypertension, microfractures
Osteophytes	Stretching of nerve endings in periosteum
Ligaments	Stretch
Enthesis	Inflammation
Joint capsule	Inflammation, distention
Periarticular muscle	Spasm
Synovium	Inflammation

synovitis or from microfractures in subchondral bone.[7] In other patients, it may reflect bone angina, caused by the distortion of medullary blood flow by the thickened subchondral trabeculae.[8] The latter may increase intraosseous pressure[9] and can cause severe intraosseous stasis. This hemodynamic abnormality is reflected in a prolongation of the emptying time after intraosseous injection of radiopaque contrast material into the femoral neck.[9] Joint instability (leading to stretching of the joint capsule, muscle spasm, enthesopathy, and bursitis) is an additional source of pain in OA.

Synovium from patients with advanced OA typically exhibits lining cell hyperplasia and marked infiltration with mononuclear cells (**Figure 3.3**).[10,11] These changes may be qualitatively and quantitatively indistinguishable from those in the synovium of patients with rheumatoid arthritis. Synovitis in OA may be due to phagocytosis of wear particles of cartilage or bone[12-15] from the abraded joint surface, release from the cartilage of soluble matrix macromolecules (eg, glycosaminoglycans, proteoglycans),[16] or the presence of crystals of calcium pyrophosphate or calcium hydroxyapatite.[17] In some cases, immune complexes containing antigens derived from cartilage matrix may be sequestered in collagenous tissue of the joint, such as the meniscus, leading to chronic low-grade synovitis.[18]

Earlier in the course of OA, however, even in the patient with joint pain and even if the articular cartilage exhibits full-thickness ulceration,[19] the synovium may be *histologically* normal (**Color Plate 10**), suggesting that the pain is due to one of the other factors mentioned earlier. Conversely, in patients with knee OA who have no joint pain, the severity of cartilage damage and synovial inflammation may be as great as that in patients with OA who *have* knee pain.[19] Among a series of patients with chronic knee pain who had only minimal radiographic changes of OA and in whom the diagnosis was confirmed arthroscopically, we found that 45% showed no evidence of inflammation in any of multiple samples of synovium, even when full-thickness cartilage ulceration was present.[19]

Thus, at least in relatively early (or mild) OA, the correlation between joint pain and synovitis is poor. This is not surprising. As noted above, joint pain in OA may be due to a variety of factors other than synovitis. The relief of joint pain achieved with a nonsteroidal anti-inflammatory drug (NSAID) may be due to its analgesic effect rather than to an anti-inflammatory effect.

The "joint pain" in patients with OA may arise from periarticular as well as articular structures. It is common for the patient with OA to develop soft tissue rheumatism in areas adjacent to the involved joint; for example:

- Anserine bursitis, in the patient with knee OA
- Trochanteric bursitis, in the patient with hip OA
- Subacromial bursitis and bicipital tendinitis, in the patient with OA of the glenohumeral or subacromial joint.

Physical Findings

Physical examination of the OA joint may reveal tenderness and bony or soft tissue swelling (**Table 5**.1). Tenderness (the sensation and/or sound of joint tissues rubbing against each other with movement of the joint) may be diffuse or localized to marginal osteophytes or to the synovium. Crepitus is characteristic of OA. It may present as the soft crepitus of fibrillated cartilage, as in the patellofemoral joint, or the harder, sharp crepitus of joints in which articular cartilage has been lost so that adjacent bony surfaces rub against each other with movement. This is particularly noticeable in OA of the thumb base and knee. Synovial effusions, when present, are usually not large, although those in the knee or shoulder may occasionally be voluminous. Palpation may reveal some warmth over the joint. In the advanced stages of OA, gross deformity, palpable bony hypertrophy, subluxation, and marked loss of joint motion, often with noticeable contracture, may be striking. Enlargement of the joint may be due to effusion, synovial thickening or osteophytes, which can significantly alter the contour of the joint. Bony swelling due to osteophytes is particularly noticeable in patients with Heberden's or Bouchard's nodes (interphalangeal joint OA of the hands) (**Figure 5.3**) and OA of the first metatarsophalangeal (bunion) joint (**Color Plate 8**). Periarticular muscle atrophy may be due to disuse (as a result of unloading of the painful extremity)[20,21] and may exaggerate the appearance of joint swelling.

The widely held notion that once symptoms appear, OA is inexorably and intractably progressive is incorrect. In many patients, the disease stabilizes. In some, especially those with OA of the knee, regression of joint pain and even of radiographic changes may occur.[22] For example, Massardo and colleagues described 31 patients with knee OA who underwent clinical and radiographic evaluation on two occasions separated by an 8-year interval. While 20% worsened over the interval and many incurred severe disability, four patients (13%) *improved* and two had striking improvement in function. Among 63 subjects in whom paired knee radiographs were obtained at a mean interval of 11 years, only 33% showed radiographic progression.[23] Notably, pain scores also tended not to worsen. Thus many subjects with knee OA do not deteriorate either radiographically or symptomatically over lengthy periods of observation. However, it is important to identify the subset of patients who do undergo more rapid progression of their disease and to direct efforts at early intervention toward that high-risk group.[24]

REFERENCES

1. Cushnaghan J, Dieppe P. Study of 500 patients with limb joint osteoarthritis. I. Analysis by age, sex, and distribution of symptomatic joint sites. *Ann Rheum Dis*. 1991;50:8-13.

2. Felson DT. Epidemiology of hip and knee osteoarthritis. *Epidemiol Rev*. 1988;10:1-28.

3. Harris WH. Etiology of osteoarthritis of the hip. *Clin Orthop*. 1986;213:20-33.

4. Wilson MG, Poss R. Osteoarthritis of the hip. In: Moskowitz RW, Howell DS, Goldberg VM, Mankin FJ, eds. *Osteoarthritis: Diagnosis and Medical/Surgical Management*. 2nd ed. Philadelphia, Pa: WB Saunders Company; 1992:621-649.

5. O'Reilly S, Doherty M. Signs, symptoms, and laboratory tests. In: Brandt KD, Doherty M, Lohmander LS, eds. *Osteoarthritis*. 2nd ed. Oxford, UK: Oxford University Press. In press.

6. Földes K, Bálint P, Gaál M, Buchanan WW, Bálint GP. Nocturnal pain correlates with effusions in diseased hips. *J Rheumatol*. 1992; 19:1756-1758.

7. Radin EL, Parker HG, Pugh JW, Steinberg RS, Paul IL, Rose RM. Response of joints to impact loading. 3. Relationship between trabecular microfractures and cartilage degeneration. *J Biomech*. 1973;6:51-57.

8. Lemperg RK, Arnoldi CC. The significance of intraosseous pressure in normal and diseased states with special reference to the intraosseous engorgement-pain syndrome. *Clin Orthop*. 1978;136:143-156.

9. Arnoldi CC, Linderholm H, Müssbichler H. Venous engorgement and intraosseous hypertension in osteoarthritis of the hip. *J Bone Joint Surg Br*. 1972;54:409-421.

10. Soren A, Cooper NS, Waugh TR. The nature and designation of osteoarthritis determined by its histopathology. *Clin Exp Rheumatol*. 1988;6:41-46.

11. Johnell O, Hulth A, Henricson A. T-Lymphocyte subsets and HLA-DR-expressing cells in the osteoarthritic synovialis. *Scand J Rheumatol*. 1985;14:259-264.

12. Evans CH, Mears DC, McKnight JL. A preliminary ferrographic survey of the wear particles in human synovial fluid. *Arthritis Rheum*. 1981;24:912-918.

13. Evans CH. Cellular mechanisms of hydrolytic enzyme release in osteoarthritis. *Semin Arthritis Rheum*. 1981;11(suppl 1):93-95.

14. Hotchkiss RN, Tew WP, Hungerford DS. Cartilaginous debris in the injured human knee. Correlation with arthroscopic findings. *Clin Orthop*. 1982;168:144-156.

15. Myers SL, Flusser D, Brandt KD, Heck DA. Prevalence of cartilage shards in synovium and their association with synovitis in patients with early and end stage osteoarthritis. *J Rheumatol*. 1992;19: 1247-1251.

16. Boniface RJ, Cain PR, Evans CH. Articular responses to purified cartilage proteoglycans. *Arthritis Rheum*. 1988;31:258-266.

17. Schumacher HR, Gordon G, Paul H, et al. Osteoarthritis, crystal deposition and inflammation. *Semin Arthritis Rheum*. 1981;11:116-119.

18. Jasin HE. Immune mechanisms in osteoarthritis. *Semin Arthritis Rheum*. 1989;18(suppl 2):86-90.

19. Myers SL, Brandt KD, Ehlich JW, et al. Synovial inflammation in patients with early osteoarthritis of the knee. *J Rheumatol*. 1990;17: 1662-1669.

20. Sirca A, Susec-Michieli M. Selective type II fibre muscular atrophy in patients with osteoarthritis of the hip. *J Neurol Sci*. 1980; 44:149-159.

21. De Andrade JR, Grant C, Dixon A St J. Joint distension and reflex muscle inhibition in the knee. *J Bone Joint Surg*. 1965;47A:313-322.

22. Brandt KD, Flusser D. Osteoarthritis. In: Bellamy N, ed. *Prognosis in the Rheumatic Diseases*. Lancaster, UK: Kluwer Academic Publishers; 1991:11-35.

23. Massardo L, Watt I, Cushnaghan J, Dieppe P. Osteoarthritis of the knee joint: an eight year prospective study. *Ann Rheum Dis*. 1989;48:893-897.

24. Spector TD, Dacre JE, Harris PA, Huskisson EC. Radiological progression of osteoarthritis: an 11 year follow up study of the knee. *Ann Rheum Dis*. 1992;51:1107-1110.

6

Pitfalls in the Diagnosis of OA

The correct diagnosis of osteoarthritis (OA) is important—misdiagnosis is likely to lead to the omission of appropriate treatment or institution of unnecessary treatment; furthermore, it may be psychologically stressful to the patient. Misinterpretation of the patient's symptoms and signs is a common pitfall in the diagnosis of OA. As indicated in previous chapters, pain is the predominant symptom in patients with OA and the pain of OA has typical characteristics. Furthermore, pain may arise not only from intra-articular structures but from periarticular muscle spasm or soft tissue rheumatism. The differentiation of articular from periarticular pain is important because periarticular pain can often be managed by local injection of a depot glucocorticoid preparation and physical therapy without systemic medication. Bálint and Szebenyi[1] have published a clear analysis of the problems underlying the diagnosis of OA and the factors that confound clinicians in this area.

Misinterpretation of Pain

Several common circumstances lead to misinterpretation of pain in the patient with OA (**Table 6.1**),[1] for example:

- The origin of pain is not the OA but some other type of arthritis, trauma, a neurologic disorder, or soft tissue rheumatism, occurring independently of OA. Rheumatic diseases are not mutually exclusive; the person with OA has no immunity from superimposed gout or staphylococcal infection of the OA joint; the person with thumb-base OA may coincidentally develop de Quervain's tenosynovitis (**Figure 6.1**).
- The pain is caused by OA, but at a remote joint site. For example, pain in the knee is commonly referred from the hip. Radiculopathy due to OA of apophyseal joints in the lumbar spine is a common cause of pain in the hip or gluteal region. Careful localization and characterization of the pain (is it burn-

TABLE 6.1 — MISINTERPRETATION OF JOINT PAIN IN PATIENTS WITH RADIOGRAPHIC EVIDENCE OF OA

The source of the pain is not osteoarthritis but...
- Some other type of arthritis
- Pathologic changes in the adjacent bone (tumor, osteomyelitis, metabolic bone disease, etc)
- Mechanical injury, pathologic fracture
- Referred pain of neuritis, neuropathy, or radiculopathy (eg, L_4 radioculopathy may cause pain in the knee or greater trochanter)
- Other neurologic disorders causing stiffness of joints (Parkinson's disease, upper motor neuron damage, etc)
- Soft tissue rheumatism independent of osteoarthritis (OA) (eg, de Quervain's tenosynovitis)

The source of the pain is osteoarthritis but not at the joint suspected, for example:
- OA of the hip causing pain localized to the knee
- OA of the cervical apophyseal joints (C4-5) causing pain in the shoulder
- OA of the acromioclavicular joint causing pain in the shoulder
- OA of the lumbar apophyseal joints causing pain in the hip, knee, or ankle

The pain is caused by secondary soft tissue rheumatism, for example:
- Ligamentous instability (especially of the knee)
- Enthesopathy
- Bursitis

Bálint G, Szebenyi B. *Drugs.* 1996;52(suppl 3):1-13.

ing? lancinating? is numbness present?) can help in making an accurate diagnosis.

- The pain is due to soft tissue rheumatism which has developed secondary to OA, eg, anserine bursitis[2] (**Figure 6.2**) or collateral ligament strain in the patient with knee OA.

FIGURE 6.1 — DE QUERVAIN'S TENOSYNOVITIS

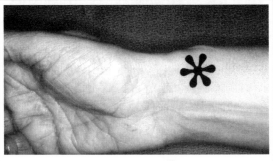

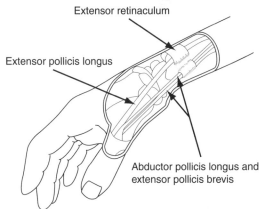

Extensor retinaculum

Extensor pollicis longus

Abductor pollicis longus and
extensor pollicis brevis

Note the swelling immediately proximal to the radial styloid (*asterisk*), reflecting inflammation of the sheath of the extensor pollicis brevis and abductor pollicis longus tendons. Diagram of underlying anatomy (*bottom*). Note that the sheath of the above tendons is proximal to the radial styloid and the first carpometacarpal joint.

Photo courtesy of Alex Mih, MD.

Diagram from Shipley M. In: *Rheumatic Diseases, Pocket Picture Guides to Clinical Medicine*. Baltimore, Md: Williams & Wilkins; 1985:1-93.

FIGURE 6.2 — SITES OF INSERTION OF THE GRACILIS, SARTORIUS, AND SEMITENDINOUS MUSCLES INTO THE PERIOSTEUM OF THE TIBIA

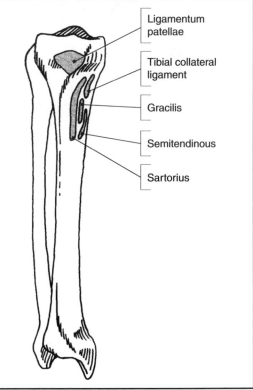

The anserine bursa is commonly a source of pain in persons with radiographic evidence of knee osteoarthritis. The bursa overlies the insertions of the gracilis, sartorius, and semitendinous muscles into the periosteum of the tibia. In patients with inflammation of the anserine bursa, examination reveals sharply localized tenderness upon palpation over the bursa.

Brandt KD. In: *Diagnostic Studies in Rheumatology*. Summit, NJ: Ciba-Geigy; 1993:1-66.

In OA, deformity is due to destruction of joint tissues, such as the articular cartilage and menisci, bony remodeling, osteophyte formation, and ligamentous damage. Deformities may be caused by diseases other than OA, some of which, like OA, may cause joint pain, gelling after periods of immobility, limitation of movement, crepitus, and bony swelling and lead to misdiagnosis. For example, hypertrophic osteoarthropathy may be confused with nodal OA of the fingers. However, clubbing of the nails and radiographic evidence of periostitis (**Figure 6.3**) differentiate this condition from OA.

In patients with psoriatic arthritis of the distal interphalangeal joint, nail changes (**Color Plate 11**) and skin lesions of psoriasis can establish the diagnosis. The skin lesions may be limited to the scalp line, perianal region, umbilicus, or external auditory canal and hence require a careful and extensive examination of the integument for their detection.

Flexion contractures of joints, particularly of fingers, knees, and hips, in elderly people may be erroneously attributed to OA when they are, in fact, due to Dupuytren's contracture (**Color Plate 12**), diabetic cheirarthropathy, trauma, or a neurologic condition. Flexion contracture of the knee may be caused by a loose body; flexion contracture of the hip may be due to osteonecrosis (avascular necrosis) of the femoral head (**Figure 6.4**).

Neuropathic arthropathy (Charcot's joint) (**Color Plate 13 and Figure 6.5**) can mimic OA. Extensive periarticular ossification, ligamentous laxity, and severe deformity, with marked bony hypertrophy and often osteochondral fractures, are characteristic and differentiate this condition from OA. Although neuropathic joint disease may be relatively painless, it is not uncommon for the neuropathic joint to be severely painful and to exhibit acute signs of inflammation, raising concern about the presence of septic arthritis. Careful neurologic examination (with particular attention paid to impairment of position sense) is important in evaluating a patient suspected of having this disorder. Arthrocentesis, with careful analysis of the synovial fluid, including a

FIGURE 6.3 — PERIOSTEAL REACTION IN THE FEMUR OF A PATIENT WITH HYPERTROPHIC OSTEOARTHROPATHY

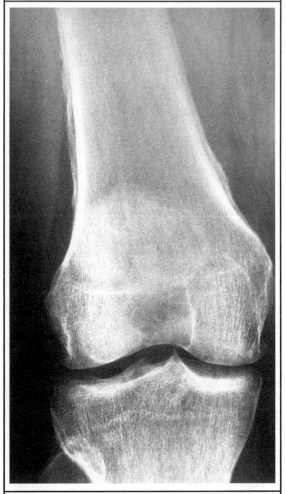

Marked periosteal reaction in the femur of a patient with hypertrophic osteoarthropy due to carcinoma of the breast which has metastasized to the lung.

FIGURE 6.4 — OSTEONECROSIS (AVASCULAR NECROSIS) OF THE HIP

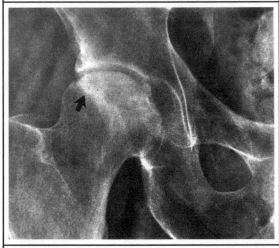

Note the slight flattening of the femoral head and patchy sclerosis and demineralization. The arrow points to an area of increased bony density, reflecting collapse and condensation of the subchondral bone.

Gram's stain and culture, may be required to exclude acute bacterial joint infection.

Misinterpretation of the Radiograph

Radiographs must be interpreted within the context of the patient's history and physical findings.[1] Misinterpretation of the radiograph is a common pitfall leading to erroneous diagnosis in patients with OA (**Table 6.2**), for example:

- The patient with radiographic evidence of OA may present with a history and physical examination that indicate a second type of arthritis having no distinguishing radiographic characteristics at the time of presentation (eg, acute gout or pseudogout without radiographic evidence of a tophus or chondrocalcinosis, respectively; or acute bacterial joint in-

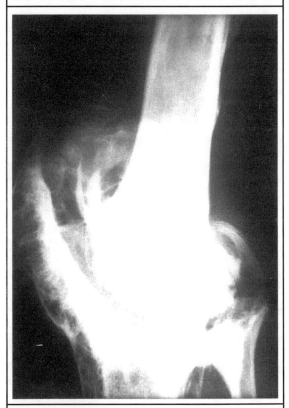

This radiograph reveals erosion and irregularity of the joint surfaces, extensive new bone formation, and soft tissue calcification and ossification. A massive amount of new bone extends anteriorly and superiorly from the anterior articulating surface of the tibia. Abundant joint detritus is present.

**TABLE 6.2 — CONDITIONS LEADING TO
MISINTERPRETATION OF THE RADIOGRAPH
RESULTING IN MISDIAGNOSIS OF OA**

- Some other type of arthritis occurring in a joint with previous OA changes
- Absence of radiographic changes in initial stages of OA
- Diffuse idiopathic skeletal hyperostosis
- Joint flexion contracture causing loss of joint space width that is misinterpreted as thinning of the articular cartilage
- Neurogenic and metabolic arthropathies

Abbreviation: OA, osteoarthritis.

Bálint G, Szebenyi B. *Drugs*. 1996;52(suppl 3):1-13.

fection before juxta-articular osteoporosis and destruction of the cortical margins have developed).

- Flexion of the knee due to pain may result in narrowing of joint space width on the conventional standing anteroposterior radiograph, which is misinterpreted as a loss of articular cartilage, when in fact, the joint is normal and the reduction in interbone distance is due only to the position of the joint.

- The patient may have diffuse idiopathic skeletal hyperostosis (**Figure 6.6**), with ossification of the anterior spinal ligament, which is misinterpreted as vertebral osteophytosis.

- The patient may have a systemic metabolic abnormality, eg, Wilson's disease, hemochromatosis, or chondrocalcinosis (**Figure 6.7**), producing radiographic changes that are misinterpreted as "garden-variety" OA.

Misinterpretation of Laboratory Results

Among the disorders that must be considered in the differential diagnosis of a patient with OA are systemic inflammatory connective tissue disease and autoimmune diseases, such as rheumatoid arthritis and systemic lupus erythematosus. Because OA is principally a disease of the

FIGURE 6.6 — DIFFUSE IDIOPATHIC SKELETAL HYPEROSTOSIS

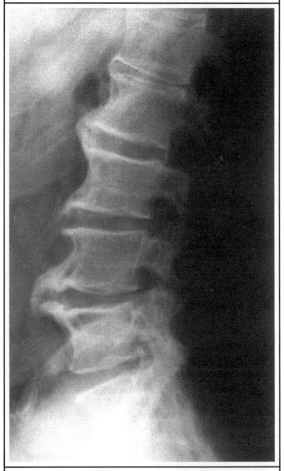

Diffuse idiopathic skeletal hyperostosis (DISH) with prominent ossification of the anterior longitudinal ligament of the spine.

Radiograph kindly provided by Kenneth Buckwalter, MD.

FIGURE 6.7 — CHONDROCALCINOSIS

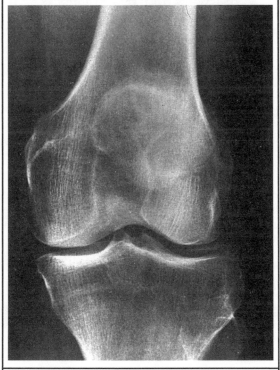

Note deposits of calcium pyrophosphate dihydrate in the menisci and articular cartilage of this patient with osteoarthritis.

elderly, it is important to recognize that the erythrocyte sedimentation rate (ESR) increases with age (**Table 6.3**); a sedimentation rate of, eg, 50 mm/hour, which would be abnormal for a person in her 20s or 30s, is consistent with age alone in an individual in her 70s.[3]

Because many patients with OA (particularly knee OA) are obese, it is notable that a higher body mass index has been found to be associated with a higher serum concentration of the acute phase reactant, C-reactive protein.[4] Furthermore, restricting the analysis to young adults (17 to 39 years of age) and excluding smokers, subjects with clini-

TABLE 6.3 — MISINTERPRETATION OF LABORATORY TEST RESULTS AS A BASIS FOR MISDIAGNOSIS OF OA

- Increase in erythrocyte sedimentation rate with age
- Increase in serum rheumatoid factor titer with age
- Increase in serum antinuclear antibody levels with age
- Increase in serum C-reactive protein levels with obesity

cally apparent inflammatory disease, cardiovascular disease, diabetes mellitus, and estrogen users, did not appreciably change the results, which suggest the presence of low-grade systemic inflammation in obese individuals.

It should also be recognized that the titers of serum rheumatoid factor and antinuclear antibodies rise with age.[5,6] In the elderly in particular, positive tests do not necessarily connote the presence of a systemic connective tissue disorder. In most cases, careful history and physical examination will differentiate these conditions from OA, obviating the need to obtain measurements of ESR, rheumatoid factor, and antinuclear antibody level in elderly subjects with OA.

Avoiding Diagnostic Pitfalls

Diagnostic pitfalls can be avoided by careful history taking, physical examination of the patient, and occasionally the use of appropriate imaging methods. These measures are also useful in differentiating the various primary and secondary forms of OA.

■ Taking a Careful History

The key to obtaining a careful patient history involves questioning the patient about:

- The prevalence of OA in the family, especially in suspected cases of generalized OA.
- The time of occurrence of initial symptoms and signs. Secondary OA due to trauma, joint laxity, joint dysplasia, osteochondromatosis, osteochondritis dissecans, metabolic disease, etc, may occur at a younger age than idiopathic (primary) OA. The joint

deformities of mucopolysaccharidoses, rickets, etc, which can mimic OA, also occur at a young age.

- The circumstances in which first symptoms and signs appeared. Were they connected to trauma that may have caused tendinous, ligamentous, meniscal, or muscular tears?
- Previous infection that might have caused septic arthritis or postinfectious arthritis.
- Underlying metabolic diseases, such as diabetes mellitus, hypothyroidism, hemochromatosis, Wilson's disease, or chondrocalcinosis, which might cause secondary OA.
- The patterns of pain and stiffness, to determine whether these are characteristic of OA.

■ Performing a Careful Physical Examination

During the physical examination, one of the most important tasks of the examiner is to elicit the pain that the patient complains of and to determine its source (ie, do active and passive movements of the joint elicit pain?).

In many cases, careful examination of the patient will permit the physician to avoid diagnostic pitfalls. For example, when it is referred from the hip, L_4 nerve root, or femoral nerve, knee pain can be elicited by movements of the hip or spine (eg, by femoral nerve stretch). Similarly, shoulder pain may originate from the cervical spine and can be provoked by movements of the neck. Pain felt at the greater trochanter may arise from the lumbar spine. Pain in the fingers or toes may be due to an entrapment neuropathy (carpal or tarsal tunnel syndrome) or nerve root irritation.

Pain in the patellofemoral joint can be elicited by pressing the patella against the femoral joint surface. Examination of the knee should include maneuvers to evoke ligamentous, meniscal, or tendoperiosteal pain and pain arising from bursae.

Tender points should be identified. In addition to, or rather than, the characteristic tenderness of joint structures, tenderness of the soft tissues may be present, eg, in patients with anserine or trochanteric bursitis.

Another important part of the physical examination is the evaluation of swelling and deformity. Bony swelling of the joint is characteristic of OA, especially around the distal interphalangeal joints (Heberden's nodes) and proximal interphalangeal joints (Bouchard's nodes) (**Figure 5.3**) and the medial and lateral tibiofemoral compartments of the knee joint. The nodes are often palpable before they can be detected on x-ray because they develop as radiolucent cartilaginous outgrowths (chondrophytes) that only later undergo ossification, when they may be recognized as radiopaque osteophytes.

Soft tissue swelling may also be a feature of OA. It may occur in addition to, or in the absence of, bony swelling. Soft tissue swelling and palpable joint effusion are often present in proximal interphalangeal and distal interphalangeal (DIP) joints and in the knee.

Palpation of crepitus may be informative. Fine crepitation felt throughout the entire range of movement is usually of capsular origin. It may occur in normal individuals and has no diagnostic significance. In contrast, coarse cracking felt with movement of the joint may be due to articular cartilage damage, in which case it is caused by the movement of uneven surfaces over each other. One or two cracks felt over the knee during movement of the joint can be a sign of a loose body or torn meniscus. Around the hip, snapping, loud crepitus is usually caused by slippage of the iliotibial ligament over the greater trochanter.[7]

Examination of joint function is an important part of the physical examination and may have diagnostic value. For example, in OA of the hip, internal rotation and abduction are initially restricted, followed by restriction of adduction, hyperextension, and external rotation. Restriction of extension without limitation of internal rotation raises the suspicion of other disorders, such as a psoas abscess or iliopectineal bursitis. Similarly, extension contracture of the knee (loss of flexion) is characteristic of spastic paresis, locking of the joint due to a loose body, or contracture resulting from immobilization but is not usually caused by OA. A flexed position of the DIP joint suggests OA or psoriatic arthritis. If free passive movement of the DIP joint exists, the flexed position is probably due to rupture of the extensor tendon.

It is important to test for abnormal passive movement of the joint due to joint laxity. These abnormalities are com-

96

COLOR PLATE 1 — ADVANCED OA OF THE KNEE

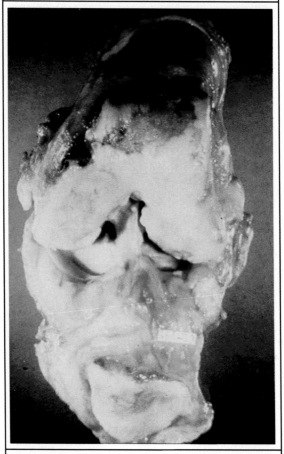

The joint has been opened anteriorly and the patella has been reflected downward. Note the large ulcerated areas of articular cartilage in the intercondylar region and on the femoral condyle surfaces and patella.

COLOR PLATE 2 — END-STAGE OA OF THE HIP

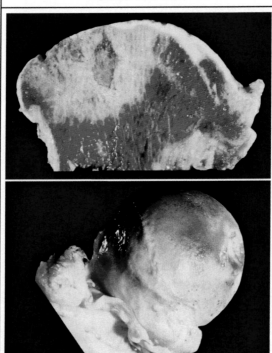

Note the thinning of the articular surface, which has resulted in full-thickness loss of the cartilage over a large portion of the femoral head. A large subchondral cyst is present centrally and osteophytes are apparent at the margin (*top*). Femoral head from another patient with end-stage OA, showing loss of cartilage with smooth, eburnated bone, simulating a billiard ball (*bottom*).

Sokoloff L. In: *The Biology of Degenerative Joint Disease.* Chicago, Ill: The University of Chicago Press; 1969:1-162.

COLOR PLATE 3 — NORMAL ARTICULAR CARTILAGE

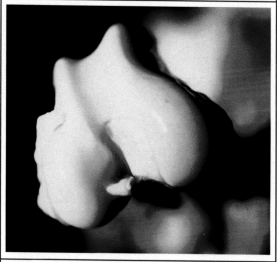

Cartilage covers the ends of the bones in every movable joint, where it transmits load from one bone to the other and provides a smooth bearing surface permitting virtually frictionless motion.

COLOR PLATE 4 — FIBRILLATION OF ARTICULAR CARTILAGE IN OA

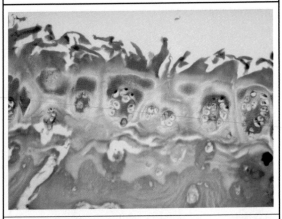

Note the disruption of surface integrity, with vertical clefts (fibrillation) extending into the depths of the cartilage. Chondrocytes have been lost in some areas. In other areas, cloning of the chondrocytes is apparent. Synthesis of DNA by the chondrocytes is increased in osteoarthritis (OA). Although cartilage chondrocytes in normal adult cartilage do not undergo cell division, chrondrocyte cloning may be prominent in OA. Clusters containing as many as 25 chondrocytes or more may be seen as a manifestation of the repair activity in the cartilage. Synthesis not only of DNA but of RNA, proteoglycans, collagen, and noncollagenous proteins is increased in OA. It is, therefore, patently incorrect to call OA a "degenerative joint disease."

COLOR PLATE 5 — DEEPER ZONE OF ARTICULAR CARTILAGE IN OA

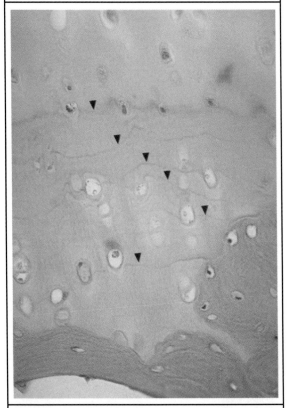

The hyaline cartilage is at the top of the section and the bony subchondral plate at the bottom. The arrows indicate the multiple tidemarks.

COLOR PLATE 6 — MARKED THICKENING OF THE SUBCHONDRAL PLATE IN OA

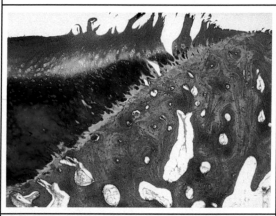

Formation and resorption of subchondral bone are both increased in osteoarthritis (OA).

COLOR PLATE 7 — SYNOVIUM FROM THE KNEE OF A PATIENT WITH ADVANCED OA

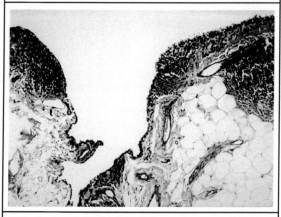

Note the hyperplasia of the lining cell layer and marked focal infiltration of lymphocytes and monocytes. In some cases of advanced OA, the intensity of the synovitis resembles that seen in patients with rheumatoid arthritis.

COLOR PLATE 8 — OA OF THE FIRST METATARSOPHALANGEAL JOINT

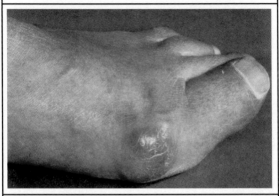

This may lead to a hallux valgus deformity with inflammation of the overlying bursa (bunion).

Shipley M. In: *Rheumatic Diseases, Pocket Picture Guides to Clinical Medicine*. Baltimore, Md: Williams & Wilkins; 1985.

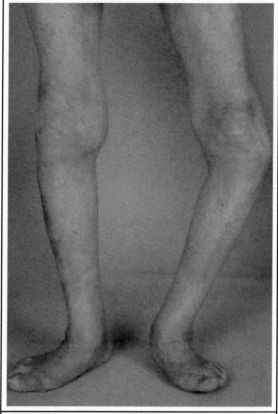

Striking bilateral genu varum deformity in a patient with advanced osteoarthritis (OA) in the medial compartment of both knees.

Shipley M. In: *Rheumatic Diseases, Pocket Picture Guides to Clinical Medicine*. Baltimore, Md: Williams & Wilkins; 1985.

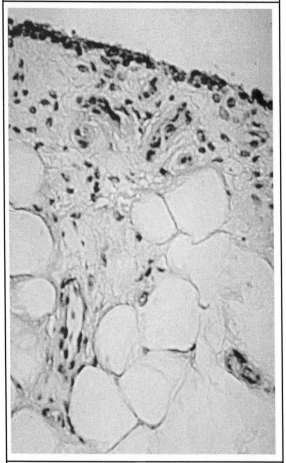

This patient had 3 years of chronic knee pain at the time the synovial biopsy was obtained. Although the knee radiograph showed only minimal changes of osteoarthritis (OA), full-thickness ulceration of the medial femoral condyle was seen.

COLOR PLATE 11 — PSORIATIC ARTHRITIS

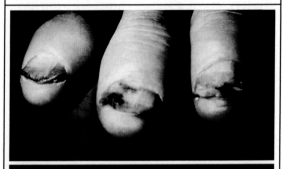

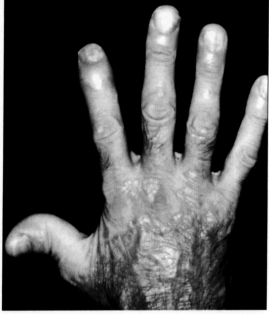

Psoriatic nail changes with swelling of the distal interphalangeal joint in a patient with psoriatic arthritis (*top*). The distal portion of the nail has separated from the bone. Fragmentation of the nail is apparent. Hand of another patient with psoriatic arthritis (*bottom*), showing hyper-

Continued

COLOR PLATE 12 — DUPUYTREN'S CONTRACTURE

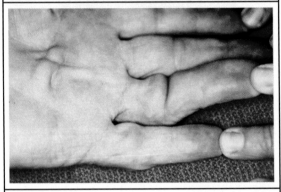

Note the thick fibrous band in the palmar fascia, causing flexion contracture of the fourth and fifth digits.

Photo courtesy of Alex Mih, MD.

COLOR PLATE 13 — NEUROPATHIC JOINT (CHARCOT'S ARTHROPATHY) IN A PATIENT WITH TABES DORSALIS

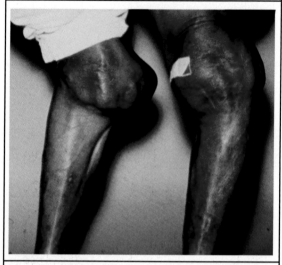

Severe destructive changes in both knees. The joints are unstable and dislocated. Varus, valgus, or recurvatum deformity may be present.

COLOR PLATE 14 — GROSS APPEARANCE OF SYNOVIAL FLUID

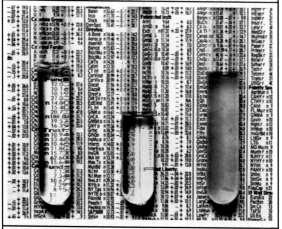

From left to right: Distilled water, sample from patient with osteoarthritis (OA), and sample from patient with rheumatoid arthritis. Note that the synovial fluid from the patient with OA, which has a low total leukocyte count, is clear; it is possible to read newsprint through the test tube. In contrast, synovial fluid from the patient with rheumatoid arthritis, in which the leukocyte count was 17,500 cells/mm³, is turbid.

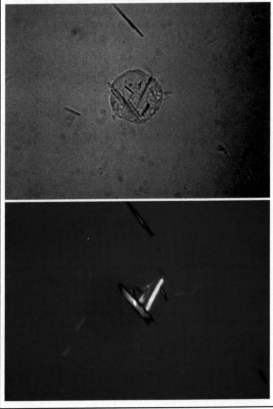

Intracellular and extracellular needle and rod-shaped crystals of monosodium urate in wet preparation of synovial fluid from a patient with gout, viewed under ordinary light × 400 (*top*). The same crystals viewed under compensated polarized light × 400 (*bottom*), showing the characteristic strongly negative birefringence of the urate crystal.

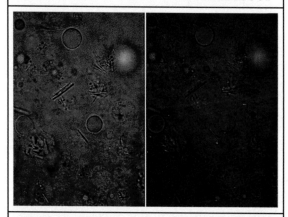

COLOR PLATE 17 — PLEOMORPHIC CLUMPS OF HYDROXYAPATITE CRYSTALS IN SYNOVIAL FLUID FROM A PATIENT WITH OA

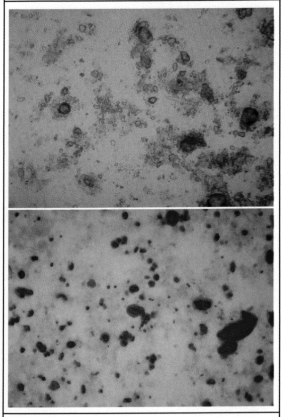

Wet preparation viewed under ordinary light × 100 (*top*). Alizarin red stain of the same fluid, wet preparation × 10 (*bottom*). The clumps of apatite stain strongly.

Schumacher HR, Reginato AJ. In: *Atlas of Synovial Fluid Analysis and Crystal Identification*. Philadelphia, Pa: Lea & Febiger; 1991.

COLOR PLATE 18 — CRYSTALS OF CHOLESTEROL MONOHYDRATE

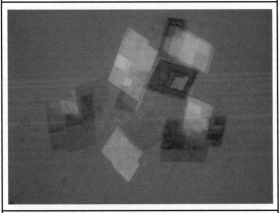

Large, plate-shaped crystals with notched corners, characteristic of cholesterol monohydrate. Cholesterol crystals are common in chronic effusions of joints and bursae of patients with rheumatoid arthritis and, occasionally, are present in the synovial fluid of patients with osteoarthritis. Compensated polarized light × 400.

Schumacher HR, Reginato AJ. In: *Atlas of Synovial Fluid Analysis and Crystal Identification*. Philadelphia, Pa: Lea & Febiger; 1991.

COLOR PLATE 19 — INHIBITION BY IBUPROFEN OF THE ANTIPLATELET EFFECT OF ASPIRIN

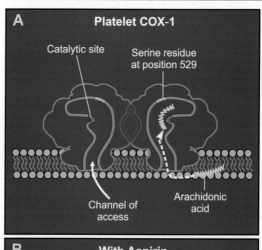

A **Platelet COX-1**

Catalytic site

Serine residue at position 529

Channel of access

Arachidonic acid

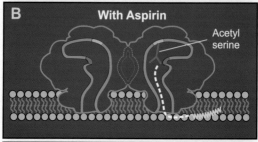

B **With Aspirin**

Acetyl serine

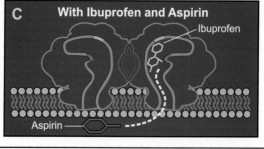

C **With Ibuprofen and Aspirin**

Ibuprofen

Aspirin

Continued

Color Plate 19 *(continued)*

Abbreviations: COX, cyclooxygenase; PGG, prostaglandin G; PGH, prostaglandin H; TBX, thromboxane; NSAID, nonsteroid anti-inflammatory drug.

The effect of aspirin alone and of ibuprofen plus aspirin on platelet COX-1. Platelet prostaglandin G/H synthase-1 (COX-1) is depicted as a dimer. The arachidonic acid substrate gains access to the catalytic site (red area) through a hydrophobic channel that leads into the core of the enzyme *(Panel A)*. Aspirin blocks the access of arachidonic acid to the catalytic site by irreversibly acetylating a serine residue at position 529 in platelet COX-1 near, but not within, the catalytic site *(Panel B)*. Interpolation of the bulky acetyl residue prevents metabolism of arachidonic acid into the cyclic endoperoxides, PGG_2, and PGH_2, for the lifetime of the platelet. Because PGH_2 is metabolized by TBX synthase into TBX A_2, aspirin thus prevents the formation of TBX A_2 by the new platelets until new platelets are generated. NSAIDs, such as ibuprofen, are reversible, competitive inhibitors of the catalytic site *(Panel C)* and result in reversible inhibition of TBX A_2 formation during the dosing interval. Prior occupancy of the catalytic site by ibuprofen prevents aspirin from gaining access to its target serine.

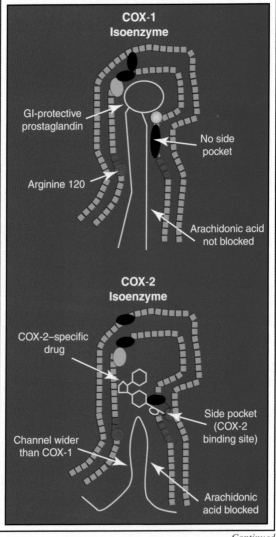

Continued

Color Plate 20 *(continued)*

Abbreviations: COX, cyclooxygenase; NSAID, nonsteroidal anti-inflammatory drug; PGE, prostaglandin E.

NSAIDs bind to the arginine at position 120 in the channel leading to the catalytic site in both COX-1 and COX-2. Therefore, they block the entrance of arachidonic acid to the catalytic site and, consequently, the production of prostaglandins by both COX-1 and COX-2. The specificity of drugs that are specific COX-2 inhibitors (ie, COX-1–sparing) is attributable to a single amino acid difference between the two isoenzymes at position 523, a site near arginine 120. In COX-1, position 523 is occupied by an isoleucine molecule. In COX-2, the isoleucine is replaced by valine, which is smaller than isoleucine by a methyl group. This creates a side pocket in the COX-2 channel, with a binding site that does not exist in COX-1. COX-2–specific agents appear to bind to the enzyme at this site, preventing arachidonic acid from reaching the catalytic site. As a result, they block the transformation of arachidonic acid to PGE_2 and other prostaglandins involved in pain, fever, and the inflammatory response. In contrast, because COX-2–specific inhibitors are unable to bind to COX-1, prostaglandins synthesized by COX-1 that are involved in normal physiologic processes, such as protection of the gastrointestinal mucosa and platelet aggregation, are not inhibited.

Hochberg MC, Katz WA, eds. *Cyclooxygenase-2 Specific Inhibition in Arthritis Therapy*. New York, NY: Center for Healthcare Education; 1999. Figure adapted from Hawkey CJ. *Lancet*. 1999;353:307-314.

COLOR PLATE 21 — X-RAY CRYSTALLOGRAPHY OF COX-1 ACTIVE SITE WITH FLURBIPROFEN AND COX-2 ACTIVE SITE WITH CELECOXIB PROTOTYPE

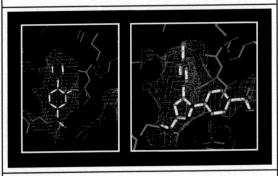

Abbreviations: COX, cyclooxygenase; NSAID, nonsteroidal anti-inflammatory drug.

X-ray crystallography shows that the channel housing the catalytic site of COX-2 allows it to accept a broader range of substrates than the channel of COX-1. The tertiary structures of the COX-1 and COX-2 isoforms are virtually identical. At the catalytic site, they are completely identical with but one exception: In COX-2, the isoleucine at position 523 is replaced by valine, which is smaller than isoleucine by a single methyl group. The presence of the smaller valine creates a side pocket in the COX-2 channel that serves as a binding site that does not exist in COX-1. COX-2–specific inhibitors bind to the enzyme at this locus. The NSAID flurbiprofen is shown at the active site of COX-1 (*left*). A prototype of celecoxib is shown at the active site of COX-2, occupying the side-pocket of the COX-2 channel (*right*).

Evolution in Arthritis Management. Focus on Celecoxib. Washington Crossing, Pa: Scientific Frontiers, Inc; 1999. Copyright Searle and Pfizer, Inc, 1999.

COLOR PLATE 22 — **CUTANEOUS AND SUBCUTANEOUS ATROPHY AFTER BADLY PLACED INJECTION OF DEPOT GLUCOCORTICOID PREPARATION IN A PATIENT BEING TREATED FOR KNEE PAIN**

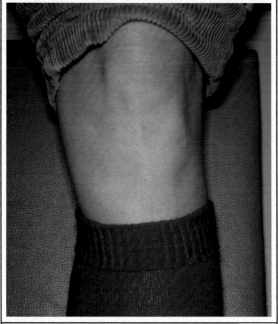

Photograph courtesy of Jeffery Travers, MD.

COLOR PLATE 23 — EVIDENCE OF PROTECTIVE EFFECT OF DOXYCYCLINE

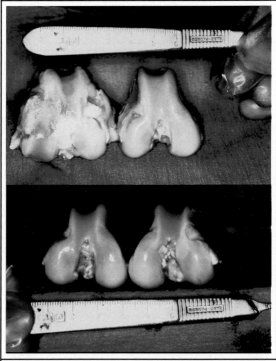

In the untreated dogs (*top*), articular cartilage on the distal femoral condyle of the unstable knee showed extensive full-thickness ulceration; cartilage from the same area of dogs (*bottom*) that received oral doxycycline was, in some cases, grossly normal, as seen in this figure; in other cases, it showed only slight pitting or thinning.

Yu LP Jr, et al. *Arthritis Rheum.* 1992;35:1150.

mon, especially in the knee and finger joints of patients with OA and are due to laxity of the capsule and ligaments. This hypermobility may cause a greater problem for the patient than restriction of movement.

Pseudothrombophlebitis, due to leakage of a popliteal (Baker's) cyst, is not an uncommon cause of diagnostic confusion in patients with knee OA. The correct diagnosis may be established either by ultrasonography (**Figure 6.8**) or by arthrography after injection of contrast material into the involved knee (**Figure 6.9**). The sensitivity of each procedure is approximately 95%. The presence of a popliteal cyst may be revealed merely by obtaining a lateral radiograph of the knee immediately after injection of 30 to 50 cc of air into the joint at the time of arthrocentesis.

In patients with knee arthritis and a popliteal cyst, a narrow connection between the cyst and the joint can be demonstrated.[8] A Bunsen-valve mechanism permits passage of synovial fluid from the knee into the cyst, but flow does not occur in the opposite direction.[9] Pressure in the cyst may exceed that in the knee[9,10] and be great enough to lead to rupture of the cyst wall. In most cases, popliteal cysts are painless. However, when they leak or rupture acutely, spilling synovial fluid into the soft tissues of the calf, they produce a clinical syndrome which may be indistinguishable from that produced by deep vein thrombosis, with swelling and tenderness of the calf, a positive Homan's sign, and, occasionally, ecchymosis around the ankle.[11-13] Rupture or leakage of a popliteal cyst often responds to bed rest, avoidance of weight bearing, and local application of heat. If a large effusion is present in the knee, an intra-articular injection of steroid may be helpful.

The patient may not readily distinguish the pain due to pseudothrombophlebitis from that due to the knee OA. Pseudothrombophlebitis should be suspected in any patient presenting with signs and symptoms of thrombophlebitis in the lower extremity, especially if a history of knee arthritis or clinical evidence of knee effusion is present. In some cases, rupture of a synovial cyst may be the initial indication of the underlying knee arthritis.[14]

It is essential to differentiate pseudothrombophlebitis from *bona fide* thrombophlebitis. Anticoagulation, which is indicated in the latter case, is contraindicated in pseudo-

6

FIGURE 6.8 — ULTRASONOGRAM OF POPLITEAL REGION WITH BAKER'S CYST

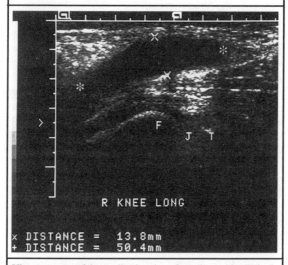

Ultrasonogram of the popliteal region of a patient with a Baker's cyst; lateral view with the patient in a prone position. The skin of the popliteal region is at the top of the figure. The large black area below the surface, delineated by asterisks, is a popliteal cyst.

Abbreviations: F, femoral condyle; J, joint line; T, tibial plateau.

Brandt KD. In: *Diagnostic Studies in Rheumatology*. Summit, NJ: Ciba-Geigy; 1993:1-66.

thrombophlebitis because it may lead to bleeding into the leg,[14,15] requiring emergency fasciotomy for treatment of an iatrogenic compartment syndrome.

FIGURE 6.9 — LATERAL PROJECTION, KNEE ARTHROGRAM

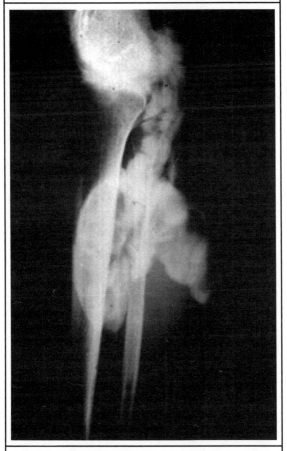

Arthrogram of a patient with a large popliteal cyst. Contrast material has been injected into the knee. Note filling of the suprapatellar bursa (top of figure) and extension of the contrast medium distally into a distended cyst. Extension and/or leakage distally into the calf is apparent.

REFERENCES

1. Bálint G, Szebenyi B. Diagnosis of osteoarthritis. Guidelines and current pitfalls. *Drugs*. 1996;52(suppl 3):1-13.

2. Brandt KD. The diagnosis of osteoarthritis: common problems and some contemporary approaches to finding solutions. In: Brandt KD, ed. *Diagnostic Studies in Rheumatology*. Summit, NJ: Ciba-Geigy; 1993:1-66.

3. Shearn MA, Kang IY. Effect of age and sex on the erythrocyte sedimentation rate. *J Rheumatol*. 1986;13:297-298.

4. Visser M, Bouter LM, McQuillan GM, Wener MH, Harris TB. Elevated C-reactive protein levels in overweight and obese adults. *JAMA*. 1999;282:2131-2135.

5. Mikkelsen WM, Dodge HJ, Duff IF, Kato H. Estimates of the prevalence of rheumatic diseases in the population of Tecumseh, Michigan, 1959-60. *J Chronic Dis*. 1967;20:351-369.

6. Cammarata RJ, Rodnan GP, Fennell RH, Cestello RJ, Creighton AS. Serologic reactions and serum protein concentrations in the aged. *Arthritis Rheum*. 1964;7:297.

7. Cardinal E, Buckwalter KA, Capello WN, Duval N. US of the snapping iliopsoas tendon. *Radiology*. 1996;198:521-522.

8. Taylor AR, Rana NA. A valve. An explanation of the formation of popliteal cysts. *Ann Rheum Dis*. 1973;32:419-421.

9. Jayson MI, Dixon AS. Valvular mechanisms in juxta-articular cysts. *Ann Rheum Dis*. 1970;29:415-420.

10. Solomon L, Berman L. Synovial rupture of knee joint. *J Bone Joint Surg Br*. 1972;54:460-467.

11. Katz RS, Zizic TM, Arnold WP, Stevens MB. The pseudothrombophlebitis syndrome. *Medicine*. 1977;56:151-164.

12. Soriano ER, Catoggio LJ. Baker's cysts, pseudothrombophlebitis, pseudo-pseudothrombophlebitis: where do we stand? *Clin Exp Rheumatol*. 1990;8:107-112.

13. Wigley RD. Popliteal cysts: variations on a theme of Baker. *Semin Arthritis Rheum*. 1982;12:1-10.

14. Eyanson S, MacFarlane JD, Brandt KD. Popliteal cyst mimicking thrombophlebitis as the first indication of knee disease. *Clin Orthop*. 1979;144:215-219.

15. Tait GBW, Bach F, Dixon A St J. Acute synovial rupture: further observations. *Ann Rheum Dis*. 1965;24:273-277.

7

Synovial Fluid Analysis

Most patients with osteoarthritis (OA) do not have a clinically apparent joint effusion or have only a small amount of intra-articular fluid detectable by physical examination. Aspiration of this fluid and synovial fluid analysis, however, can be very useful diagnostically.[1-5] As much may be learned from careful analysis of a few drops of joint fluid as from the study of 50 cc.

The characteristics of the synovial effusion from an OA joint are consistent with the presence of only a low grade of synovial inflammation. Typically, the fluid is clear—newsprint can be read through a test tube containing fluid from an OA joint (**Color Plate 14**). The total white cell count is uniformly <2,000 cells/mm^3 and often <500 cells/mm^3 (**Table 7.1**). Only about 15% of the cells are polymorphonuclear leukocytes. A good mucin test is characteristic of OA. The synovial fluid glucose concentration approximates that of the simultaneous blood glucose concentration.

The *real* value of synovial fluid analysis in the patient with a joint effusion and x-ray evidence of OA lies in its ability to reveal additional, coexisting joint pathology. Thus a synovial fluid leukocyte count in excess of 2,000/mm^3—even if the joint exhibits classical x-ray findings of OA—indicates the presence of some inflammatory joint disease *in addition to* OA.

Examination by polarization microscopy of fluid from an OA joint may reveal crystals of monosodium urate (**Color Plate 15**) or calcium pyrophosphate dihydrate (**Color Plate 16**), leading to a diagnosis of gout or pseudogout, respectively. In other cases, very weakly bire-fringent crystals of calcium hydroxyapatite may be present (**Color Plate 17**). These can be easily visualized with an alizarin red stain of the joint fluid. Apatite crystals may be an incidental finding in synovial fluid from patients with OA, but are occasionally seen in patients with rapidly progressive OA who undergo rapid loss of their articular cartilage. Occasionally, cholesterol crystals may be seen. These

TABLE 7.1 — CHARACTERISTICS OF SYNOVIAL FLUID IN OA AND OTHER COMMON RHEUMATIC DISEASES*

Diagnosis	Appearance	Viscosity	White Cell Count/mm³	% of Polymorphonuclear Leukocytes	Mucin Test	Crystals	Difference in Glucose Concentration (Blood and Synovial Fluid mg/dL)
Normal	Clear yellow	Normal	< 200	7	Good	—	0
Osteoarthritis	Clear or turbid	Decreased	600	13	Good	†	5
Traumatic arthritis	Clear or bloody	Decreased	1500	20	Good	—	5
Gout	Turbid	Decreased	21,500	70	Poor	Monosodium urate	11
Pseudogout	Slightly turbid	Slightly decreased	14,200	68	Fair	Calcium pyrophosphate dihydrate (CPPD)	—
Rheumatoid arthritis	Turbid	Decreased	1900	66	Fair-poor	Rare	30
Acute bacterial joint infection	Very turbid	Decreased	80,000	90	Poor	—	91

Abbreviation: OA, osteoarthritis.

* Modified from: Krey PR, Lazaro DM. In: *Diagnostic Studies in Rheumatology*. 1992:74-85; Ropes MW, Bauer W. *Synovial Changes in Joint Disease*. 1953; and Cohen AS, et al. In: *Laboratory Diagnostic Procedures in the Rheumatoid Diseases*. 2nd ed. 1975:1-62.

† As many as 70% of fluids from patients with osteoarthritis contain crystals of CPPD, calcium hydroxyapatite, or both.

are most common in chronic effusions and are asymptomatic (**Color Plate 18**). Bacteria may be seen in the Gram's stain or culture of fluid from the OA joint, providing definite evidence of a bacterial joint infection. Finally, it is important to exclude artifacts, such as talc crystals from the gloves of the physician performing the aspiration.

In addition to the value of synovial fluid analysis in establishing a diagnosis of OA, the procedure may be helpful in the patient already known to have OA who develops a new effusion or an increase in joint pain that requires explanation. In such instances, whenever the cause of the joint effusion is not certain, arthrocentesis and synovial fluid analysis should be performed.

REFERENCES

1. Krey PR, Lazaro DM. Analysis of synovial fluid. In: Brandt KD, ed. *Diagnostic Studies In Rheumatology*. Summit, NJ: Ciba-Geigy; 1992:74-85.

2. Ropes MW, Bauer W. *Synovial Changes in Joint Disease*. Cambridge, Mass: Harvard University Press; 1953.

3. Krey PR, Bailen DA. Synovial fluid leukocytosis. A study of extremes. *Am J Med*. 1979;67:436-442.

4. Cohen AS, Brandt KD, Krey PR. Synovial fluid. In: Cohen AS, ed. *Laboratory Diagnostic Procedures in the Rheumatoid Diseases*. 2nd ed. Boston, Mass: Little, Brown and Company, Inc; 1975:1-62.

5. Schumacher HR, Reginato AJ. *Atlas of Synovial Fluid and Crystal Identification*. Philadelphia, Pa: Lea and Febiger; 1991.

8 Radiography

The diagnosis of osteoarthritis (OA) is usually based on clinical and radiographic features. In the early stages of the disease, x-rays may be normal, but as articular cartilage is lost, narrowing of the interbone distance becomes evident (**Figure 8.1**). Other characteristic x-ray findings include subchondral cysts, subchondral sclerosis, and marginal osteophytes, which represent the response of the bone to the increased mechanical load resulting from cartilage degeneration (**Figure 8.2**). Although some investigators have suggested that the primary abnormality in OA is in the bone and that the changes in the overlying cartilage are secondary, this represents a minority opinion.

Disparity between severity of radiographic findings and severity of symptoms or functional impairment in subjects with OA is common. While some x-ray evidence of OA in weight-bearing joints is present in >90% of people over the age of 40, only about 30% will have symptoms.[1] For example, among men with advanced x-ray changes of hip OA, nearly 50% may not have joint pain.[2] As noted in Chapter 2, *Epidemiology*, risk factors for pain and disability in OA are different from those related to joint pathology.

A knee x-ray taken while the subject is standing is more likely to exhibit joint-space narrowing—the surrogate of articular cartilage thinning—than one obtained in the supine position.[3,4] However, when we examined the relationship between articular cartilage degeneration and joint-space narrowing in standing anteroposterior knee radiographs of patients with chronic knee pain, most of whom had x-ray findings of only mild OA, we found 33% of those with tibiofemoral joint-space narrowing had *grossly normal* cartilage at arthroscopy and, therefore, a "false-positive" radiograph.[5] Joint-space narrowing in these patients with chronic knee pain and relatively mild x-ray changes of OA did *not* predict the status of the articular cartilage.

In some cases, the poor correlation between radiographic joint space narrowing and degeneration of articu-

FIGURE 8.1 — OA OF THE KNEE

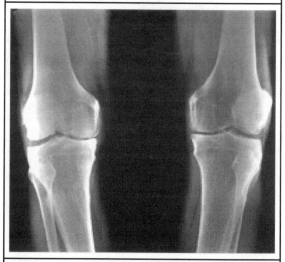

Note the narrowing of the medial tibiofemoral joint space bilaterally. This is generally considered to be due to loss of articular cartilage, although "false-positives" are common. For example, a minor degree of knee flexion can result in significant narrowing of the tibiofemoral joint space. Small osteophytes are present on the medial border of the medial-tibial plateau in both knees.

lar cartilage in the knee may be due to the fact that the radiographic joint-space loss is due to meniscal extrusion[6]; in others, it may be due to the fact that knee pain may limit the patient's ability to fully extend the knee, reducing the interbone distance.[7] Although it remains the gold standard for assessing progression of OA, the conventional standing knee radiograph is not a sensitive technique for identifying articular cartilage changes in OA.

The grading scale that has been employed most widely for assessment of the severity of OA, the Kellgren and Lawrence (K&L) Scale[8,9] (**Table 8.1**, **Figure 8.3**), was developed prior to the demonstration that the standing knee x-ray is more sensitive for assessment of joint-space narrowing than a radiograph taken with the patient supine. It permits a diagnosis of definite OA in the presence of osteophytosis alone, ie, in the absence of joint-space nar-

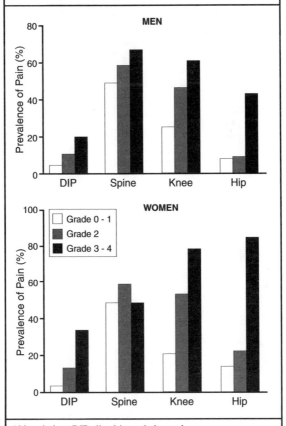

FIGURE 8.2 — PREVALENCE OF PAIN AT VARIOUS JOINT SITES IN RELATIONSHIP TO THE RADIOGRAPHIC SEVERITY OF OA BASED ON THE KELLGREN AND LAWRENCE GRADE

Abbreviation: DIP, distal interphalangeal.

O'Reilly S, Doherty M. In: *Osteoarthritis*. Oxford, UK: Oxford University Press; 1998:197-217.

TABLE 8.1 — KELLGREN AND LAWRENCE GRADING CRITERIA FOR RADIOGRAPHIC SEVERITY OF KNEE OA

Grade	OA Severity	Radiographic Findings
Grade 0	None	No features of OA
Grade I	Doubtful	Minute osteophyte, doubtful significance
Grade II	Minimal	Definite osteophyte, unimpaired joint space
Grade III	Moderate	Moderate diminution of joint space
Grade IV	Severe	Joint space greatly impaired with sclerosis of subchondral bone

Abbreviation: OA, osteoarthritis.

Kellgren JH, Lawrence JS. *Ann Rheum Dis.* 1957;16:494-501; and Department of Rheumatology and Medical Illustration, University of Manchester. *The Epidemiology of Chronic Rheumatism.* Atlas of Standard Radiographs of Arthritis. Philadelphia, Pa: FA Davis Company; 1973;2:1-15.

FIGURE 8.3 — KELLGREN AND LAWRENCE GRADING OF RADIOGRAPHIC SEVERITY OF OA

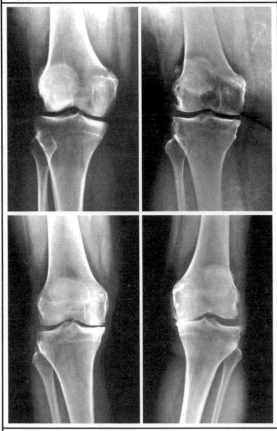

Normal knee radiograph, Kellgren and Lawrence (K&L) grade 0 (*top*, *left*); mild but definite osteophyte formation, with essentially normal joint-space width, K&L grade II (*top*, *right*); osteophytosis with marked narrowing of the joint space in the medial tibiofemoral compartment, K&L grade III (*bottom*, *left*); and complete loss of joint space in the medial tibiofemoral compartment with prominent osteophytes and subchondral sclerosis of medial tibial plateau, K&L grade IV (*bottom*, *right*).

8

rowing. As indicated, however, loss of articular cartilage, not osteophytosis, is the predominant pathologic feature of OA. Indeed, in the absence of joint-space narrowing or other bony changes, osteophytosis may be due to aging, not to OA. [10,11]

Furthermore, all semiquantitative scoring systems, including the K&L Scale, suffer from two limitations, which are based on the following assumptions:

- That the change in any radiographic feature (eg, joint-space narrowing, osteophytes) is linear and constant during the course of the disease
- That the relationship between the different radiographic features of OA is constant.

Neither of these assumptions is valid. In most cases, the rate of progression of x-ray severity is not constant but advances in a stepwise fashion, and the individual radiographic features of OA do not progress at comparable rates. In some patients, for example, the rate of joint-space loss may be much greater than the rate of osteophyte growth, or *vice versa*. The essential point is that neither osteophytosis nor joint-space narrowing provides an accurate assessment of the intra-articular pathology in patients with relatively early OA.

While serial radiography may be essential in a clinical trial evaluating a drug or biologic agent for its potential to modify structural damage in OA, in clinical practice serial x-rays of the patient with OA are seldom indicated.[12] At the initial clinic visit, it is reasonable to obtain an x-ray of the involved joint to assess the degree of pathology and exclude other causes of the patient's joint pain (eg, rheumatoid disease, crystal deposition disease, infection), but repeat x-rays of the OA joint are generally not necessary unless the patient becomes a candidate for joint surgery or the rate of progression of the disease accelerates markedly.

REFERENCES

1. Lawrence JS, Bremmer JM, Bier F. Osteo-arthrosis. Prevalence in the population and relationship between symptoms and x-ray changes. *Ann Rheum Dis.* 1966;25:1-24.

2. Lawrence JS. Osteoarthrosis. In: *Rheumatism in Populations.* London: Heinemann; 1977;98-155.

3. Ahlbach S. Osteoarthritis of the knee: a radiographic investigation. *Acta Radiol.* 1986;277:7-61.

4. Leach RE, Gregg T, Siber FJ. Weight-bearing radiography in osteoarthritis of the knee. *Radiology.* 1970;97:265-268.

5. Fife RS, Brandt KD, Braunstein EM, et al. Relationship between arthroscopic evidence of cartilage damage and radiographic evidence of joint space narrowing in early osteoarthritis of the knee. *Arthritis Rheum.* 1991;34:377-382.

6. Adams JG, McAlindon T, Dimasi M, Carey J, Eustace S. Contribution of meniscal extrusion and cartilage loss to joint space narrowing in osteoarthritis. *Clin Radiol.* 1999;54:502-506.

7. Mazzuca SA, Brandt KD, Lane KA, Katz BP. Knee pain reduces joint space width in conventional standing anteroposterior radiographs of osteoarthritic knees. *Arthritis Rheum.* 2002;46:1223-1227.

8. Kellgren JH, Lawrence JS. Radiologic assessment of osteoarthritis. *Ann Rheum Dis.* 1957;16:494-501.

9. Department of Rheumatology and Medical Illustration, University of Manchester. *The Epidemiology of Chronic Rheumatism.* Atlas of Standard Radiographs of Arthritis. Philadelphia, Pa: FA Davis Company; 1973;2:1-15.

10. Danielsson L, Hernborg J. Clinical and roentgenological study of knee joints with osteophytes. *Clin Orthop.* 1970;69:302-312.

11. Hernborg J, Nilsson BE. The relationship between osteophytes in the knee joint, osteoarthritis and aging. *Acta Orthop Scand.* 1973; 44:69-74.

12. O'Reilly S, Doherty M. Clinical features of osteoarthritis and standard approaches to the diagnosis. Signs, symptoms and laboratory tests. In: Doherty M, Lohmander LS, Brandt KD, eds. *Osteoarthritis.* 2nd ed. Oxford, UK: Oxford University Press. In press.

8

9

Nonmedicinal Therapy for OA Pain

Exercise

Osteoarthritis (OA) limits physical activity and the amount of exercise that a subject can perform. Because of their inactivity, people with OA of weight-bearing joints are at increased risk for hypertension, obesity, diabetes, and cardiovascular disease.[1] In considering OA, we need to address not only the problem within a specific joint, but we must consider how the disease affects the ability of the individual to live within society, ie, disability and handicap must be taken into account.

Disability may be ascertained by interrogation of the patient or by observing the patient during the performance of common activities. It reflects the consequences of the impairment (ie, the objective changes as seen in an x-ray or measurement of range of motion of the joint) with respect to the patient's ability to carry out activities of daily living, such as feeding, dressing, cleaning oneself, and going shopping. As discussed by Liang,[2] disability is determined not only by people's physical capacity, but also by their will and needs; a concert pianist with an adduction contracture of the thumb due to trapeziometacarpal joint OA may be severely handicapped, while a blue-collar worker with the same hand impairment may have no handicap.

Handicap refers to the disadvantage imposed on the patient by the disease and the effect of the disease on the patient's role in society. It is affected by the patient's perception of how one is doing within the context of their environment. Notably, it may bear little relationship to the score the patient might provide on a standardized questionnaire about function.

The disability of patients with OA arises as a result of the disease, the aging process, and inactivity. In OA, the value of exercise extends beyond management of the joint disease itself and is derived to a considerable extent from

113

the fact that exercise modifies inactivity. Exercise is effective, economical, and safe and is underprescribed in management of the patient with OA. Much of the following discussion on exercise reflects comments made by Dr. Marian Minor in a recent workshop, "Controversies and Practical Issues in the Management of Osteoarthritis."[3]

The approach of most physicians to management of OA today is aimed at reducing joint pain pharmacologically. Exercises are prescribed much less often than drugs.[4] However, *nonpharmacologic* measures—not drugs—are the cornerstone of management of the patient with symptomatic OA. Analgesics and anti-inflammatory drugs are adjuncts, not alternatives, to nonmedicinal measures. Because the benefits of nonpharmacologic measures and drugs are additive, use of the former often permits a reduction in the dose of drug, thereby decreasing the risk of adverse events and the cost of therapy. This chapter describes a variety of nonpharmacologic measures that are useful in symptomatic treatment of the patient with OA.

Unfortunately, prescribed exercises for OA generally focus only on the impairment (muscle weakness, loss of motion, pain) in and around the involved joint. However, because OA can result in severe functional limitation and disability, effective management requires more than attention to only the localized impairment. The prescribed exercise regimen must also address functional limitations and disability arising from inactivity. As noted by Minor,[5] the goals of an exercise program for the patient with OA should be:

- Reduction of impairment and improvement of function; ie, reduction of joint pain, increases in range of motion (ROM) and strength, normalization of gait, and improvement in performance of daily activities
- Protection of the OA joint from further damage by reducing stress on the joint, attenuating joint forces, and improving biomechanics
- Prevention of disability and poor health secondary to inactivity by increasing the daily level of physical activity and improving physical fitness.

Exercise programs for patients with OA should be individualized. In the patient with significant weakness or reduction in joint motion, the initial aim should be to:

114

- Reduce the impairment
- Improve function
- Prepare for increased activity.

For the patient with good strength and ROM, the exercise program should focus on joint-protection strategies and general conditioning.

For knee OA, a combination of exercises, including ROM, strengthening, and low-impact aerobic exercise, is appropriate. However, two precautions should be considered before implementation of the exercise program:

- First, exercise of an acutely inflamed or significantly swollen joint should be deferred until the acute inflammation has subsided.
- Second, before initiation of an aerobic exercise program, an exercise stress test should be performed to identify cardiac disease; the objective of the proposed aerobic program should be to achieve 60% to 80% of the target heart rate.[6]

Patients who do not have mechanical instability of the knee may tolerate walking without an increase in symptoms if they begin slowly and gradually increase their walking time to approximately 30 minutes 3 days a week. Each session should be preceded by a warm-up period consisting of ROM and strengthening exercises and followed by a cool-down period of stretching exercises.[7] Because compliance with an exercise regimen is likely to decrease if pain increases, it is important to ascertain how much exercise is necessary to obtain the desired results and how much can be performed without producing significant pain.

Daily exercise, which includes full, active ROM and periods of weight-bearing exercise, appears necessary to maintain the integrity of articular cartilage. Even with preservation of ROM, loss of contraction of periarticular muscles will lead to cartilage atrophy.[8] Even when loading of the joint is contraindicated, attention to ROM may help maintain some cartilage integrity.

Many physicians fail to appreciate that the patient with OA is often able to tolerate load-bearing exercises and that an exercise program may decrease joint pain as much as treatment with a drug. Several studies have shown that a

115

patient with hip or knee OA can participate safely in appropriate conditioning exercise programs to improve fitness and health without increasing joint pain.[9-14] Furthermore, subject retention in such studies has been excellent and exercise behaviors have been maintained long after completion of the study protocol.

Recent epidemiologic evidence indicates that exercise for health maintenance need not be as intensive as was previously believed.[9] An effective exercise program can be designed even for those with significant joint disease.

Aerobic Exercise

Regular physical activity is important for patients with knee OA. A subject with OA is less active and tends to be less fit with respect to both musculoskeletal and cardiovascular status than normal age- and sex-matched control subjects.[10,15,16] The health benefits of aerobic exercise include:

- Increased aerobic capacity, muscle strength, and exercise endurance
- Less exertion at a given workload
- Weight loss.

■ OA and the Risks of Inactivity

Recent data from the Behavioral Risk Factor Surveillance System of the Centers for Disease Control indicate that people with arthritis are much less active than those who do not have arthritis.[1] Only 24% of people with arthritis report a level of physical activity sufficient to achieve or maintain health; 76% are doing nothing or are not sufficiently active. Arthritis is *the* major reason that elderly individuals limit their activity (**Figure 9.1**).[17] It is a greater factor in limiting activity than heart disease, hypertension, blindness, or diabetes.[18]

Studies of cardiovascular health have shown that the aerobic capacity (cardiovascular fitness) of men with severe knee OA is more than 30% lower than that of men of comparable age who do not have OA.[17] Among subjects who were characterized as high risk, moderate risk, or low risk on the basis of body weight, smoking history, and participation in exercise, those in the high-risk group became disabled (ie, reported difficulty with performance of activities

116

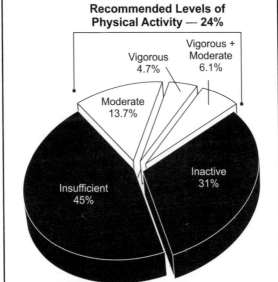

FIGURE 9.1 — LEVELS OF PHYSICAL ACTIVITY REPORTED BY PEOPLE WITH ARTHRITIS

Recommended Levels of Physical Activity — 24%

Vigorous + Moderate 6.1%

Vigorous 4.7%

Moderate 13.7%

Inactive 31%

Insufficient 45%

Only 24% of people with arthritis report achieving levels of physical activity that are recommended for health. The remainder are essentially inactive or insufficiently active.

Ries MD, et al. *Clin Orthop Rel Res.* 1995;313:169-176.

of daily living) some 7 years earlier than those in the low-risk group (**Figure 9.2**).[19]

Disability in patients with OA may have more to do with their ability to remain active and physically fit and to maintain their body weight than with the pathologic changes in the OA joint. Subjects with knee OA expend more energy to walk—even at a slow speed—than age- and sex-matched controls. People with knee OA work against much more than the OA present in the knee; the mechanics not only of the knee but also of the ankle, foot, hip, and low back are affected.

Even if we cannot cure OA, we can cure inactivity. In a longitudinal study of men in their 40s, 50s, and 60s who

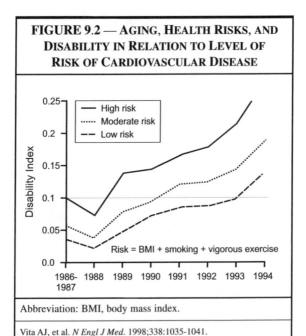

FIGURE 9.2 — AGING, HEALTH RISKS, AND DISABILITY IN RELATION TO LEVEL OF RISK OF CARDIOVASCULAR DISEASE

Risk = BMI + smoking + vigorous exercise

Abbreviation: BMI, body mass index.

Vita AJ, et al. *N Engl J Med*. 1998;338:1035-1041.

were assessed at 5-year intervals, Blair and colleagues[20] found that those in their 40s who were not performing sufficient physical activity and had low scores on a treadmill test had remarkably higher death rates than those who were fit. However, among those who were not fit at the outset but *became fit*, the risk of mortality decreased by 44%. Each 1-minute increase in time on a treadmill at maximal effort was accompanied by a decrease of about 8% in mortality risk.

■ **Exercise Dosing**

What dose of exercise is required? The amount of *aerobic conditioning* (eg, walking, cycling, aquatic exercise) necessary for cardiovascular fitness is not so great that it cannot be achieved by people with hip or knee OA. Subjects with OA of lower extremity joints who are able to perform moderate to vigorous exercise, ie, 70% to 85% of maximal heart rate (an intensity that permits the subject to talk while exercising continuously) for 20 to 60 minutes at least 3 days per week, can improve their fitness and health without exacerbating their joint pain or increasing their need for analgesic drugs. People with OA who exercise consistently at this level report decreases in joint pain and disability while improving their cardiovascular fitness by 25% to 30% and their muscular fitness (strength and endurance) by as much as 100%. They also report improvement in function and in quality of life and exhibit improved gait and walking speed. Thus there is no question that conditioning exercise for people with OA is safe and effective. However, many of the patients with OA whom we encourage to walk and to increase their level of physical activity in order to improve their level of fitness may require some mechanical intervention to assist them in meeting that objective (see below).

In a trial of aerobic exercise in patients with symptomatic hip or knee OA, patients were randomized into three treatment groups for a 12-week program of aerobic walking, aerobic pool exercises, or nonaerobic ROM exercises.[13] Both aerobic exercise groups showed significant gains in aerobic capacity in comparison with the controls, and all three groups showed similar improvement in joint pain and tenderness. Notably, none of the three groups increased their use of pain medication during the study.

A randomized, controlled trial of fitness walking in patients with knee OA employed an 8-week walking program that included flexibility and strengthening exercises as a warm-up and gradual progression of walking under supervision for 5 to 30 minutes three times per week. The control group received only a weekly telephone call.[14] In comparison with controls, the walking group showed significant improvement in walking distance, self-reported physical activity, and joint pain.

Aerobic exercises that may be recommended include:
- Walking
- Biking
- Swimming
- Aerobic dance
- Aerobic pool exercises.

Swimming and pool exercises cause less joint stress than the other forms of aerobic exercise. Each aerobic session should be preceded by a warm-up period consisting of ROM exercises and should be followed by a cool-down period of stretching. If walking or jogging results in an increase in symptoms, the patient should reduce the intensity of the activity or change to another form of aerobic exercise. Proper footwear is important and exercise on soft surfaces should be encouraged. To increase aerobic capacity, patients need to sustain a heart rate that is 60% to 80% of their target heart rate for 20 to 30 minutes three to four times weekly. Because maximum loading of the hip and knee occurs during stair climbing and descent,[21,22] even though stair climbing is an excellent aerobic exercise, it may be inadvisable for a patient with OA affecting these joints.

Range of Motion and Strengthening Exercises

Although aerobic exercise can increase aerobic power and reduce fatigue, it does not appear to improve muscle strength or functional capacity. Stretching or ROM exercises for a patient with OA[7] may be helpful symptomatically, but controlled clinical trials have not been performed to document their value.

In the presence of knee OA, knee extensor strength may be diminished by as much as 60%.[10,15,23] Exercise programs aimed at strengthening the knee extensors can result in:

- Significant gains in strength
- Reduction of joint pain[11]
- Improvement in gait.[12]

For strengthening, isometric exercises are recommended initially, because they employ less joint motion and are less likely to aggravate symptoms.[16,24] Isometric quadriceps exercises, followed by progressive resistance exercises (which are superior for maintaining or increasing function), will reduce joint pain and increase function in patients with knee OA.

Tables 9.1 and 9.2 contain instructions for isometric quadriceps exercises for patients with knee OA. The exercise that focuses on the vastus medialis obliquus muscle may be particularly helpful for the patient with lateral subluxation of the patella.

120

An exercise program aimed at strengthening knee extensors should include training to increase contraction velocity and endurance as well as isometric and isotonic strength. Improvement in endurance and speed will result in much greater functional improvement than improvement in strength alone.[10] Even in older subjects with OA, a program of resistive strengthening of hip, knee, and ankle, coupled with postural control exercises, can significantly improve strength and gait.[12]

The benefits of quadriceps-strengthening exercise and aerobic exercise for patients with knee OA have been confirmed in the Fitness Arthritis and Senior Trial,[25] in which patients with mild disability due to knee OA were randomized to either an aerobic exercise group, a resistance (muscle-strengthening) exercise group, or an education/attention control group. In comparison with the controls, both exercise groups exhibited modest but significant improvement that notably was sustained over an 18-month period.

Most of the information available about therapeutic exercise has been derived from patients with knee OA and relates to strength training. However, therapeutic exercise goes far beyond muscle strengthening. In studies that employed four to ten instructional sessions followed by 6 months of self-directed home exercise (in which patients initially exercised up to 5 days per week),[26,27] with recommendations to decrease the frequency over 6 months to 2 days per week, compliance was excellent. Little equipment was required, and the results showed not only significant improvement in lower extremity strength, but decreases in pain, anxiety, depression, endurance, proprioception, functional status, and disability. Thus with fairly minimal intervention and self-directed exercise, people with OA can achieve—and are able to maintain—important gains.

Contractures

Chronic joint pain may lead to muscle atrophy, weakness, deconditioning, and flexion contracture, resulting in inefficient gait patterns. Adduction contracture of the hip may increase forces in the acetabulum[28] and increase valgus forces at the knee and ankle. Furthermore, contractures of the hip may have a profound effect on function. Sitting,

TABLE 9.1 — QUADRICEPS-STRENGTHENING EXERCISE

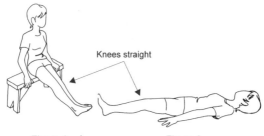

Figure 1   Figure 2

1. Sit on a firm surface (Figure 1) or lie flat in bed (Figure 2).

2. Perform this exercise in either of the following positions:

   a. Sit in a chair (Figure 1) with your legs straight, heels on the floor or on a footstool. Squeeze your thigh muscles, pushing your knees downward toward the floor.

   b. Lie in bed (Figure 2) with your legs straight and squeeze your thigh muscles, pushing the back of your knees into the bed.

3. Hold this position for a full 5 seconds. Use a clock or watch with a second hand, or count: one-one thousand, two-one thousand, three-one thousand, four-one thousand, five-one thousand.

4. Relax the muscles.

5. Begin your strengthening program with 10 repetitions, holding each contraction for a full 5 seconds. Perform this exercise seven times daily and increase the number of repetitions you perform with each set by three to five daily during the first week.

6. By the end of the week, you should be able to perform 15 repetitions per set. This is the maximum number of repetitions you should perform in a set. (Total per day = 15 repetitions per set × 7 sets = 105.)

7. If your arthritis is causing knee pain, apply heat to your knees for 15 or 20 minutes prior to performing your exercises.

Caution: In most patients, these knee exercises will not cause joint pain or increase the pain from your arthritis. If, however, you have significant pain lasting more than 20 minutes after you perform these exercises, decrease the number of repetitions by five per set. Maintain this number of repetitions until your knee discomfort subsides. Then, each day thereafter, increase the number of repetitions by three per set until you reach a maximum of 15 per set.

Rheumatology Division, Indiana University School of Medicine; 1993.

gait, personal hygiene, and sexual function may all be affected. Preventive posturing (eg, prone lying) may be helpful. Stand-up exercises to help maintain strength in hip and knee extensors can be programmed, beginning with standing up from a high seat surface, that is then progressively lowered as the activities are completed successfully. For patients unable to exercise in full gravity, exercising under water will reduce the load.

Contractures of soft tissues and tendons surrounding a joint, persistent poor posture, or imbalance between agonist and antagonist muscle groups may limit joint motion. Maintenance of a flexed position, while minimizing intra-articular pressure and reducing pain, may result in flexion contracture. Patients with a knee flexion contracture should not sleep with pillows under the knee. Contracture may be prevented or reduced by application of deep heat (eg, via ultrasound [see below]), followed by passive ROM, stretching, and active ROM exercises to maintain functional range. Serial casting may help reduce contracture.

OA involving only a single joint (eg, hip or knee) is a multijoint problem. Patients with knee OA, for example, exhibit decreased ROM not only in the involved joint but

TABLE 9.2 — QUADRICEPS-STRENGTHENING EXERCISE CONCENTRATING ON THE VASTUS MEDIALIS OBLIQUE MUSCLE

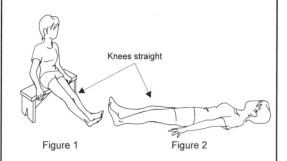

Knees straight

Figure 1   Figure 2

1. Sit on a firm surface (Figure 1) or lie flat in bed (Figure 2).

2. Cross your ankles, with right leg above and left leg below. Legs should be stretched out straight.

3. With your heels on the floor or on the bed, push down with right leg, push up with left leg, squeezing your ankles together. (Pretend that you're crushing a walnut between your ankles.) There should be little actual movement except for the muscle tightening.

4. Hold this position for a full 5 seconds. Use a clock or watch with a second hand, or count: one-one thousand, two-one thousand, three-one thousand, four-one thousand, five-one thousand.

5. Relax the muscles.

6. Reverse the position of the legs so that the leg that was on top is now on the bottom.

7. Repeat steps 1, 2, and 3.

8. Begin your strengthening program with 10 repetitions, holding each contraction for a full 5 seconds. Perform this exercise seven times daily and increase the number of repetitions you perform with each set by three to five daily during the first week.

9. By the end of the week, you should be able to perform 15 repetitions per set. This is the maximum number of repetitions you should perform in a set. (Total per day = 15 repetitions per set × 7 sets = 105.)

7. If your arthritis is causing knee pain, apply heat to your knees for 15 or 20 minutes prior to performing your exercises.

Caution: In most patients, these knee exercises will not cause joint pain or increase the pain from your arthritis. If, however, you have significant pain lasting more than 20 minutes after you perform these exercises, decrease the number of repetitions by five per set. Maintain this number of repetitions until your knee discomfort subsides. Then, each day thereafter, increase the number of repetitions by three per set until you reach a maximum of 15 per set.

Rheumatology Division, Indiana University School of Medicine; 1993.

also in the ipsilateral hip and ankle and contralateral hip, knee, and ankle.[21,29] For this reason, active motion in functional positions should be assessed in *all* joints of *both* lower extremities. The motion actually used in gait, stair climbing, and arising from a chair should be observed for symmetry and smoothness. Stair climbing requires the greatest velocity of knee flexion[21] and is an excellent activity with which to assess knee function. The functional requirements for ROM of lower extremity joints for walking, stair climbing, and arising from a chair are useful treatment goals (**Table 9.3**).

Although ankle OA is uncommon, limited ROM and reduction of ankle strength are common in patients with hip or knee OA. Lower extremity pain and loss of motion in the large joints result in diminished push-off and decreased limb loading at heel strike, leading to deconditioning of calf

TABLE 9.3 — FUNCTIONAL RANGE OF MOTION OF LOWER EXTREMITY JOINTS REQUIRED FOR LOCOMOTOR ACTIVITIES

Joint	Motion	Range (in degrees) Needed for…		
		Level Walking	Climbing Stairs	Arising From a Chair
Hip	Extension	15	7	0
	Flexion	37	67	112
	Abduction	7	8	20
	Adduction	5	—	—
	Internal rotation	4	—	—
	External rotation	9	10	17
Knee	Extension	0	0	0
	Flexion	70	83	93
Ankle	Dorsiflexion	10	15	15
	Plantar flexion	15	10	—

Minor MA. *Arthritis Care Res.* 1994;7:198.

muscles and loss of ankle motion.[21,29] Adequate joint motion, strength, and endurance are crucial for gait, balance, stair climbing, and arising from a chair (**Table 9.3**). Changes in the ankle can account for loss of these parameters in patients with hip or knee OA.

Exercise and Joint Protection

Periarticular muscles are of major importance in attenuating shock to the joint.[30] Attenuation of impact by neuromuscular mechanisms depends upon an adequate mass of conditioned muscle and the ability to generate force quickly for an eccentric contraction. Muscle mass, contractile velocity, force production, endurance for repetitive motions, and motor skill all may be compromised by pain or inactivity in patients with knee OA. To optimize a patient's neuromuscular capacity in order to protect the joint from sudden-impact loading and attenuate load, exercises to improve concentric and eccentric strength and endurance at functional speeds and motor-skill learning should be included in the exercise program.

Because muscles are important shock absorbers and help stabilize the joint, periarticular weakness may result in progression of structural damage to the joint in OA. In addition to the decrease in joint pain that exercise regimens that strengthen lower extremity muscles may achieve,[10,11] they may slow the progression of joint damage in patients with knee OA. Insufficient loading of a joint will lead to atrophy of both the articular cartilage and subchondral bone.[8] Control of joint loading is especially important when the joint capsule is weakened, instability exists, or muscle weakness is severe enough to distort weight-bearing forces. In these instances, pool therapy will allow rotary torques to be generated in a buoyancy-assisted environment in which the load may be controlled.

With respect to joint protection, the objectives of an exercise program are to reduce stress on the involved joint, improve shock attenuation during exercise and activities of daily living, and improve active joint motion and alignment.

To control joint loading while preserving function, appropriate shoes, compliant walking surfaces (cinders, wood), and, at times, use of a cane, walker, or crutches can all be

127

helpful (see below). In hip OA, use of a cane in the contralateral hand has been shown to reduce joint reaction forces by as much as 50%.[31] Although such measurements have not been made in patients with knee OA, the results should be similar. Furthermore, unloading the knee joint by the above technique is often associated with a decrease in joint pain.

Forces at the knee may be reduced also by walking at a speed that does not increase mechanical stress. Faster walking speeds and running will increase stress on the knee. Subjects with knee OA should walk at speeds that do not increase joint pain or swelling. Even though an increase in walking speed is generally considered a measure of improvement in patients with OA, if insufficient attention is paid to joint biomechanics, gains in walking speed may be detrimental. In a clinical trial in patients who had knee OA with varus deformity due to medial tibiofemoral compartment disease, although treatment with a nonsteroidal anti-inflammatory drug (NSAID) resulted in a reduction in the severity of joint pain and an increase in walking speed, these benefits were accompanied by an increase in adductor moment at the knee and greater loading of the damaged cartilage, in comparison with values obtained after an NSAID washout, ie, when the patient had greater pain.[32] This increase in loading and increased stress on supporting structures of the lateral aspect of the knee could, in the long run, outweigh the advantage of the increase in speed.

Table 9.4 contains some general principles of joint protection for patients with knee OA.

Ambulatory Assistive Devices (Canes, Walkers)

Canes and walkers can be used to support gait in patients with painful OA of a lower extremity joint. In addition, if stability is a problem, a cane may be used for balance. If a cane is used to relieve weight-bearing in a patient with unilateral OA of a lower extremity joint, it should be placed in the contralateral hand. By increasing the base of support on the uninvolved side, this will allow the patient's weight to be shifted toward that side.

The cane should be fitted properly. When the cane is placed vertically alongside the toes, the top of the cane should be aligned with the patient's ulnar styloid process. This will produce 20° to 30° of elbow flexion when the cane is held properly (**Figure 9.3**). The force on the cane should be exerted directly downward. If the patient has significant OA of interphalangeal joints or thumb base, the handle of the cane may be padded to decrease stress on those joints.

Instability in Knee OA

Rehabilitation programs for patients with knee OA have focused largely on restoration of joint mobility and strengthening. However, exercise programs that focus only on improving the above impairments may be inadequate for optimal restoration of function and slowing progression of joint damage in some patients with knee OA.

People with knee OA often experience episodes of instability (ie, "giving way" or buckling) during weight bearing. This may be caused by pain, changes in lower extremity muscle function, and/or laxity of the joint capsule or ligaments. Sharma and associates[33] have shown that an increase in knee laxity may reduce the magnitude of the relationship between lower extremity muscle strength and function in patients with knee OA. Addition of a knee-stability program to a standardized muscle-strengthening exercise program may improve dynamic knee stability in patients with OA.

Patients with knee OA are similar to those who develop knee instability as a result of a ligamentous injury, insofar as both exhibit a reduction in knee flexion/extension during weight bearing[34,35] and cocontraction of the quadriceps and hamstring muscles. Although these changes may represent an attempt to increase knee stability, the reduced excursion of the joint and cocontraction of agonists/antagonists reduces the area of loading across the articular surface, increasing compressive stresses across the joint. Therefore, exercise therapy for patients with knee OA may be more effective if it includes measures that address knee instability.

Controlled exposure of a patient to movements that challenge stability may help prepare the neuromuscular system to react rapidly and efficiently when the need arises to

TABLE 9.4 — JOINT PROTECTION FOR PATIENTS WITH KNEE OA

Recent studies show that protecting your arthritic knee from joint stress will decrease joint pain and protect your cartilage. Research has shown that ordinary walking transmits $3\frac{1}{2}$ times body weight across your knee cartilage; doing a squat puts a stress as high as nine times body weight across your knee cartilage.

It is important that you protect your knees even if you are not experiencing joint pain. Sometimes, only simple adjustments are needed to improve your level of comfort and protect your joints. These are a few suggestions to help you protect your knees:

1. Wear properly fitted shoes with well-cushioned soles, such as Reeboks or Rockports. Sometimes, special inserts are needed to readjust alignment and reduce stress on the knee. Your rheumatologist or physical therapist can help you decide what you need regarding footwear.

2. Sit, rather than stand, for activities lasting longer than 10 minutes. When working at a counter for a lengthy period of time, sit on a high stool rather than stand. If you must stand, take at least a 5-minute break every hour.

3. When arranging your work space, keep items that you use frequently where you can reach them easily without squatting or kneeling.

4. A long-handled reacher can be used to pick up objects from the floor. This item can be obtained from the Occupational Therapy Department, a drug store that carries convalescent aids, or the Sears Home Health Catalog.

5. Park your car close to your destination.

6. Activities that jar your knees may further damage your cartilage. Swimming and walking will place much less stress on your knees than tennis, jogging, or racquetball.

7. Use ramps or elevators. If you must use stairs, taken them one at a time, stopping occasionally to rest.

8. Patients with knee arthritis should avoid:

   a. Low chairs. Sit on a high, firm chair or use a pillow for elevation. Blocks can also be anchored under chair legs. This will put less stress on your knees and requires less energy when you stand up.

   b. Low beds. Blocks can be anchored under bed legs to increase the height of the bed.

   c. Low toilet seats. Elevated toilet seats, which will make getting up much easier, can be obtained from medical supply companies.

   d. Bathtubs. A shower with shower chair, if necessary, is a much better alternative.

   e. Kneeling, squatting, or sitting cross-legged on the floor. All of these will put undue stress on your knee cartilage.

Rheumatology Division, Indiana University School of Medicine; 1993.

maintain joint stability during performance of daily activities. Such stability training programs, which are commonly employed for younger, physically active individuals with knee instability due to ligamentous damage,[36,37] may be helpful also in patients with knee OA.

Techniques for improving stability and balance can be readily employed within the context of functional tasks. Agility training techniques focus on rapid stopping, starting, twisting, and changes in direction. Balance training may include the perturbation of stability on tilt and roller boards. In applying these techniques to patients with knee OA, however, the intensity of effort must be reduced to prevent overloading of the joint. If this is done, improvement in stability and balance can be achieved without exacerbating symptoms or signs of joint inflammation.

FIGURE 9.3 — PROPER USE OF CANE BY PATIENT WITH OA

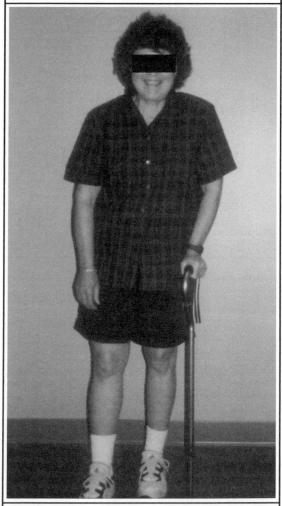

A patient with OA of a lower extremity joint should hold the cane in the contralateral hand.

Photo kindly provided by Marilyn Sissel.

Weight Loss

Chapter 2, *Epidemiology*, emphasizes the importance of obesity as a risk factor for knee OA. Weight reduction in patients who are obese may result in a reduction in pain and improvement in function of weight-bearing joints.[38] Even a small amount of weight loss may be beneficial in patients with knee OA.[39]

Thermal Modalities

Applications of heat, cold, or both have been widely employed for short-term pain relief in many musculoskeletal conditions, including OA. However, no controlled clinical trials of the application of superficial heat or cold to OA joints have been reported.

■ Heat

Most modalities for application of superficial heat can elevate the temperature of the soft tissues 3° at a depth of 1 cm beneath the surface. Because infrared heat penetrates the skin only a few millimeters, superficial heat does not penetrate deeper joints, such as the hip or knee. By diverting blood flow to more superficial tissues, it may lower the intra-articular temperature slightly.[40] In contrast, use of a heat mitten for 30 minutes may increase the temperature in the superficial small joints of the hand.[41]

Moist heat produces greater elevation of the subcutaneous temperature than dry heat and is often preferable for relief of joint pain. Care must be taken to avoid burning, particularly over bony prominences.[42] **Table 9.5** provides some practical instructions and precautions for a patient applying heat to an arthritic joint at home.

A patient with painful Heberden's nodes may find that dipping the hand into a paraffin bath, prepared by mixing hot paraffin wax with mineral oil at 47.5° to 52° C, soothing and analgesic. Comparable results, however, may be obtained simply by immersing the hand in warm tap water. Therapy in a heated pool permits simultaneous treatment of multiple painful joints and muscles. Furthermore, the buoyancy of the water is particularly useful in assuring that minimal stress will be applied to the joint during ROM exercises.

TABLE 9.5 — APPLICATION OF HEAT TO A JOINT

The objective of applying heat to your arthritic joint is to reduce muscle spasm and joint pain. This may permit you to perform your joint exercises more effectively. You may find moist heat more effective than dry heat, although either can be used. Consider what is most convenient for you. You may use a shower or bath once a day and use a heating pad for the other heat applications.

Observe the following rules for safe and effective application of heat to your joints:

1. Apply heat to the affected area for no more than 15 to 20 minutes at a time.

2. Avoid lying on a heating pad, since your body weight will decrease the circulation to that area and increase the risk of a burn.

3. Before using a heating pad, wash off any liniment on the skin, since this could cause a burn.

4. Use the heating pad only on low or medium temperature settings (not on high).

5. Do not apply heat to any region in which you have had an artificial joint implanted.

Deep heat is also useful. In contrast to superficial heat, it can affect the viscoelastic properties of collagen. Because tension is applied to the tissues as they are stretched, an increase in "creep" (the plastic stretch of ligaments under tension) occurs.[43] Application of deep heat prior to stretching exercises will enhance the efficacy of the exercises.

Diathermy can be employed as either shortwave or microwave electromagnetic irradiation or by ultrasound, in which high-frequency sound waves are converted to heat.[44] Ultrasound penetrates more deeply than either shortwave or microwave diathermy; among these three forms of deep heat, it alone can raise the intra-articular temperature of the hip joint.[45] Joint pain in patients with OA of the hip or knee can be significantly reduced by either ultrasound or shortwave diathermy, especially if these are combined with an analgesic or NSAID.[46]

Deep heat is contraindicated in a patient with a local malignancy or bleeding diathesis[47] and after laminectomy. The risk of thermal injury with use of any of the above heat modalities is increased if the circulation is poor, the patient sedated, or sensation impaired.

■ **Cold**

Cold is often recommended to relieve muscle aching after strenuous exercise. It may be delivered by ice packs, ice massage, or local spray. Superficial cooling can decrease muscle spasm and increase the pain threshold.[48,49] Use of vapocoolant sprays over areas of painful trigger points may be effective.[50] Fluoromethane, which is not flammable, is preferable to ethyl chloride.[51]

Cold applications should not be used in patients with Raynaud's phenomenon, cold hypersensitivity, cryoglobulinemia, or paroxysmal cold hemoglobinuria.[52]

Periodic Phone Calls

Incorporation of simple periodic contact measures may be a valuable adjunct to pharmacologic therapy in patients with OA. When patients with knee OA who had relatively poor social support were randomized into two groups—one that received a telephone call monthly from a trained lay person and the other that did not receive the phone calls—improvement in joint pain and mobility among those who received the phone calls was as great as that seen in clinical trials of NSAIDs.[53] In this study, the phone calls were "second-line therapy," insofar as all of the subjects were taking an NSAID throughout the period of the study. Notably, the calls did not focus on medical education issues, such as might be dealt with by a doctor or nurse, but on general issues, relevant to the daily lives of the patients, such as: Do you have food in the refrigerator? Do you remember the date of your next clinic visit? Do you have transportation to the clinic?

Functional Knee Braces

In patients with knee OA who have significant varus deformity, specifically designed functional knee braces (valgus braces)—although they are relatively cumbersome and their acceptance by female patients, in particular, may be low—may decrease joint pain and improve function and quality of life.[54-57] By producing a valgus thrust, they unload the medial tibiofemoral compartment. It has been suggested that neuromuscular effects may also contribute to their efficacy.

As noted below, elastic bandages have been shown to improve proprioception in patients with knee OA who were tested in a non–weight-bearing position.[58] However, the effects of bracing on proprioception are unknown and the clinical relevance of proprioceptive impairment to weight-bearing activities, such as postural control, is unclear. In a study of 20 patients with varus malalignment due to medial compartment knee OA, a valgus brace produced a small, albeit statistically significant, improvement in proprioception, but this had no effect on postural control.[59] These results bring into question the clinical importance of the small changes in proprioception achieved with bracing and suggest that the improvement in pain, function, and quality of life that may result from bracing are related more to mechanical factors, such as alteration of the adductor moment and of compressive stresses about the knee, than to changes in proprioception.

Patellar Taping

Osteoarthritis of the patellofemoral compartment can cause severe pain, especially with kneeling, squatting, or climbing stairs. Although no controlled clinical trials have been performed to support this recommendation, taping the patella to pull it medially, followed by quadriceps exercises, has been recommended for treatment of chondromalacia patellae, ie, patellofemoral joint pain in young subjects.[60,61]

Cushnaghan and colleagues reported a controlled clinical trial of knee taping to realign the patella in 14 subjects with patellofemoral OA.[62] Taping was accomplished with a strip of Leukotape P (Beiersdorf, UK). Significant reduction in pain occurred with medial taping in comparison with taping in the lateral or neutral position. Furthermore, patient preference favored medial taping over the other positions.

The taping procedure is simple and patients can learn to apply their own tape after minimal instruction. The treatment is inexpensive. The prompt relief of symptoms that may be achieved by taping may be maintained by concurrent isometric exercises to strengthen the vastus medialis obliquus component of the quadriceps muscle, facilitating realignment of the patella on a long-term basis.[61,63,64]

Splinting for Hand OA

If a distal interphalangeal (DIP) joint becomes so painful that it interferes with hand function, a rigid, custom-molded, thermoplastic cylindric orthosis or tri-point splint that blocks flexion can reduce pain, improve overall hand function, and reduce muscular guarding by allowing the patient to use the hand without fear of pain (**Figure 9.4**, *top*).[65] Rigid immobilization can be employed also for severe pain of the proximal interphalangeal (PIP) joint but is generally not an acceptable option because it limits hand function and can result in shortening of the collateral ligaments, reducing the mobility of the PIP joint.

Two studies[66,67] have indicated that approximately 80% of patients with trapeziometacarpal joint (TMJ) OA who were referred for surgery found that splinting provided sufficient symptomatic relief so that they did not require the operation. A short opponens splint that permits wrist motion has greater patient acceptance than a long opponens splint that restricts the wrist and appears to be as effective. A custom-fitted thermoplastic immobilization splint that provides a C-bar to stabilize the TMJ in abduction but permits full mobility of the thumb IPJ and wrist can be helpful (**Figure 9.4**, *center*). Melvin[65] evaluated this splint with a protocol that required continuous use for 2 to 3 weeks and, once the patient became pain free for as long as 3 hours without the splint, use of the splint only during stressful activities. In a 3-month follow-up study of 35 patients, 80% complied with instructions regarding splint usage, 17% were pain free after treatment, and another 68% reported significant reduction in pain. Seven patients reduced their dose of NSAID or discontinued NSAID use.

Several commercially available TMJ splints do not include a C-bar over the web space. These permit adduction

FIGURE 9.4 — IMMOBILIZATION SPLINTS

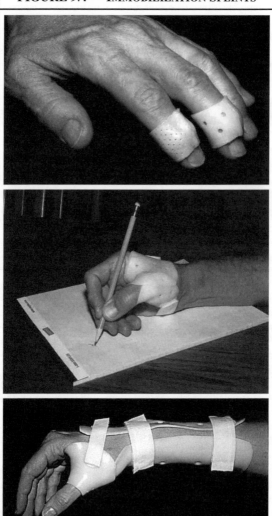

(Top) Immobilization splint for the distal interphalangeal joint (made of Aquaplast): one is pre-perforated and the other has been perforated manually. Use of a simple cylinder splint can

Continued

138

of the thumb at the TMJ and may not sufficiently immobilize the TMJ to adequately treat inflammation. Pantrapezial OA requires a splint that immobilizes the wrist as well as the TMJ (**Figure 9.4,** *bottom*).

Elastic Bandages for Patients With Knee OA

Elastic bandages may afford pain relief for patients with knee OA and reduce the feeling of "giving way" of the knee and fear of falling, although there is little information from randomized controlled trials to support this treatment. In a crossover study of patients with symptomatic knee OA who were assigned to wear either a standard-size bandage or a slightly looser bandage and were then given a bandage of the opposite size 2 weeks later,[59] the more loosely fitting bandage significantly reduced knee pain and improved postural sway, although it did not affect proprioception. In contrast, the more tightly fitting bandage had no effect on joint pain, proprioception, or sway. In both cases, improvement was lost rapidly upon removal of the bandage.

It is possible that the reduction in knee pain while the bandage was worn was due to stimulation of large type $A\delta$ sensory fibers carrying impulses from skin mechanoreceptors, leading to a reduction in the central transmission of pain signals.[68] In addition, movement of the bandage on the skin may have influenced proprioceptive activity and thereby resulted in improvement in sway, with a secondary benefit on joint pain.

Although the difference between the results with the looser-fitting and those with the more tightly fitting bandage is surprising at first glance, it is possible that cutaneous receptors adapted rapidly to the constant pressure and duration of the stimulus produced by the tighter wrap. As suggested by the authors,[59] the looser bandage may have generated a greater number of recurrent new stimuli and elicited a greater and more persistent response from cutaneous receptors. Although these results require confirmation and the relevance of the improvement in postural sway to daily function is not clear (will it reduce the incidence of falls or feeling of giving way?), if a simple inexpensive elastic bandage helps in the control of knee OA pain, it is a useful addition to the treatment program.

Tidal Irrigation of the Knee

The concept that perfusing an arthritic joint with a volume of physiologic fluid can sometimes lead to lasting clinical improvement, and thus be worthy of considering as a therapeutic intervention, originated in the writings of the first American arthroscopists. Burnam and colleagues,[69] describing their initial observations after knee arthroscopy in 30 subjects, noted: "It was in this group of arthritic cases that we had the pleasant surprise of seeing a marked improvement of the joint following arthroscopy." One of the patients who underwent arthroscopy had such a good result that "he begged us to do the same for the other knee." This patient had undergone arthroscopy to determine whether his chronically swollen knee might harbor infection with tubercle bacilli and to decide upon further surgical management with synovectomy or arthrodesis.

Several studies have examined the effects of knee lavage, performed without arthroscopy with the use of a large-bore needle, in treatment of OA.[70] Guidelines for management of OA of the knee published in 1995 by the American College of Rheumatology stated: "Most individuals who require more than three to four intra-articular injections of steroid per year to control symptoms are probably candidates for joint lavage or surgical intervention."[71] An update of those guidelines published 5 years later recognized the large placebo response that may accompany tidal irrigation

(TI) and pointed out that results of properly controlled studies of this procedure were not available at that time.[72] A recent randomized controlled trial of TI in 180 patients with knee OA, half of whom underwent a sham-irrigation procedure, led to the conclusion that "...most, if not all, of the effect of TI..." can be attributed to the placebo effect.[73]

Wedged Insoles

Wedged insoles may be useful in conservative treatment of OA of the medial tibiofemoral compartment.[74,75] The insole changes the spatial position of the lower limb so that the mechanical axis becomes more nearly upright and the calcaneal axis is shifted to a valgus position with respect to the tibiotalar joint. On the basis of two-dimensional analysis, it was concluded that these changes reduced excessive loading on the medial compartment of the knee and strain on the lateral collateral ligament.[74]

In a comparative study of 107 patients with OA in which 67 were treated with both the wedged insole and indomethacin and 40 with indomethacin alone,[75] the insole group showed significantly greater improvement. The insole was significantly more effective in patients with mild OA than in those with more advanced disease. The data suggest that the wedged insole represents an effective, conservative treatment for early, medial compartment knee OA. Keating and associates,[76] on the other hand, in an uncontrolled study, found lateral heel and sole wedges effective in treatment of medial compartment knee OA even in patients with complete loss of joint space on the knee radiograph. Fifty percent of the 85 patients who were evaluated (121 knees) showed an improvement in pain score of a magnitude corresponding to a "good" result from total knee arthroplasty. Although Maillefert and colleagues[77] failed to demonstrate significant short-term symptomatic benefit of lateral wedged insoles in patients with medial tibiofemoral OA, use of the insoles resulted in a significant decrease in NSAID consumption. Furthermore, compliance with wear of the lateral wedges was significantly greater than that of neutrally wedged insoles (employed as a control), suggesting a beneficial effect. A polypropylene mesh shoe-type insole is practical, inexpensive, and washable and will last approximately 2 years, ie, approximately twice as long as a leather insole.

Several studies suggest that patients tolerate foot orthotics well. Donatelli and associates[78] reported that 94% of patients who responded to a survey about their use of their orthotic reported they were still wearing the orthotic at the time of the survey. The majority believed they had derived pain relief exclusively from use of the orthotic. More than half would "not leave home without the orthotic." Although data from prospective controlled clinical trials evaluating the tolerability of orthotics are not available, retrospective data and clinical experience suggest they are well tolerated and that patients feel they are useful.

Wedged insoles may offer an additional benefit in patients with medial compartment knee OA because the external adductor moment appears to be important in the progression of medial compartment knee OA[79-81] and lateral wedges significantly reduce the external adductor moment of the knee. In addition to being of symptomatic benefit, they could, theoretically, slow the progression of structural damage in patients with knee OA. This possibility has not been examined in clinical trials.

Patient Education

A number of studies have shown that patient education programs offer benefits beyond those that can be achieved with an NSAID in symptomatic treatment of patients with OA. A meta-analysis found that patient education interventions provided additional benefit 20% to 30% as great as that of NSAID treatment alone.[82] We have shown that self-care education for inner-city patients with knee OA (ie, a group with relatively poor social support), delivered as an adjunct to primary care, resulted in preservation of function and control of knee pain.[83] For effective management of many patients with OA, encouragement, reassurance, advice about exercise, and recommendation of measures to unload the arthritic joint, such as a cane and proper footwear, may be all that is required.

Acupuncture

Ezzo and colleagues[84] recently reviewed controlled clinical trials of acupuncture in patients with knee OA and concluded that *verum* acupuncture was more effective than sham acupuncture in relieving OA pain but that the evidence that functional improvement was greater with real acupuncture than with the sham procedure was inconclusive. The authors also noted that the evidence was insufficient to determine how the results of acupuncture compare with those of physical therapy, to ascertain which aspects of acupuncture treatment might be conducive to positive results, to determine the optimal treatment protocol, or to determine whether maintenance acupuncture treatments prolong the effect in those who respond to the initial treatment.

9

REFERENCES

1. Centers for Disease Control. Prevalence of leisure-time physical activity among persons with arthritis and other rheumatic conditions—United States, 1990-1991. *Morb Mortal Wkly Rep.* 1997;46:389-393.

2. Liang M. Evaluation of the status of the OA patient and assessment of outcomes in the clinical setting. In: Brandt KD, Doherty M, Raffa RB, et al. Proceedings of symposium: controversies and practical issues in the management of osteoarthritis. *J Clin Rheum.* 2003;9(suppl): S1-S39.

3. Minor MA. The utility and importance of nonpharmacologic therapy for the patient with OA. In: Brandt KD, Doherty MA, Raffa RB, et al. Symposium proceedings: controversies and practical issues in the management of osteoarthritis. *J Clin Rheum.* 2003;9(suppl):S1-S39.

4. Moskowitz RW, Goldberg VM. Osteoarthritis: clinical features and treatment. In: Schumacher HR Jr, ed. *Primer on the Rheumatic Disease.* 10th ed. Atlanta, Ga: Arthritis Foundation; 1993:188-190.

5. Minor MA. Exercise in the management of osteoarthritis of the knee and hip. *Arthritis Care Res.* 1994;7:198-204.

6. Kasper MJ, Robbins L, Root L, Peterson MG, Allegrante JP. A musculoskeletal outreach screening, treatment, and education program for urban minority children. *Arthritis Care Res.* 1993;6:126-133.

7. Semble EL, Loeser RF, Wise CM. Therapeutic exercise for rheumatoid arthritis and osteoarthritis. *Semin Arthritis Rheum.* 1990;20: 32-40.

8. Palmoski MJ, Colyer RA, Brandt KD. Joint motion in the absence of normal loading does not maintain normal articular cartilage. *Arthritis Rheum.* 1980;23:325-334.

143

9. Blair SN, Kohl HW, Gordon NF, Paffenbarger RS Jr. How much physical activity is good for health? *Annu Rev Public Health.* 1992;13:99-126.

10. Fisher NM, Pendergast DR, Gresham GE, Calkins E. Muscle rehabilitation: its effect on muscular and functional performance of patients with knee osteoarthritis. *Arch Phys Med Rehabil.* 1991;72:367-374.

11. Chamberlain MA, Care G, Harfield B. Physiotherapy in osteoarthrosis of the knees. A controlled trial of hospital versus home exercises. *Int Rehabil Med.* 1982;4:101-106.

12. Judge JO, Underwood M, Gennosa T. Exercise to improve gait velocity in older persons. *Arch Phys Med Rehabil.* 1993;74:400-406.

13. Minor MA, Hewett JE, Webel RR, Anderson SK, Kay DR. Efficacy of physical conditioning exercise in patients with rheumatoid arthritis and osteoarthritis. *Arthritis Rheum.* 1989;32:1396-1405.

14. Kovar PA, Allegrante JP, Mackenzie CR, Peterson MG, Gutin B, Charlson ME. Supervised fitness walking in patients with osteoarthritis of the knee. A randomized, controlled trial. *Ann Intern Med.* 1992; 116:529-534.

15. Lankhorst GJ, Van de Stadt RJ, Van der Korst JK. The relationships of functional capacity, pain, and isometric and isokinetic torque in osteoarthrosis of the knee. *Scand J Rehabil Med.* 1985;17:167-172.

16. Minor MA, Hewett JE, Webel RR, Dreisinger TE, Kay DR. Exercise tolerance and disease related measures in patients with rheumatoid arthritis and osteoarthritis. *J Rheumatol.* 1988;15:905-911.

17. Ries MD, Philbin EF, Groff GD. Relationship between severity of gonarthrosis and cardiovascular fitness. *Clin Orthop.* 1995;313:169-176.

18. CDC. Prevalence and impact of arthritis among women – United States 1989-1991. *Morb Mortal Wkly Rep.* 1995;44:329-334.

19. Vita AJ, Terry R B, Hubert HB, Fries JF. Aging, health risks, and cumulative disability. *N Engl J Med.* 1998;338:1035-1041.

20. Blair SN, Kohl HW 3rd, Barlow CE, Paffenbarger RS Jr, Gibbons LW, Macera CA. Changes in physical fitness and all-cause mortality. A prospective study of healthy and unhealthy men. *JAMA.* 1995;273: 1093-1098.

21. Jevsevar DS, Riley PO, Hodge WA, Krebs DE. Knee kinematics and kinetics during locomotor activities of daily living in subjects with knee arthroplasty and in healthy control subjects. *Phys Ther.* 1993;73: 229-242.

22. Krebs DE, Elbaum L, Riley PO, Hodge WA, Mann RW. Exercise and gait effects on *in vivo* hip contact pressures. *Phys Ther.* 1991;71:301-309.

23. Lankhorst GJ, van de Stadt RJ, van der Korst JK, Hinlopen-Bonrath E, Griffioen FM, de Boer W. Relationship of isometric knee extension torque and functional variables in osteoarthrosis of the knee. *Scand J Rehabil Med.* 1982;14:7-10.

144

24. Epstein WV, Yelin EH, Nevitt M, Kramer JS. Arthritis: a major health problem in the elderly. In: Moskowitz R, Haug M, eds. *Arthritis and the Elderly*. New York, NY: Springer; 1986:5-17.

25. Ettinger WH Jr, Burns R, Messier SP, et al. A randomized trial comparing aerobic exercise and resistance exercise with a health education program in older adults with knee osteoarthritis. The Fitness Arthritis and Seniors Trial (FAST). *JAMA*. 1997;277:25-31.

26. O'Reilly SC, Muir KR, Doherty M. Effectiveness of home exercise on pain and disability from osteoarthritis of the knee: a randomised controlled trial. *Ann Rheum Dis*. 1999;58:15-19.

27. Hurley MV, Scott DL. Improvements in quadriceps sensorimotor function and disability of patients with knee osteoarthritis following a clinically practicable exercise regime. *Br J Rheumatol*. 1998;37:1181-1187.

28. Leivseth G, Torstensson J, Reikeras O. Effect of passive muscle stretching in osteoarthritis of the hip. *Clin Sci*. 1989;76:113-117.

29. Messier SP, Loeser RF, Hoover JL, Semble EL, Wise CM. Osteoarthritis of the knee: effects on gait, strength, and flexibility. *Arch Phys Med Rehabil*. 1992;73:29-36.

30. Radin EL, Yang KH, Riegger C, Kish VL, O'Connor JJ. Relationship between lower limb dynamics and knee joint pain. *J Orthop Res*. 1991;9:398-405.

31. Neumann DA. Biomechanical analysis of selected principles of hip joint protection. *Arthritis Care Res*. 1989;2:146-155.

32. Schnitzer TJ, Popovich JM, Andersson GB, Andriacchi TP. Effect of piroxicam on gait in patients with osteoarthritis of the knee. *Arthritis Rheum*. 1993;36:1207-1213.

33. Sharma L, Hayes KW, Felson DT, et al. Does laxity alter the relationship between strength and physical function in knee osteoarthritis? *Arthritis Rheum*. 1999;42:25-32.

34. Gyory AN, Chao EY, Stauffer RN. Functional evaluation of normal and pathologic knees during gait. *Arch Phys Med Rehabil*. 1976;57: 571-577.

35. Snyder-Mackler L, Ladin Z, Schepsis AA, Young JC. Electrical stimulation of the thigh muscles after reconstruction of the anterior cruciate ligament. Effects of electrically elicited contraction of the quadriceps femoris and hamstring muscles on gait and on strength of the thigh muscles. *J Bone Joint Surg*. 1991;73:1025-1036.

36. Snyder-Mackler L, Delitto A, Bailey SL, Stralka SW. Strength of the quadriceps femoris muscle and functional recovery after reconstruction of the anterior cruciate ligament. A prospective, randomized clinical trial of electrical stimulation. *J Bone Joint Surg*. 1995;77: 1166-1173.

37. Ihara H, Nakayama A. Dynamic joint control training for knee ligament injuries. *Am J Sports Med*. 1986;14:309-315.

9

145

38. Felson DT, Anderson JJ, Naimark A, Walker AM, Meenan RF. Obesity and knee osteoarthritis. The Framingham Study. *Ann Intern Med.* 1988;109:18-24.

39. Felson DT, Chaisson CE. Understanding the relationship between body weight and osteoarthritis. *Baillières Clin Rheumatol.* 1997;11:671-681.

40. Hollander JL, Horvath SM. Changes in joint temperature produced by diseases and by physical therapy. *Arch Phys Med Rehabil.* 1949;30: 437-440.

41. Mainardi CL, Walter JM, Spiegel PK, Goldkamp OG, Harris ED Jr. Rheumatoid arthritis: failure of daily heat therapy to affect its progression. *Arch Phys Med Rehabil.* 1979;60:390-393.

42. Hicks J, Nicholas JJ. Treatments utilized in rehabilitative rheumatology. In: Hicks J, Nicholas JJ, Swezey R, eds. *Handbook of Rehabilitative Rheumatology.* Atlanta, Ga: American College of Rheumatology; 1989:45.

43. Lehmann JF, Masock AJ, Warren CG, Koblanski JN. Effect of therapeutic temperatures on tendon extensibility. *Arch Phys Med Rehabil.* 1970;51:481-487.

44. Schwan HP, Piersol GM. The absorption of electromagnetic energy on body tissues: a review and critical analysis. II. Physiological and clinical aspects. *Am J Phys Med.* 1955;34:425-448.

45. Lehman JF. Diathermy. In: Krusen FH, Kottke FJ, Ellwood PM, eds. *Handbook of Physical Medicine and Rehabilitation.* 2nd ed. Philadelphia, Pa: WB Saunders Company; 1971:273-375.

46. Svarcová J, Trnavský K, Zvárová J. The influence of ultrasound, galvanic currents and shortwave diathermy on pain intensity in patients with osteoarthritis. *Scand J Rheumatol.* 1987;67:83-85.

47. Lahmann JF, Krusen FH. Biophysical effects of ultrasonic energy on carcinoma and their possible significance. *Arch Phys Med Rehabil.* 1955;36:452-459.

48. Miglietta O. Action of cold on spasticity. *Am J Phys Med.* 1973;52: 198-205.

49. Benson TB, Copp EP. The effects of therapeutic forms of heat and ice on the pain threshold of the normal shoulder. *Rheumatol Rehabil.* 1974;13:101-104.

50. Travell J. Ethyl chloride spray for painful muscle spasm. *Arch Phys Med.* 1952;33:291-298.

51. Mennel JM. Spray and stretch treatment for myofascial pain. *Hosp Phys.* 1973;12:47-50.

52. Olson JE, Stravino VD. A review of cryotherapy. *Phys Ther.* 1972;52: 840-853.

53. René J, Weinberger M, Mazzuca SA, Brandt KD, Katz BP. Reduction of joint pain in patients with knee osteoarthritis who have received monthly telephone calls from lay personnel and whose medical treatment regimens have remained stable. *Arthritis Rheum.* 1992;35:511-515.

54. Matsuno H, Kadowaki KM, Tsuji H. Generation II knee bracing for severe medial compartment osteoarthritis of the knee. *Arch Phys Med Rehabil*. 1997;78:745-749.

55. Lindenfeld TN, Hewett TE, Andriacchi TP. Joint loading with valgus bracing in patients with varus gonarthrosis. *Clin Orthop*. 1997;344: 290-297.

56. Hewett TE, Noyes FR, Barber-Westin SD, Heckmann TP. Decrease in knee joint pain and increase in function in patients with medial compartment arthrosis: a prospective analysis of valgus bracing. *Orthopedics*. 1998;21:131-138.

57. Kirkley A, Webster-Bogaert S, Litchfield R, et al. The effect of bracing on varus gonarthrosis. *J Bone Joint Surg*. 1999;81:539-548.

58. Hassan BS, Mockett S, Doherty M. Influence of elastic bandage on knee pain, proprioception, and postural sway in subjects with knee osteoarthritis. *Ann Rheum Dis*. 2002;61:24-28.

59. Birmingham TB, Kramer JF, Kirkley A, Inglis JT, Spaulding SJ, Vandervoort AA. Knee bracing for medial compartment osteoarthritis: effects on proprioception and postural control. *Rheumatology*. 2001;40:285-289.

60. McConnell J. The management of chondromalacia patellae: a long-term solution. *Aust J Physiother*. 1986;32:215-223.

61. McConnell JS. Training the vastus medialis oblique in the management of patellofemoral pain. *Proceedings of the 10th International Congress WCPT*. Sydney, Australia; 1987.

62. Cushnaghan J, McCarthy C, Dieppe P. Taping the patella medially: a new treatment for osteoarthritis of the knee joint? *BMJ*. 1994;308: 753-755.

63. Marks R. Quadriceps strength training for osteoarthritis of the knee: a literature review and analysis. *Physiotherapy*. 1993;79:13-18.

64. Doucette SA, Goble EM. The effect of exercise on patellar tracking in lateral patellar compression syndrome. *Am J Sports Med*. 1992;20: 434-440.

65. Melvin JL. Occupational therapy. In: Brandt KD, Doherty M, Lohmander SL, eds. *Osteoarthritis*. 2nd ed. Oxford, UK; Oxford University Press. In press.

66. Swigart CR, Eaton R G, Glickel SZ, Johnson C. Splinting in the treatment of arthritis of the first carpometacarpal joint. *J Hand Surg*. 1999;24:86-91.

67. Dell PC, Brushart TM, Smith RJ. Treatment of trapeziometacarpal arthritis: results of resection arthroplasty. *J Hand Surg*. 1978;3:243-249.

68. Guyton AC, Hall JE. Somatic sensation: I. General organization; the tactile and position senses. In: Guyton AC, Hall JE, eds. *Textbook of Medical Physiology*. Philadelphia, PA: Saunders; 1996:595-607.

69. Burnam MS, Finkelstein FH, Mayer L. Arthroscopy of the knee joint. *J Bone Joint Surg*. 1934;16A:255.

70. Ike RW. Joint lavage. In: Brandt KD, Doherty M, Lohmander LS, eds. *Osteoarthritis*. Oxford, UK: Oxford University Press; 1998:359-377.

71. Hochberg MC, Altman RD, Brandt KD, et al. Guidelines for the medical management of osteoarthritis. Part II. Osteoarthritis of the knee. American College of Rheumatology. *Arthritis Rheum*. 1995;38:1541-1546.

72. American College of Rheumatology Subcommittee on Osteoarthritis Guidelines. Recommendations for the medical management of osteoarthritis of the hip and knee: 2000 update. *Arthritis Rheum*. 2000;43:1905-1915.

73. Bradley JD, Heilman DK, Katz BP, G'sell P, Wallick JE, Brandt KD. Tidal irrigation as treatment for knee osteoarthritis: a sham-controlled, randomized, double-blinded evaluation. *Arthritis Rheum*. 2002;46:100-108.

74. Yasuda K, Sasaki T. The mechanics of treatment of the osteoarthritic knee with a wedged insole. *Clin Orthop*. 1987;215:162-172.

75. Sasaki T, Yasuda K. Clinical evaluation of the treatment of osteoarthritic knees using a newly designed wedged insole. *Clin Orthop*. 1987;221:181-187.

76. Keating EM, Faris PM, Ritter MA, Kane J. Use of lateral heel and sole wedges in the treatment of medial osteoarthritis of the knee. *Orthop Rev*. 1993;22:921-924.

77. Maillefert JF, Hudry C, Baron G, et al. Laterally elevated wedged insoles in the treatment of medial knee osteoarthritis: a prospective randomized controlled study. *Osteoarthritis Cartilage*. 2001;9:738-745.

78. Donatelli R, Hurlbert C, Conaway D, St Pierre R. Biomechanical foot orthotics: a retrospective study. *J Orthop Sports Phys Ther*. 1988;10:205-212.

79. Baliunas AJ, Hurwitz DE, Ryals AR, et al. Increased knee joint loads during walking are present in subjects with knee osteoarthritis. *Osteoarthritis Cartilage*. 2002;10:573-579.

80. Sharma L, Hurwitz DE, Thonar EJ, et al. Knee adduction moment, serum hyaluronan level, and disease severity in medial tibiofemoral osteoarthritis. *Arthritis Rheum*. 1998;41:1233-1240.

81. Weidenhielm L, Svensson OK, Brostrom LA, Mattsson E. Adduction moment of the knee compared to radiological and clinical parameters in moderate medical osteoarthrosis of the knee. *Ann Chir Gynaecol*. 1994;83:236-242.

82. Superio-Cabuslay E, Ward MM, Lorig KR. Patient education interventions in osteoarthritis and rheumatoid arthritis: a meta-analytic comparison with nonsteroidal antiinflammatory drug treatment. *Arthritis Care Res*. 1996;9:292-301.

83. Mazzuca SA, Brandt KD, Katz BP, Chambers M, Byrd D, Hanna M. Effects of self-care education on the health status of inner-city patients with osteoarthritis of the knee. *Arthritis Rheum*. 1997;40:1466-1474.

84. Ezzo J, Hadhazy V, Birch S, et al. Acupuncture for osteoarthritis of the knee: a systematic review. *Arthritis Rheum*. 2001;44:819-825.

10   Acetaminophen

Efficacy of ACET in Palliation of OA Pain

Despite the voluminous literature comparing one non-steroidal anti-inflammatory drug (NSAID) with another or with placebo in treatment of OA, until relatively recently, no reports were available comparing the efficacy of an NSAID with that of an analgesic essentially devoid of any anti-inflammatory effect (eg, acetaminophen [ACET], dextropropoxyphene) in treatment of OA pain. As discussed below, the evidence now indicates that a simple analgesic is as effective as an NSAID in symptomatic treatment of many patients with OA.

For example, in a study of patients with chronic knee pain and moderately severe radiographic changes of OA treated for 4 weeks with either an anti-inflammatory dose or an analgesic dose of ibuprofen (2400 mg/d, 1200 mg/d, respectively) or with ACET (4000 mg/d), Bradley and colleagues found no superiority of either the anti-inflammatory dose or the lower dose of ibuprofen in comparison with ACET.[1]

Despite the fact that American and European guidelines for management of OA continue to advocate ACET as the initial drug for treatment of symptomatic OA, until recently only a single study comparing ACET with placebo in treatment of patients with OA had been published.[2] All other studies that were taken into account in the formulation of OA management guidelines compared ACET to an active control (NSAID). Furthermore, the study referred to above[2] involved only 25 subjects with knee OA. It is notable, therefore, that on the basis of a randomized double-blind placebo-controlled trial of diclofenac 75 mg bid vs ACET 1000 mg qid, Case and colleagues recently concluded that diclofenac was effective in symptomatic treatment of knee OA but ACET was not.[3]

However, this study involved only 82 subjects (25 randomized to diclofenac, 29 to ACET, and 28 to placebo). The diagnosis of OA was based on a radiographic assessment in which joint-space narrowing is weighted as heavily as osteophytosis.[4] (This radiographic grading may be problematic insofar as joint-space narrowing alone may be due to meniscus damage or extrusion[5] or to knee pain, limiting the ability of the patient to fully extend the knee for the anteroposterior view that was employed in this study.[6]) The authors' conclusions, furthermore, were based on an analysis in which the results of the last observation were used to compute results for subsequent visits, an approach of questionable validity because 20% to 30% of subjects in each of the three treatment groups did not complete the study. Furthermore, baseline pain scores were 17% higher in the diclofenac group than in the ACET group, suggesting that improvement in the former may have been due, at least partly, to regression to the mean. Indeed, at week 2, the difference between diclofenac and ACET vs diclofenac and placebo reached statistical significance only in patients with the lowest baseline pain scores (**Table 10.1**). Similarly, the results with diclofenac were not significantly different from those with either ACET or placebo in subjects with more severe radiographic changes of OA at baseline (**Table 10.2**), although the small number of subjects in this study limits the power of subgroup analysis.

Do Clinical Signs of Inflammation Predict a Better Response to an NSAID Than to ACET?

Should an NSAID be considered as the initial drug of choice in OA patients with signs of joint inflammation? There are essentially no data to support that view. Neither joint swelling, effusion, synovial tenderness,[7] nor the severity of inflammation in a synovial biopsy[8] predict a better response to an anti-inflammatory dose of NSAID than to ACET. However, prospective randomized controlled trials have not been performed in patients who were stratified at the outset on the basis of severity of inflammation in the OA joint. Such information would be very helpful in

TABLE 10.1 — STRATIFICATION OF WOMAC RESPONSE AT WEEK 2 IN THE DICLOFENAC TREATMENT GROUP BASED ON BASELINE PAIN SEVERITY

Baseline Variable	Comparison	P Value*	
		WOMAC Pain Score	Total WOMAC Score
Pain tertile			
Lowest (n = 27)	Diclofenac with ACET	.05	.03
	Diclofenac with placebo	.04	.05
Middle (n = 28)	Diclofenac with ACET	.49	.06
	Diclofenac with placebo	.23	.07
Highest (n = 27)	Diclofenac with ACET	.11	.11
	Diclofenac with placebo	.09	.37

Abbreviations: ACET, acetaminophen; WOMAC, Western Ontario and McMasters Universities Arthritis Index.

* Using ANOVA (analysis of variance).

Modified from: Case JP, et al. *Arch Intern Med.* 2003;163:174.

10

TABLE 10.2 — STRATIFICATION OF WOMAC RESPONSE AT WEEK 2 IN THE DICLOFENAC TREATMENT GROUP BASED ON RADIOGRAPHIC SEVERITY OF OA AT BASELINE

Baseline Variable	Comparison	P Value*	
		WOMAC Pain Score	Total WOMAC Score
Kellgren-Lawrence Grade[†]			
1 or 2 (n = 47)	Diclofenac with ACET	.002	<.001
	Diclofenac with placebo	.003	.001
3 or 4 (n = 24)	Diclofenac with ACET	.85	.42
	Diclofenac with placebo	.37	.46
Medial Joint-Space Narrowing			
0 or 1 (n = 34)	Diclofenac with ACET	.005	<.001
	Diclofenac with placebo	.002	<.001
2 or 3 (n = 34)	Diclofenac with ACET	.63	.47
	Diclofenac with placebo	.29	.56

Abbreviations: ACET, acetaminophen; OA, osteoarthritis; WOMAC, Western Ontario and McMasters Universities Arthritis Index.

* Using ANOVA (analysis of variance).
[†] Modified to weight joint space narrowing as heavily as osteophytes (see text).

Modified from: Case JP, et al. *Arch Intern Med.* 2003;163:174.

ascertaining whether synovitis predicts a better response to an NSAID than to a simple analgesic. Given the differences between ACET and NSAIDs with respect to safety and cost, the question is important. Clearly, some patients with OA find an NSAID more efficacious than ACET. It is impossible to predict, however, *which* OA patient will do better with an NSAID than with ACET.

The above results should not have been unanticipated. Previous evidence had indicated that ibuprofen, in a daily dose of only 1200 mg (which, as noted earlier, provides minimal anti-inflammatory effect),[9] was as effective as several other NSAIDs, including the very potent anti-inflammatory drug phenylbutazone, in relieving joint pain in patients with OA, even when the others were given in anti-inflammatory doses.[10,11]

In further support of the evidence suggesting that an analgesic may be as effective as an anti-inflammatory dose of an NSAID in symptomatic treatment of OA, in a double-blind crossover study of patients with OA, pain scores and the duration of inactivity stiffness were no better after treatment with the NSAID ketoprofen than with an ACET-propoxyphene analgesic preparation.[12] Furthermore, the daily dose of ACET in that study was only about half as great as that in the study by Bradley and associates.[1] Similarly, few differences were noted between patients with knee OA who were treated with diclofenac for 2 years and those treated with matching placebo.[13]

Does Greater Severity of OA Pain Predict a Better Response to an NSAID Than to ACET?

In a retrospective analysis by Bradley and colleagues,[14] severity of joint pain at baseline did not predict a better response to an NSAID than to ACET. However, a *post hoc* analysis of the results of a clinical trial comparing ACET with a diclofenac/misoprostol formulation suggested that although the difference in efficacy between the NSAID and ACET was negligible in patients with mild symptoms, the NSAID was more efficacious than ACET in those with more severe OA pain.[15]

Felson[16] has suggested that the failure of the earlier trials to demonstrate a difference in efficacy between ACET and an NSAID may have been due, in part, to relatively small sample sizes and the modest effect of the treatments. He concluded that this study[15] and a multicenter clinical trial with similar findings[17] supported the recommendation that an NSAID merits consideration as first-line therapy in patients with more severe OA pain. The latter study, which has been presented only as an abstract, was a 6-day trial in which an analgesic dose of ibuprofen (1200 mg/d) was statistically superior to ACET 4000 mg/d in subjects with knee OA who had moderately severe to severe knee pain at baseline, but not in those with mild to moderate pain. The brief duration of this study,[17] however, imbues it with features of an acute pain model, in which pharmaco-dynamic and pharmacokinetic differences between analge-sics may be accentuated. The relevance of the results to management of the chronic pain of OA is questionable. Pro-spective data from clinical trials in which patients are strati-fied at the outset on the basis of pain severity and ran-domized to treatment with an NSAID vs ACET are needed.

For the reasons stated above and because of concern about serious adverse effects of NSAIDs, recent American College of Rheumatology guidelines for management of OA[18-20] have recommended ACET (up to 4000 mg/d) as the initial drug of choice for symptomatic treatment of OA. Similarly, European League Against Rheumatism guidelines for management of knee OA state: "paracetamol (ie, ACET) is the oral analgesic to try first and, if successful, is the preferred long-term oral analgesic."[21] Guidelines of the American Geriatric Society for management of chronic pain in older persons similarly conclude: "For most patients with mild to moderate pain from degenerative joint disease (ie, OA), ACET provides satisfactory pain relief with a much lower risk of side effects than with NSAID drugs."[22]

Mechanism of Action of ACET

The mechanism of action of ACET is unknown, but the prevailing evidence suggests it involves a central com-ponent. Several possible actions have been proposed on the basis of *in vitro* studies. The merits of these claims are still being evaluated.

The oldest proposal is that ACET inhibits cyclooxygenase (COX)-1 in the central nervous system (rather than in the periphery).[23] Another suggestion is that ACET inhibits a specific type of COX-2 activity, such as that present in murine J774.2 (transformed monocyte/macrophage) cells undergoing NSAID-induced apoptosis.[24] However, the activity of this COX-2 variant is highly cell-specific, since it is not prominent in J774.1 cells and is essentially absent in A549 cells.[24]

Recently, another form of COX (ie, COX-3) has been identified, and the suggestion has been made that it may be the target on which ACET acts to exert its analgesic and antipyretic effect.[25] COX-3 is the product of the COX-1 gene and appears to be a distinct isoenzyme. In human tissues, expression of COX-3 appears to be greatest in heart and brain. Notably, COX-3 is considerably more sensitive to inhibition by ACET than either COX-1 or COX-2, tempting speculation that inhibition of COX-3 in the central nervous system may explain the mechanism of action of ACET as an analgesic and antipyretic.

COX-3 is susceptible also to inhibition by nonselective NSAIDs (eg, aspirin, diclofenac, ibuprofen, indomethacin) and is much more susceptible to inhibition by them than by ACET. However, the *differential* sensitivity of COX-3 to inhibition by ACET, relative to COX-1 and COX-2, suggests the possibility that highly selective COX-3 inhibitors could be developed.

An implication of the above study is that a number of COX isoenzymes could be derived from the two COX genes, providing a continuum of enzymes and products. As suggested by Warner and Mitchell,[26] these early findings raise the interesting possibility that the clinical observation that individual patients appear to benefit from different NSAIDs is due to the fact that these drugs inhibit different variants of COX to different degrees.

Some reports suggesting that receptor mechanisms are involved in the mechanism of action of ACET[27,28] relate to recent work by Raffa and associates[29,30] demonstrating spinal-supraspinal self-synergy of ACET. These studies involved administration of ACET to mice by three different routes: directly into the brain (intracerebroventricular), directly into the spinal cord (intrathecal), or into brain and spinal cord simultaneously,[29] following which antinociception (analgesia) was assessed using a standard abdominal constriction test in which a chemical irritant (acetylcholine) was injected into the peritoneum. Inhibition of the behavioral response was equated with antinociception.

Administration of ACET only into the brain produced minimal antinociception, while administration of ACET only into the spinal cord produced dose-related antinociception, but only to about 60% of the maximum effect. In contrast, administration of ACET simultaneously into brain and spinal cord produced a dose-related and full analgesic effect. The dose-response curve for combined administration fell to the left of the single-site dose-response curves (**Figure 10.1**), reflecting enhancement of the antinociceptive effect. Mathematical analysis revealed a significant synergistic analgesic interaction between spinal and supraspinal administration. These findings and subsequent work[30] suggest that ACET has a direct action at the level of the spinal cord and also stimulates a supraspinal system that releases neurotransmitters that are active at the level of the spinal cord.

Adverse Effects of ACET

■ Hepatotoxicity

Adverse effects of ACET are uncommon and generally mild. Although in the case of overdose, ACET can cause hepatotoxicity and even acute hepatic necrosis with fulminant hepatic failure, this has generally been seen with daily doses exceeding 10 g, ie, 2.5 times the maximum recommended therapeutic dose for adults.[31]

The possibility that a genetic basis for ACET-induced hepatotoxicity exists is provided by the recent study by Zhang and colleagues,[32] who identified the xenobiotic (constitutive androstane receptor [CAR]) as a key regulator of ACET metabolism and hepatotoxicity. Known activators of the receptor and high doses of ACET induced expression of ACET-metabolizing enzymes in wild-type but not in CAR-null mice, which were resistant to ACET hepatotoxicity. Inhibition of CAR activity by administration of

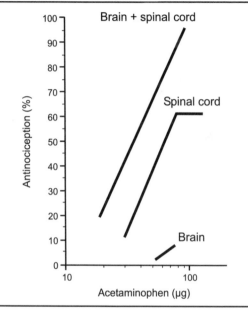

FIGURE 10.1 — ANTINOCICEPTION PRODUCED IN MICE BY ADMINISTRATION OF ACETAMINOPHEN INTO THE SPINAL CORD, BRAIN, OR BOTH SIMULTANEOUSLY

Combined administration produced a synergistic antinociceptive effect (self-synergy).

Modified from: Raffa RB, et al. *J Pharmacol Exp Ther*. 2000;295:291-294.

the inverse agonist ligand, androstanol, after administration of ACET blocked hepatotoxicity in wild-type but not in CAR-null mice. It is possible that an inverse agonist for human CAR could provide a novel approach to treatment of ACET hepatotoxicity.

The toxicity of *N*-acetyl-p-benzoquinoneimine (NAPQI) is due to its covalent binding to cellular macromolecules, which results in the generation of reactive oxygen species.[33,34] At subtoxic doses, NAPQI is inactivated by glutathione S-transferases (GSTs) through conjugation with reduced glutathione (GSH). However, when GSH levels are depleted, NAPQI accumulates. The GSTPi isoforms of the GSTs are particularly effective in inactivating NAPQI. Knockout mice that lack both GSTPi isoforms have been shown to be relatively resistant to ACET hepatotoxicity because of a decreased rate of GSH depletion.[35]

Alcohol and ACET Hepatotoxicity

A chronic high intake of alcohol appears to increase the risk of liver toxicity from ACET when the recommended dose has been exceeded. Regular consumption of alcohol lowers the threshold for ACET-induced liver damage by inducing the enzymes that catalyze metabolism of the drug, leading to an increase in concentration of the toxic metabolite NAPQI (**Figure 10.2**).

Furthermore, in alcoholics, stores of glutathione, to which NAPQI is conjugated, may be depleted.[36] The syndrome is characterized by a striking elevation of the serum aspartate aminotransferase (AST) level and a fatality rate of approximately 20%.[37]

Although fatal hepatic injury has been documented in patients reported to drink only moderate amounts of alcohol and to use ACET only in recommended doses, the accuracy of reports of the level of alcohol intake in such cases is often highly uncertain and the dose of ACET underestimated, as judged by extrapolation of the serum concentration measured when treatment is initiated. In an analysis of cases from a registry of drug-induced hepatic injury and review of the literature, Zimmerman and Maddrey[37] found that among 261 cases of liver damage in patients taking ACET with therapeutic intent, only 8% had an alcohol intake <6 g/d (equivalent to four glasses of wine, a six-pack of beer, or three mixed drinks containing hard liquor). Kuffner and colleagues[38] found no difference between mean serum AST, alanine aminotransferase (ALT), or international normalized ratio (INR) levels in alcoholics treated with ACET, 4 g/d for 2 consecutive days, and those treated with placebo. Nonetheless, it is prudent to discourage regular use of any analgesic in patients who consume alcohol regularly and to encourage use of the lowest possible dose of analgesics by those who use them regularly.[36]

In a recent study evaluating the association of alcohol use and of fasting with ACET hepatotoxicity, 49 patients

FIGURE 10.2 — PATHWAYS FOR METABOLISM OF ACETAMINOPHEN

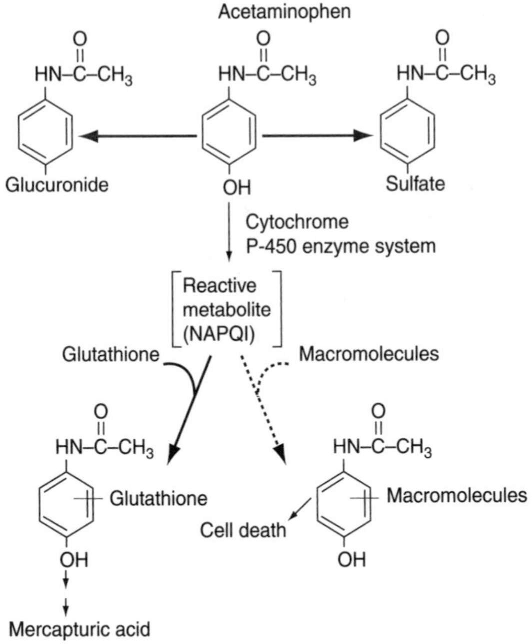

While most of the drug is conjugated with glucuronide or sulfate in the liver, some is metabolized through the cytochrome P-450 enzyme system, producing the highly reactive metabolite *N*-acetyl-p-benzoquinoneimine (NAPQI). In the presence of adequate stores of glutathione, a harmless metabolite is produced. However, if NAPQI concentrations are increased or a relative deficiency of glutathione exists, NAPQI interacts with intracellular macromolecules, resulting in cell damage and death. Glucuronidation may be impaired by glycogen depletion (eg, in starvation), diverting more metabolism along the potentially toxic P-450 pathway. Glutathione stores may be decreased by alcoholism.

with ACET hepatotoxicity (defined as an AST concentration >1,000 U/L) were identified, 21 of whom had ingested the drug for therapeutic purposes.[39] All patients with hepatotoxicity took more than the recommended limit of 4 g/d. Among those who developed hepatotoxicity after an ACET dose of 4 to 10 g/d, recent fasting was more common than alcohol use, while alcohol use was more common in those who took more than 10 g/d for therapeutic purposes. However, this study has two significant limitations: First, because it was not hospital based, it was dependent on accurate reporting of ACET ingestion and alcohol use by the patient or a family member. Second, it required that the terms "hepatotoxicity" and "ACET" or a similar expression be dictated into the medical record. Although a prospective study would overcome some of these disadvantages, the rarity of hepatotoxicity due to ingestion of ACET for therapeutic reasons would make a prospective clinical trial extremely difficult.

An editorial that accompanied the above article concluded that, even in alcoholics and fasting patients "ACET remains the over-the-counter analgesic of choice. If such patients were to switch from ACET to a salicylate or (other) NSAID, the number of cases of ACET-induced hepatotoxicity prevented would be dwarfed by the number of excess deaths from gastrointestinal (GI) bleeding."[40]

■ Renal Disease

Few reports exist of ACET-induced renal disease, presumably because of the absence of peripheral inhibition of prostaglandin synthesis. Acute ACET nephrotoxicity has been documented only with overdoses,[41,42] when it is most often secondary to acute hepatic failure.[43,44] A case-control study showed no association between analgesic use and end-stage renal disease.[45] Sandler and associates, however, have suggested that chronic ingestion of ACET increases the risk of chronic renal disease.[46] Among daily users of ACET, this increased risk was reflected by an odds ratio of 3:2. However, methodologic flaws (eg, in patient selection and disproportionate use of proxies to obtain histories of analgesic abuse from patients, in comparison with controls) severely limit the conclusions that can be drawn from that study.[47]

In a case-control study of the use of over-the-counter (OTC) analgesics as a risk factor for end-stage renal disease, Perneger and colleagues[48] concluded that average use of ACET in quantities greater than one pill per day and medium-to-high cumulative ACET intake (more than 1,000 pills in a lifetime) both doubled the odds of end-stage renal disease. In contrast, no association was found with aspirin use. However, as noted in an editorial accompanying the above article,[49] because the drugs under study were OTC medications, an epidemiologic study could not match prescription records with records of morbidity and mortality. Furthermore, the telephone sampling method used in the study was limited by the interviewers' lack of assurance of the accuracy of information about the extent of drug exposure, the diagnosis of underlying kidney disease, and the absence of renal insufficiency in the controls. Also, case-control studies are subject to recall bias (ie, better recall of drug intake by patients than by controls because of repeated earlier interrogation of patients about drug-consumption habits). Finally, analysis of ACET use in the above study was not confined to the period surrounding the onset of renal disease. Rather, the date of initiation of chronic dialysis was chosen as the index date, with no evidence that exposure to ACET preceded the onset of renal failure. This presents a significant problem because analgesic drugs may have been taken to relieve symptoms caused by, rather than resulting from, the renal disease bias (see comment below on protopathic bias).

Recently, Fored and associates[50] published the results of a nationwide, population-based case-control study of early-stage chronic renal failure (CRF) in Sweden and concluded that their findings were "...consistent with the existence of exacerbating effects of ACET and aspirin on CRF." The authors acknowledged, however, that they were unable to rule out the possibility of bias due to the triggering of analgesic use by predisposing conditions. Their record review, which was supplemented by face-to-face interviews of 926 patients and 998 controls, indicated that regular use of analgesics was twice as common in subjects with CRF as in the controls. The relative risk of CRF appeared to be similar between regular users of ACET and of aspirin.

This paper highlights the problem of differentiating an *association* between ACET use and a clinical outcome from *causality* and exemplifies the problems of confounding by indication and protopathic bias. Several points should be noted:

- The distribution of underlying diseases leading to CRF (eg, diabetic nephropathy, glomerulonephritis) among chronic users of ACET or aspirin was similar to that among nonusers. Subjects with CRF were much more likely than controls to report the onset of pain within 5 years of the interview, and about 50% of the cases, but only 29% of the controls, had begun regular analgesic use within the previous 5 years. Thus, in many instances, subjects with CRF were likely taking analgesics for prodromal symptoms of the renal disease that predisposed them to CRF (protopathic bias).

- With respect to confounding by indication (or contraindication), because of the well-recognized adverse effects of NSAIDs on renal hemodynamics and salt and water homeostasis—especially in subjects with intrinsic renal disease— there is high likelihood that when such patients require an analgesic, physicians are likely to recommend ACET and to proscribe the use of NSAIDs.

- Although a variety of OTC analgesics other than ACET are available, including aspirin, ibuprofen, and naproxen, physicians commonly counsel patients with renal insufficiency to avoid aspirin and other NSAIDs because of the risks of bleeding and changes in renal hemodynamics caused by inhibition of prostaglandin synthesis. Therefore, use of ACET as an analgesic is far greater than that of NSAIDs in patients with renal insufficiency and some association between ACET use and end-stage renal disease is to be expected. However, for the reasons cited above, the above study does not establish ACET as a significant cause of end-stage renal disease.

Although Perneger and colleagues[48] suggested that aspirin be used as an alternative to ACET in patients with renal disease who require an analgesic, the data do not support that recommendation. The rate of complications related to effects of aspirin on platelets, the GI mucosa, and renal blood flow would be substantial. Although ingestion of large quantities of ACET should be discouraged, caution is required in recommending restriction of modest doses, which might induce habitual ACET users to change to other medications, such as NSAIDs, whose safety is more questionable than that of ACET. Indeed, it must be considered that ACET is the OTC analgesic of choice for patients with renal disease. This view is consistent with recommendations expressed in a National Kidney Foundation position paper: "ACET remains the non-narcotic analgesic of choice for episodic use in patients with underlying renal disease" but "habitual consumption of ACET should be discouraged [and when] indicated medically, long-term use of this drug should be supervised by a physician."[51] It is important to bear in mind that a variety of nonpharmacologic measures may be effective in diminishing joint pain in OA (see Chapter 9, *Nonmedicinal Therapy for OA Pain*), reducing the need for analgesics and permitting use of a lower dose when an analgesic is required.

10

■ **ACET and Upper GI Ulcers**

Although two recent reports have raised a question about the risks of upper GI bleeding,[52,53] a previous meta-analysis by Lewis and colleagues[54] showed no increase in the incidence of GI bleeding among ACET users across a range of countries, regardless of dose (**Figure 10.3**). Although the frequency of dyspepsia and/or other minor non-specific GI complaints has been reported to be higher in subjects treated with ACET than in the placebo group,[55,56] an increase in the rate of serious GI adverse events has not been noted previously. For example, in a case-control study of the use of OTC NSAIDs and ACET in more than 600 patients enrolled in the American College of Gastroenterology GI Bleeding Registry and a similar number of procedure-matched controls,[57] the risk of GI bleeding was increased 2- to 3-fold among recent users of aspirin and other NSAIDs, but no excess risk was seen among those who used ACET. Other epidemiologic studies[58-62] had similarly provided estimates ranging from 0.2-1.9 (mean = 1.4, 95% CI = 1.0-2.0) for the relative risk (RR) of upper GI com-

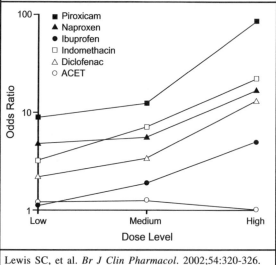

Lewis SC, et al. *Br J Clin Pharmacol.* 2002;54:320-326.

plications associated with use of ACET in any dose. Only one of these studies reported an increased risk of upper GI complications with ACET doses >1 g/d (RR = 2.6).[61]

In view of the above, it was surprising that García Rodríguez and Hernández-Díaz[52] recently concluded that ACET intake >2 g/d results in a greater relative risk of an upper GI complication than a low/medium dose of NSAID. This conclusion was reached from an analysis of the population-based United Kingdom General Practice Research Database, in which physicians store diagnoses and prescription records. However, it may not be clear from this database whether a diagnosis (eg, gastritis) preceded or followed prescription of ACET. Thus analysis of the data was confounded by a lack of adequate knowledge of the condition for which ACET was prescribed. Furthermore, although a number of risk factors for an upper GI bleed are recognized even among individuals who do not take ACET, the above report does not take into account the severity of underlying illness. The point is important: sicker patients are more likely to receive ACET than an alternative analgesic and comorbidity (eg, coronary artery disease, which frequently leads to use of low-dose aspirin) increases the risk of an upper GI complication. The bias inherent in this approach is obvious; as indicated above, ACET is likely to be prescribed preferentially for patients who would be at high risk for adverse effects if treated with the most common alternative analgesics (ie, aspirin or other NSAIDs).

Notably, the authors suggested that the increased incidence of upper GI complications observed with high doses of ACET may have been due to inhibition of prostaglandin synthesis.[52] However, Cryer and Feldman[63] found that clinically relevant concentrations of neither celecoxib, rofecoxib, nor ACET inhibited cyclooxygenase (COX)-1 synthesis by gastric mucosa *ex vivo*, whereas naproxen 100 μm produced inhibition >90%.

In the other paper linking ACET use to upper GI complications, Rahme and associates[53] found that subjects at higher risk (eg, older subjects, regular aspirin users, patients taking warfarin) were more likely to be taking ACET than alternative analgesics. In addition, two thirds of the subjects who experienced an upper GI complication while taking ACET had been taking the drug for <14 days. Therefore, if they had a preexisting ulcer due to, eg, *Helicobacter pylori* or recent NSAID use, their upper GI bleeding may have been due to that cause rather than to recent-onset ACET use.

It is important to note that Rahme and colleagues[53] defined the incidence of upper GI events by either dyspepsia, hospitalization for a GI complication, or a diagnosis of ulcer because after adjustment for risk susceptibility, *dyspepsia*—not ulcers, ulcer complications, or hospitalization—was chiefly responsible for the observed increase in GI toxicity attributed to ACET. Furthermore, dyspepsia was more prevalent in NSAID users than in ACET users, likely explaining the 4-fold greater use of gastroprotective agents (eg, proton pump inhibitors) in the former group, which may have decreased the risk of an upper GI bleed in NSAID users.

Thus this study was confounded by the greater incidence of risk factors in ACET users than in controls, ie, subjects who bled were likely to have had a greater incidence of GI bleeding even if they had not used ACET. In summary, the conclusion reached in both of these recent studies[52,53] (that ACET use increases the risk of an upper GI complication) must be viewed with considerable caution, insofar as both were confounded by indication and by inherent biases in the patient populations studied.

Rahme and colleagues[53] recognized the inevitability of confounding by indication in observational studies such as this, ie, that ACET use was a surrogate for greater risk of upper GI complications from NSAID use and acknowledged that their effort to control for known risk factors for upper GI complications would not have eliminated such bias. Furthermore, they recognized that their use of a computerized prescription database may have resulted in underascertainment of OTC drug use. Wilcox and colleagues[64] have emphasized that upper GI bleeding may be more common with OTC use of aspirin than with prescription doses.

The possibility has been suggested that higher doses of ACET may inhibit COX-1 in the gastric lining. However, Cryer and Feldman[63] recently reported preliminary data from a study in which they measured gastric COX activity in endoscopically obtained biopsies of gastric mucosa from 20 healthy humans who had not been recently exposed to NSAIDs. The biopsies were incubated *ex vivo* with celecoxib, rofecoxib, naproxen, or ACET. Naproxen 100 μm, inhibited gastric COX-1 synthesis >90%, while ACET had no effect at any drug concentration tested. These data, therefore, do not support the contention that inhibition of gastric COX-1 by ACET accounts for the results of the database analysis noted above.[65]

■ Interaction of ACET With Warfarin

The anticoagulant effect of warfarin can be potentiated by ACET in a dose-dependent fashion. For patients who reported taking the equivalent of at least four regular-strength (325-mg) tablets per day for longer than 1 week, the odds of having an international normalized ratio (INR) >6.0 were increased 10-fold relative to those for subjects not taking ACET. The risk decreased with a lower intake of ACET and reached the background level of risk with six or fewer 325-mg tablets per week.[66]

Although ACET is generally preferred to NSAIDs as an analgesic because it does not inhibit platelet function or increase the risk of gastric mucosal damage, these data should lead physicians to counsel their patients who are taking warfarin about the use of ACET. INR levels should be monitored closely in patients taking warfarin who also require a sustained high dose of ACET.

The above caution notwithstanding, the risk of bleeding appears to be much lower with ACET than that in patients taking a nonselective NSAID or coxib, making ACET the nonopioid analgesic of choice in such cases. Reports of clinically important bleeding with prolongation of the INR related to use of ACET by patients taking warfarin are rare; on the other hand, it is well established that use of aspirin, other nonselective NSAIDs, or coxibs by patients taking warfarin can be associated with serious bleeding. The package inserts for both celecoxib and rofecoxib caution against their use in patients taking warfarin.

Notably, whereas Cryer and Feldman[67] found that a clinically relevant dose of ACET does not affect COX-1 activity in the gastric mucosa, Catella-Lawson and associates[68] found that administration of a single 1000-mg dose of ACET inhibited serum thromboxane B_2 levels by 44 ± 14%, indicating some effect of ACET on COX-1 *in the platelet*. However, this degree of inhibition of COX is too low to inhibit platelet aggregation—an effect not seen until thromboxane inhibition reaches a level of about 95%. Notably, in these studies ACET also inhibited COX-2 activity *ex vivo*; a single oral dose of 1000 mg produced 53 ± 8% inhibition of lipopolysaccharide-stimulated prostaglandin E_2 (PGE_2) levels in a whole-blood assay 2 hours after dosing. Thus these data indicate that ACET is a weak, reversible, isoform-nonspecific COX inhibitor. The lack of effect of ACET on *gastric* COX-1 while it modestly inhibited *platelet* COX-1 raises the possibility that thromboxane generation by the platelet is mediated, at least in part, not by COX-1 but by a COX-1 variant (?COX-3) (see above).

In any case, the results of Catella-Lawson and colleagues[68] indicate also that although ibuprofen competitively inhibits access of aspirin to the acetylation site in platelet COX-1, no such effect is seen with ACET.

REFERENCES

1. Bradley JD, Brandt KD, Katz BP, Kalasinski LA, Ryan SI. Comparison of an antiinflammatory dose of ibuprofen, an analgesic dose of ibuprofen, and acetaminophen in the treatment of patients with osteoarthritis of the knee. *N Engl J Med*. 1991;325:87-91.

2. Amadio P Jr, Cummings DM. Evaluation of acetaminophen in the management of osteoarthritis of the knee. *Curr Ther Res*. 1983; 34:59-66.

3. Case JP, Baliunas AJ, Block JA. Lack of efficacy of acetaminophen in treating symptomatic knee osteoarthritis: a randomized, double-blind, placebo-controlled comparison trial with diclofenac sodium. *Arch Intern Med*. 2003;163:169-178.

4. Felson DT, Zhang Y, Hannan MT, et al. The incidence and natural history of knee osteoarthritis in the elderly. The Framingham Osteoarthritis Study. *Arthritis Rheum*. 1995;38:1500-1505.

5. Adams JG, McAlindon T, Dimasi M, Carey J, Eustace S. Contribution of meniscal extrusion and cartilage loss to joint space narrowing in osteoarthritis. *Clin Radiol*. 1999;54:502-506.

6. Mazzuca SA, Brandt KD, Lane KA, Katz BP. Knee pain reduces joint space width in conventional standing anteroposterior radiographs of osteoarthritic knees. *Arthritis Rheum*. 2002;46:1223-1227.

7. Bradley JD, Brandt KD, Katz BP, Kalasinski LA, Ryan SI. Treatment of knee osteoarthritis: relationship of clinical features of joint inflammation to the response to a nonsteroidal antiinflammatory drug or pure analgesic. *J Rheumatol*. 1992;19:1950-1954.

8. Hugenberg ST, Myers SL, Brandt KD, et al. Synovitis does not predict response to nonsteroidal anti-inflammatory drug therapy in knee osteoarthritis. *Arthritis Rheum*. 1991;34:S84.

9. Huskisson EC, Hart FD, Shenfield GM, Taylor RT. Ibuprofen. A review. *Practitioner*. 1971;207:639-643.

10. Cimmino MA, Cutolo M, Samantà E, Accardo S. Short-term treatment of osteoarthritis: a comparison of sodium meclofenamate and ibuprofen. *J Int Med Res*. 1982;10:46-52.

11. Moxley TE, Royer GL, Hearron MS, Donovan JF, Levi L. Ibuprofen versus buffered phenylbutazone in the treatment of osteoarthritis: double blind trial. *J Am Geriatr Soc*. 1975;23:343-349.

12. Doyle DV, Dieppe PA, Scott J, Huskisson EC. An articular index for the assessment of osteoarthritis. *Ann Rheum Dis*. 1981;40:75-78.

13. Dieppe P, Cushnaghan J, Jasani MK, McCrae F, Watt I. A two-year, placebo-controlled trial of non-steroidal anti-inflammatory therapy in osteoarthritis of the knee joint. *Br J Rheumatol*. 1993;32:595-600.

14. Bradley JD, Katz BP, Brandt KD. Severity of knee pain does not predict a better response to an antiinflammatory dose of ibuprofen than to analgesic therapy in patients with osteoarthritis. *J Rheumatol*. 2001;28:1073-1076.

15. Pincus T, Koch GG, Sokka T, et al. A randomized, double-blind, crossover clinical trial of diclofenac plus misoprostol versus acetaminophen in patients with osteoarthritis of the hip or knee. *Arthritis Rheum*. 2000;44:1587-1598.

16. Felson DT. The verdict favors nonsteroidal antiinflammatory drugs for treatment of osteoarthritis and a plea for more evidence on other treatments. *Arthritis Rheum*. 2001;44:1477-1480.

17. Altman RD. The IAP Study Group. Ibuprofen, acetaminophen and placebo in osteoarthritis of the knee: a six-day double-blind study. *Arthritis Rheum*. 1999;42(suppl 9):S403. Abstract.

18. Hochberg MC, Altman RD, Brandt KD, et al. Guidelines for the medical management of osteoarthritis: Part I. Osteoarthritis of the hip. American College of Rheumatology. *Arthritis Rheum*. 1995;38:1535-1540.

19. Hochberg MC, Altman RD, Brandt KD, et al. Guidelines for the medical management of osteoarthritis: Part II. Osteoarthritis of the knee. American College of Rheumatology. *Arthritis Rheum*. 1995; 38:1541-1546.

20. American College of Rheumatology Subcommittee on Osteoarthritis Guidelines. Recommendations for the medical management of osteoarthritis of the hip and knee: 2000 update. *Arthritis Rheum*. 2000;43:1905-1915.

21. Pendleton A, Arden N, Dougados M, et al. EULAR recommendations for the management of knee osteoarthritis: report of a task force of the Standing Committee for International Clinical Studies Including Therapeutic Trials (ESCISIT). *Ann Rheum Dis*. 2000;59:936-944.

22. American Geriatrics Society Panel on Chronic Pain in Older Persons. The management of chronic pain in older persons: AGS Panel on Chronic Pain in Older Persons. American Geriatrics Society. *J Am Geriatr Soc*. 1998;46:635-651.

23. Flower RJ, Vane JR. Inhibition of prostaglandin synthetase in brain explains the anti-pyretic activity of paracetamol (4-acetamidophenol). *Nature*. 1972;240:410-411.

24. Simmons DL, Botting RM, Robertson PM, Madsen ML, Vane JR. Induction of an acetaminophen-sensitive cyclooxygenase with reduced sensitivity to nonsteroid antiinflammatory drugs. *Proc Natl Acad Sci (USA)*. 1999;96:3275-3280.

25. Chandrasekharan NV, Dai H, Roos KL, et al. COX-3, a cyclooxygenase-1 variant inhibited by acetaminophen and other analgesic/antipyretic drugs: cloning, structure, and expression. *Proc Natl Acad Sci (USA)*. 2002;99:13926-13931.

26. Warner TD, Mithcell JA. Cyclooxygenase-3 (COX-3): filling in the gaps toward a COX continuum? *Proc Natl Acad Sci (USA)*. 2002;99:13371-13373.

27. Pelissier T, Alloui A, Paeile C, Eschalier A. Evidence of a central antinociceptive effect of paracetamol involving spinal 5-HT$_3$ receptors. *Neuroreport*. 1995;6:1546-1548.

28. Pelissier T, Alloui A, Caussade F, et al. Paracetamol exerts a spinal antinociceptive effect involving an indirect interaction with 5-hydroxytryptamine$_3$ receptors: in vivo and in vitro evidence. *J Pharmacol Exp Ther*. 1996;278:8-14.

29. Raffa RB, Stone DJ Jr, Tallarida RJ. Discovery of "self-synergistic" spinal/supraspinal antinociception produced by acetaminophen (paracetamol). *J Pharmacol Exp Ther*. 2000;295:291-294.

30. Raffa RB, Stone DJ Jr, Tallarida RJ. Unexpected and pronounced antinociceptive synergy between spinal acetaminophen (paracetamol) and phentolamine. *Eur J Pharmacol*. 2001;412:R1-R2.

31. Farrell GC. The hepatic side-effects of drugs. *Med J Aust*. 1986;145:600-604.

32. Zhang J, Huang W, Chua SS, Wei P, Moore DD. Modulation of acetaminophen-induced hepatotoxicity by the xenobiotic receptor CAR. *Science*. 2002;298:422-424.

33. Rogers LK, Moorthy B, Smith CV. Acetaminophen binds to mouse hepatic and renal DNA at human therapeutic doses. *Chem Res Toxicol*. 1997;10:470-476.

34. Lores Arnaiz S, Llesuy S, Cutrín JC, Boveris A. Oxidative stress by acute acetaminophen administration in mouse liver. *Free Radic Biol Med*. 1995;19:303-310.

35. Henderson CJ, Wolf CR, Kitteringham N, Powell H, Otto D, Park BK. Increased resistance to acetaminophen hepatotoxicity in mice lacking glutathione S-transferase Pi. *Proc Natl Acad Sci (USA)*. 2000;97:12741-12745.

36. Acetaminophen, NSAIDS and alcohol. *Med Lett Drugs Ther*. 1996;38:55-56.

37. Zimmerman HJ, Maddrey WC. Acetaminophen (paracetamol) hepato-toxicity with regular intake of alcohol: analysis of instances of thera-peutic misadventure. *Hepatology*. 1995;22:767-773.

38. Kuffner EK, Dart RC, Bogdan GM, Hill RE, Casper E, Darton L. Ef-fect of maximal daily doses of acetaminophen on the liver of alco-holic patients: a randomized, double-blind, placebo-controlled trial. *Arch Intern Med*. 2001;161:2247-2252.

39. Whitcomb DC, Block GD. Association of acetaminophen hepatotox-icity with fasting and ethanol use. *JAMA*. 1994;272:1845-1850.

40. Strom BL. Adverse reactions to over-the-counter analgesics taken for therapeutic purposes. *JAMA*. 1994;272:1866-1867.

41. Kincaid-Smith P. Effects of non-narcotic analgesics on the kidney. *Drugs*. 1986;32(suppl 4):109-128.

42. Jones AF, Vale JA. Paracetamol poisoning and the kidney. *J Clin Pharm Ther*. 1993;18:5-8.

43. Kaysen GA, Pond SM, Roper MH, Menke DJ, Marrama MA. Com-bined hepatic and renal injury in alcoholics during therapeutic use of acetaminophen. *Arch Intern Med*. 1985;145:2019-2023.

44. Kritharides L, Fassett R, Singh B. Paracetamol-associated coma, metabolic acidosis, renal and hepatic failure. *Intensive Care Med*. 1988;14:439-440.

45. Murray TG, Stolley PD, Anthony JC, Schinnar R, Hepler-Smith E, Jeffreys JL. Epidemiologic study of regular analgesic use and end-stage renal disease. *Arch Intern Med*. 1983;143:1687-1693.

46. Sandler DP, Smith JC, Weinberg CR, et al. Analgesic use and chronic renal disease. *N Engl J Med*. 1989;320:1238-1243.

47. Analgesic use and chronic renal disease. *N Engl J Med*. 1989; 321:1125-1127. Comment.

48. Perneger TV, Whelton PK, Klag MJ. Risk of kidney failure associ-ated with the use of acetaminophen, aspirin, and nonsteroidal antiin-flammatory drugs. *N Engl J Med*. 1994;331:1675-1679.

49. Ronco PM, Flahault A. Drug-induced end-stage renal disease. *N Engl J Med*. 1994;331:1711-1712.

50. Fored CM, Ejerblad E, Lindblad P, et al. Acetaminophen, aspirin, and chronic renal failure. *N Engl J Med*. 2001;345:1801-1808.

51. Henrich WL, Agodoa LE, Barrett B, et al. Analgesics and the kid-ney: summary and recommendations to the Scientific Advisory Board of the National Kidney Foundation from an Ad Hoc Committee of the National Kidney Foundation. *Am J Kidney Dis*. 1996;27: 162-165.

52. García Rodríguez LA, Hernández-Díaz S. Relative risk of upper gastrointestinal complications among users of acetaminophen and nonsteroidal anti-inflammatory drugs. *Epidemiology.* 2001;12:570-576.

53. Rahme E, Pettitt D, LeLorier J. Determinants and sequelae associated with utilization of acetaminophen versus traditional nonsteroidal antiinflammatory drugs in an elderly population. *Arthritis Rheum.* 2002;46:3046-3054.

54. Lewis SC, Langman MJ, Laporte JR, Matthews JN. Rawlins MD, Wiholm BE. Dose-response relationships between individual nonaspirin nonsteroidal anti-inflammatory drugs (NANSAIDs) and serious upper gastrointestinal bleeding: a meta-analysis based on individual patient data. *Br J Clin Pharmacol.* 2002;54:320-326.

55. Bradley JD, Brandt KD, Katz BP, Kalasinski LA, Ryan SI. Comparison of an antiinflammatory dose of ibuprofen, an analgesic dose of ibuprofen, and acetaminophen in the treatment of patients with osteoarthritis of the knee. *N Engl J Med.* 1991;325:87-91.

56. Le Parc JM, Van Ganse E, Moore N, Wall R, Schneid H, Verriere F. Comparative tolerability of paracetamol, aspirin and ibuprofen for short-term analgesia in patients with musculoskeletal conditions: results in 4291 patients. *Clin Rheumatol.* 2002;21:28-31.

57. Blot WJ, McLaughlin JK. Over the counter non-steroidal anti-inflammatory drugs and risk of gastrointestinal bleeding. *J Epidemiol Biostat.* 2000;5:137-142.

58. Laporte JR, Carné X, Vidal X, Moreno V, Juan J. Upper gastrointestinal bleeding in relation to previous use of analgesics and non-steroidal anti-inflammatory drugs. *Lancet.* 1991;337:85-89.

59. Holvoet J, Terriere L, Van Hee W, Verbist L, Fierens E, Haulekeete ML. Relation of upper gastrointestinal bleeding to non-steroidal anti-inflammatory drugs and aspirin: a case-control study. *Gut.* 1991;32: 730-734.

60. Nobili A, Mosconi P, Franzosi MG, et al. Non-steroidal anti-inflammatory drugs and upper gastrointestinal bleeding: a postmarketing surveillance case-control study. *Pharmacoepidemiol Drug Saf.* 1992;1:65-72.

61. Savage RT, Moller PW, Ballantyne CL, Wells JE. Variation in the risk of peptic ulcer complications with nonsteroidal antiinflammatory drug therapy. *Arthritis Rheum.* 1993;36:84-90.

62. Langman MJ, Weil J, Wainwright P, et al. Risks of bleeding peptic ulcer associated with individual non-steroidal anti-inflammatory drugs. *Lancet.* 1994;343:1075-1078.

63. Cryer B, Feldman M. Comparison of effects of celecoxib, rofecoxib, naproxen and acetaminophen on gastric COX inhibition. *Am J Gastroenterol.* 2002;97(suppl):S57.

64. Wilcox CM, Shalek KA, Cotsonis G. Striking prevalence of over-the-counter nonsteroidal anti-inflammatory drug use in patients with upper gastrointestinal hemorrhage. *Arch Intern Med*. 1994; 154:42-46.

65. García Rodríguez LA, Hernández-Díaz S. Relative risk of upper gastrointestinal complications among users of acetaminophen and nonsteroidal anti-inflammatory drugs. *Epidemiology*. 2001;12:570-576.

66. Hylek EM, Heiman H, Skates SJ, Sheehan MA, Singer DE. Acetaminophen and other risk factors for excessive warfarin anticoagulation. *JAMA*. 1998;279:657-662.

67. Cryer B, Feldman M. Effects of very low dose daily, long-term aspirin therapy on gastric, duodenal, and rectal prostaglandin levels and on mucosal injury in healthy humans. *Gastroenterology*. 1999; 117:17-25.

68. Catella-Lawson F, Reilly MP, Kapoor SC, et al. Cyclooxygenase inhibitors and the antiplatelet effects of aspirin. *N Engl J Med*. 2001;345:1809-1817.

10

11 Nonselective NSAIDS

Nonsteroidal anti-inflammatory drugs (NSAIDs) are analgesic, anti-inflammatory, and antipyretic and have as their predominant mechanism of action the inhibition of prostaglandin biosynthesis. The adverse effects of this class of drugs on, eg, the gastrointestinal (GI) tract, kidney, and platelets are also due to prostaglandin inhibition. As discussed extensively in Chapter 12, *NSAIDs That Are Selective Inhibitors of COX-2*, it is now recognized that two isoforms of cyclooxygenase (COX) exist and that the adverse effects of NSAIDs are due predominantly (although not exclusively) to inhibition of the synthesis of one isoform and the beneficial effects are due to inhibition of synthesis of the other isoform. This chapter deals with nonselective NSAIDs that are not specific inhibitors of either COX isoform but which, in fact, in many instances preferentially inhibit COX-1 relative to COX-2.

Short-Term Efficacy of NSAIDs in OA

Use of NSAIDs has reduced joint pain and improved mobility for millions of people with OA. There is ample evidence that these drugs are superior to placebo for symptomatic treatment of OA.[1-5] However, NSAIDs are only modestly effective in OA; control of symptoms is rarely complete. For example, in many of the studies documenting the superiority of an NSAID over placebo, a visual analog scale (VAS) has been used to quantitate individual changes and mean group changes in pain and/or function. In a representative double-blind study comparing ibuprofen with benoxaprofen,[6] in both treatment groups, the mean level of overall pain derived from a 100-mm VAS, was 55 at baseline and 34 after 4 weeks of treatment—an improvement of about 21%. Other studies documenting the superiority of an NSAID over placebo have typically shown an improvement of about 20% with active treatment, relative to baseline, and a difference between NSAID and placebo of 15% to 20%, with baseline values ranging between 40 and 60 on a VAS scale of 0-100 and post-treatment values ranging from 25 to 45.[3,7,8] Some studies, however, have shown improvement of somewhat greater magnitude.[9-11]

Long-Term Efficacy of NSAIDs in OA

Most clinical trials of NSAID efficacy in OA have been only 1 to 3 months in duration, although many patients with OA take these drugs for years. In a 2-year trial, Dieppe and associates[12] randomized 89 patients who had been taking NSAIDs chronically for knee OA to diclofenac 100 mg daily or placebo. Patients were permitted to take acetaminophen (ACET), up to 4 g/d, as "rescue" medication. Only 57% completed the study. Twenty-seven percent of the placebo group and 7% of the diclofenac group withdrew because of lack of efficacy, primarily within the first 3 months of the trial. Some 30% of the noncompleters were withdrawn because of side effects and 15% because of poor compliance, but there was no significant difference between the two treatment groups in this respect. Among subjects still in the trial at the end of 2 years, 52% of those randomized to diclofenac reported they were better; 16%, the same; and 32%, worse. The respective distributions among those in the placebo group were similar—45%, 25%, and 30%. Those who received placebo consumed an average of ACET 2 g/d, compared to 1.7 g by those given diclofenac.

In another 2-year study, Williams and colleagues[13] randomized 178 patients with knee OA who had not been on long-term NSAID therapy to naproxen 750 mg daily or ACET 2600 mg daily. Only 35% of these patients completed the 2-year trial, 31% of those randomized to ACET and 39% of those in the naproxen group. Withdrawals due to adverse effects were slightly more common among naproxen (23%) than ACET (18%) recipients; however, withdrawals due to lack of efficacy and other reasons were less common in the naproxen group (16% vs 22%; 22% vs 30%, respectively). For those who remained in the trial 2 years, efficacy of both drugs was modest and few differences between the treatment groups were apparent, although naproxen appeared to be slightly more effective.

These trials demonstrate that OA patients find the long-term effectiveness of NSAIDs and ACET far from satisfactory. They also suggest that although NSAIDs are superior to placebo, for many patients they are not clearly superior to ACET, a finding supported also by shorter-term studies.[14] Indeed, the study by Dieppe and associates indicates that a substantial proportion of OA patients receiving chronic NSAID therapy may do as well with withdrawal of their NSAID and use of ACET only as needed.[12] It is not surprising that only about 15% of patients with OA for whom an NSAID is prescribed are still using the same NSAID 12 months later.[15]

Efficacy of Various NSAID Dosing Regimens

Little information is available on NSAID dosing schedules other than daily administration. However, because OA pain may be intermittent or may vary in intensity, other schedules may be more appropriate. In treatment of chronic malignant and nonmalignant pain, it has been recommended that opioid analgesics be administered on a fixed-dosing schedule.[16] However, for most patients with OA it is reasonable to prescribe NSAIDs on an as-needed basis, rather than in a fixed daily dose; pain control may be comparable and toxicity will be lower.[8] Furthermore, an as-needed schedule encourages self-efficacy, permits patients to feel more in control of their symptoms, and emphasizes to the patient that these drugs are useful only for palliation of symptoms and do not treat the underlying arthritis. If this approach is ineffective, the NSAID may then be given in a fixed daily dose. Use of a supplementary analgesic during episodic increases in joint pain, rather than an increase in NSAID dose, should be considered.

Kvien and colleagues[8] compared a standard, fixed-dosing regimen of naproxen (500 mg, 750 mg, or 1000 mg daily, as determined by patient and physician) to a variable-dosing regimen (maximum of 1000 mg daily, with individual doses and timing determined by the patient) in patients with hip or knee OA. Efficacy was similar to that reported in other trials, and no difference was observed between the two groups. However, those assigned to the variable-dose regimen consumed less naproxen (mean daily dose at 8 weeks, 450 mg vs 1335 mg) and had significantly fewer withdrawals due to adverse effects than those on the fixed-dose regimen (12% vs 17%).

In many clinical trials of NSAIDs, patients are permitted to take a supplementary analgesic, most often ACET, but the benefit is seldom evaluated. In a small crossover study in patients with hip OA, Seideman and associates[17] found that naproxen plus ACET was more effective than the same dose of naproxen alone and that the effect of naproxen 500 mg/d combined with ACET 4 g/d is similar to that of 1000 mg naproxen alone.

Thus ACET may be used both as a supplementary analgesic for patients whose OA pain is not adequately controlled by NSAIDs and as NSAID-sparing therapy, permitting reduction in the patient's NSAID dose, thereby reducing the risk of adverse effects and cost of therapy.

Major Adverse Effects of Nonselective NSAIDs

■ **NSAID Gastroenteropathy**

Much of the current ambivalence of physicians with respect to NSAID administration in OA is related to concern about the adverse effects of these agents, especially those related to the GI tract.[18,19] Prospective controlled studies have shown a relative risk of about 1.5 for perforation or hemorrhage of an NSAID-related peptic ulcer[20,21]; in case-control studies, the relative risk has been three to four times higher.[22] Notably, those at greatest risk for OA (ie, the elderly) are also at greatest risk for:

- GI symptoms
- Ulceration
- Hemorrhage
- Death.[23,24]

Among elderly individuals, the annual rate of hospitalization for peptic ulcer disease (PUD) among those currently using a nonselective NSAID is 16/1000—four times greater than that for subjects not taking an NSAID.[25] The risk increases with the dose; the annual hospitalization rate rises from 4/1000 for those who did not use NSAIDs to more than 40/1000 for those using the highest doses. Based on prospective data from the Arthritis, Rheumatism and Aging Medical Information System, the risk of serious GI complications among patients with OA who take an NSAID for 1 year is 7.3 per 1000.[26] It was estimated in 1999 that 16,500 NSAID-related deaths occur annually among patients with rheumatoid arthritis or OA in the United States, a number similar to that of deaths from acquired immune deficiency syndrome and considerably greater than the death toll from multiple myeloma, asthma, cervical cancer, or Hodgkin's disease (**Figure 11.1**).[27] Among people age 65 years and older, as many as 30% of all hospitalizations and deaths related to PUD have been attributed to NSAID use.[22,28,29]

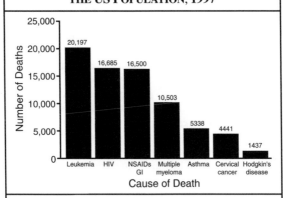

FIGURE 11.1 — NUMBER OF DEATHS ASSOCIATED WITH NSAID-INDUCED GASTROINTESTINAL DAMAGE COMPARED WITH THOSE FROM OTHER CAUSES IN THE US POPULATION, 1997

Abbreviations: GI, gastrointestinal; HIV, human immunodeficiency virus; NSAID, nonsteroidal anti-inflammatory drug; US, United States.

A total of 16,500 patients with rheumatoid arthritis or osteoarthritis died from GI effects of NSAIDs.

Singh G, Triadafilopoulos G. *J Rheumatol*. 1999;26(suppl 56):18-24.

Although dyspepsia is common with NSAID use, it correlates poorly with the presence of endoscopically visualized lesions or clinical episodes of GI bleeding.[30,31] Most patients who incur a serious GI complication from NSAID use have not had prior GI symptoms.[32]

In addition to age and dose, risk factors associated with NSAID-induced peptic ulcer complications include:

- History of prior ulcer, GI hemorrhage, dyspepsia, and/or previous NSAID intolerance[33-35]
- Use of corticosteroids[33,34,36,37]
- Use of anticoagulants[38,39]
- Poor general health (comorbidity)[35,36,40]
- Concomitant use of more than one NSAID
- Alcohol use[41]
- Smoking.[41]

Helicobacter pylori

The relevance of *Helicobacter pylori* infection to NSAID-related gastric ulceration is somewhat unclear. NSAID-induced ulcerations may occur in the absence of *H pylori*.[42] Graham and associates[43] found the prevalence of *H pylori* infection in NSAID users with and without ulcers to be comparable, as was the prevalence of NSAID-induced ulcers in patients with and without *H pylori* infection.[44] However, it has been suggested that a subset of patients with preexisting *H pylori*–induced erosions may be at greater risk for acquiring ulcers with NSAID treatment.[45]

Does eradication of *H pylori* prior to NSAID treatment decrease the risk of ulcer? Chan and colleagues[46] noted that the incidence of ulcers decreased from 26% to 3% if *H pylori* was eradicated prior to institution of NSAID therapy. On the other hand, Hawkey and associates[47] concluded that NSAID ulcers were less likely to recur in the presence of *H pylori*.

H pylori and NSAIDs appear to constitute independent risk factors for ulcers. While the issue remains controversial, the current literature does not unequivocally support the view that *H pylori* infection potentiates the development of either NSAID-associated ulcers or ulcer complications.[48,49]

Concomitant Aspirin Use

With respect to the risk associated with use of anticoagulants, not only warfarin but aspirin—even in the low doses used for cardiovascular prophylaxis—may present problems.

Regardless of the dose or formulation, aspirin increases the risk of gastric mucosal damage, ulcers, and ulcer complications. Virtually all normal subjects will show evidence of gastric mucosal injury after aspirin ingestion.[50] Weil and colleagues[51] reported that the odds ratio for an upper GI adverse event in patients taking daily aspirin was 2.3 with a dose of 75 mg, 3.2 with a dose of 150 mg, and 3.9 with a dose of 300 mg. In a placebo-controlled study of >2000 ulcer-free patients, gastric and duodenal ulcers developed about 10 times more frequently in those who received aspirin 1 g/d than in controls.[52] In a meta-analysis of 21 primary and secondary myocardial infarction (MI) and stroke prevention trials, the Antiplatelet Trialists Collaboration found the risk of significant GI bleeding and hospitalization for ulcer was approximately 2-fold greater in patients treated with aspirin (75–1500 mg/d) than in those receiving placebo.[53]

Because OA affects primarily the elderly (ie, a segment of the population at risk for cardiovascular events, such as MI and stroke) in whom low-dose aspirin prophylaxis for primary and secondary prevention is being utilized with increasing frequency, it is important to recognize that the combination of aspirin and an NSAID is particularly damaging to the gastric mucosa. In a study from Denmark[54] in which the incidence rate ratio of GI bleeding with low-dose aspirin was 2.6, the rate was twice as high among patients who were also taking an NSAID. Notably, in the Celecoxib Long-term Arthritis Safety Study (CLASS)[55] the incidence of upper GI complications, with or without symptomatic ulcers, in aspirin users was no lower in those receiving celecoxib than in those receiving diclofenac or ibuprofen (see Chapter 12, *NSAIDs That Are Selective Inhibitors of COX-2*).

In a study evaluating the long-term effects of very low daily doses of aspirin on the GI tract and on platelet-derived serum thromboxane (TBX) levels in normal volunteers, aspirin 10 mg daily significantly reduced gastric mucosal prostaglandin levels to about 40% of the baseline value and induced significant gastric injury (**Figure 11.2**).[56] A dose of 325 mg/d also resulted in injury to the duodenum. Although a 10-mg dose did not significantly reduce duodenal mucosal prostaglandin levels, 81 mg and 325 mg resulted in reductions to about 40% of the baseline value. Serum TBX levels were inhibited by 62%, 90%, and 98%, with a daily dose of 10 mg, 81 mg, and 325 mg aspirin, respectively. Thus even 10 mg aspirin per day may lead to GI complications.

FIGURE 11.2 — EFFECTS OF ASPIRIN TREATMENT ON ENDOSCOPIC INJURY SCORES IN THE STOMACH, DUODENUM, AND RECTUM

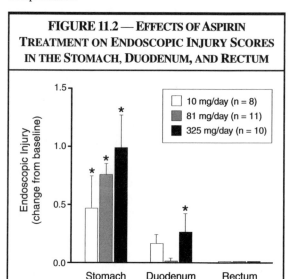

* $P \leq 0.05$ vs baseline by the Wilcoxon's signed rank test.

Effects of aspirin treatment at 10, 81, and 325 mg/day on endoscopic injury scores in the stomach, duodenum, and rectum expressed as change ($\pm$ SEM) from the baseline value. Data obtained after 1.5 months and 3 months were averaged. For the rectum, n = 7 for each aspirin dose. No rectal biopsies were performed at 1.5 months.

Cryer B, Feldman M. *Gastroenterology*. 1999;117:17-25.

Gastric Acid Suppression

Lai and colleagues[57] have examined the role of gastric acid suppression in preventing recurrence of ulcer complications after eradication of *H pylori* in patients taking long-term low-dose aspirin. After elimination of *H pylori* infection by standard treatment, 123 such patients were randomized to treatment with lansoprazole 30 mg/d or placebo, in addition to aspirin 100 mg/d for 12 months. Nine of the 61 patients in the placebo group (14.8%) but only 1 of the 62 in the lansoprazole group (1.6%) had a recurrence of ulcer complications (adjusted hazard ratio, 9.6; 95% CI, $1.2 - 76.1$, $P = 0.008$). Four of these patients had evidence of recurrent *H pylori* infection and two had taken an NSAID before the onset of ulcer complications.

Histamine$_2$ (H$_2$) antagonists reduce the incidence of endoscopically diagnosed NSAID-induced duodenal ulcer.[40] Omeprazole reduced the incidence of NSAID-induced gastric ulcer, and misoprostol, a prostaglandin E$_1$ analogue, reduced the incidence of both.[58,59] That this decrease in endoscopically recognizable ulcers may be accompanied by a decrease in the rate of GI perforation, hemorrhage, and death is suggested by the results of a 6-month, randomized, double-blind, placebo-controlled trial involving nearly 9000 patients with rheumatoid arthritis in which misoprostol reduced the risk of serious upper GI complications of NSAID use by 40% in comparison with placebo.[35] However, it is not clear that the level of NSAID intake throughout the study was comparable in the two treatment groups, and despite the large number of subjects enrolled, the reduction in risk afforded by misoprostol barely reached statistical significance ($P = 0.049$).

The *routine* coprescription of misoprostol with NSAIDs is controversial.[60] Misoprostol is expensive, and as indicated above, efficacy is by no means complete. Furthermore, the drug often does not relieve NSAID-induced dyspepsia, and diarrhea is relatively common with misoprostol.[35,61] Therefore, the daily quality of life of patients taking misoprostol and an NSAID may be worse than that of those taking an NSAID alone.[62] Certainly, for that subgroup of OA patients who are at high risk for ulcer complications and in whom symptomatic benefit from an NSAID is significantly greater than that from a nonacetylated salicylate or an analgesic, it is reasonable to prescribe misoprostol. However, many patients will not tolerate the recommended dose of 200 μg qid. Although a dose of 200 μg bid is better tolerated, it affords significantly less protection from gastric ulcers than the higher dose.[61]

As an alternative to misoprostol, an H_2-receptor antagonist (eg, famotidine) or proton pump inhibitor (eg, omeprazole) may be used. Both have been shown by endoscopy to be effective in treating and preventing NSAID-induced ulcers,[63-65] although the protective effect of neither has been assessed in large-scale clinical trials, as was done with misoprostol. However, in usual doses, H_2-blockers were not as effective as misoprostol in treatment of existing ulcers,[64] whereas omeprazole 20 mg/d or 40 mg/d, was as effective as a 200-μg-bid dose of misoprostol, better tolerated, and associated with a lower relapse rate.[65]

Differences in GI Complication Rates Among Various NSAIDs

Rates of GI complications vary among NSAIDs, but differences between NSAIDs are usually not statistically significant. Whether relative differences in serious toxicity observed among NSAIDs are attributable to differences in the drugs themselves, in the patients taking these drugs, in dosing, or in compliance is unknown. Nonetheless, it is reasonable to attempt to avoid use of those NSAIDs that consistently rank higher than others with respect to serious GI toxicity (eg, piroxicam, ketoprofen, tolmetin),[41] especially when additional risk factors for ulcer disease are present. It is also reasonable, especially in the elderly, to avoid NSAIDs that have other frequent, bothersome side effects, such as indomethacin (central nervous system) and meclofenamate (diarrhea). Endoscopic evidence suggests that nabumetone may have less GI toxicity than other NSAIDs.[59]

Gastrointestinal hemorrhage is associated not only with use of prescription NSAIDs but also with use of over-the-counter (OTC) products.[66] In a recent study of 421 patients who were evaluated for upper GI hemorrhage, use of an OTC aspirin or nonaspirin NSAID during the week prior to admission was reported by 35% and 9%, respectively, while use of a prescription nonaspirin NSAID or aspirin was reported in much lower proportions, 14% and 6%, respectively.

Given the high frequency with which these OTC agents were used (often for nonmedicinal purposes), short-term NSAID use may be a major cause of ulcer-related hemorrhage.

Not only serious and life-threatening adverse GI events, such as perforation, ulceration, and upper GI hemorrhage, but also nonspecific GI adverse events, such as dyspepsia, abdominal pain, and diarrhea, are associated with NSAID use. The latter, even if not life-threatening, are important because they affect compliance with prescribed NSAID dosing, result in the use of additional therapies for treatment of the symptoms, and lead to expensive radiographic and/or endoscopic investigations to rule out the presence of ulcer or malignancy, thereby increasing the cost of managing the disease and, at times, producing additional adverse effects.

Meloxicam

Meloxicam (Mobic), an enolcarboxamide that is structurally related to piroxicam,[13] has been shown to inhibit COX-2 with greater selectivity than many other NSAIDs and to a level similar to that seen with celecoxib (**Table 11**.1).[67-69] It is structurally different from both celecoxib and rofecoxib and may not work by binding to the COX-2 side pocket in the channel of the enzyme but by exploiting the flexibility that exists at the apex of the COX-2 channel, which is greater than that of the COX-1 channel.[70] Clinical trials have suggested that the efficacy of meloxicam is comparable to that of other NSAIDs but that it may be associated with a lower incidence of nonspecific GI adverse events.

In a study involving 8600 patients with symptomatic hand, hip, knee, or spine OA who were treated for 28 days with meloxicam 7.5 mg/d or with piroxicam 20 mg/d (the Safety and Efficacy Large-Scale Evaluation of COX-Inhibitors Therapies [SELECT] trial), efficacy of the two treatments was comparable, while the incidence of adverse events was lower in the meloxicam group (22.5% vs 27.9% in the piroxicam group, P <0.001), chiefly because of a lower incidence of GI adverse events (10.3% vs 15.4%, P <0.001).[71] Dyspepsia, nausea, vomiting, and abdominal pain all were significantly less common with meloxicam (**Figure 11**.3). Furthermore, 16 patients in the piroxicam

11

TABLE 11.1 — CLASSIFICATION OF NSAIDS ACCORDING TO THEIR SELECTIVITY IN INHIBITING COX-1 AND COX-2

NSAID	Ratio*
Flurbiprofen	10.27
Ketoprofen	8.16
Fenoprofen	5.14
Tolmetin	3.93
Aspirin	3.12
Oxaprozin	2.52
Naproxen	1.79
Indomethacin	1.78
Ibuprofen	1.69
Ketorolac	1.64
Piroxicam	0.79
Nabumetone, 6-MNA	0.64
Etodolac	0.11
Celecoxib	0.11
Meloxicam	0.09
Mefenamic acid	0.08
Diclofenac	0.05
Rofecoxib	0.05
Nimesulide	0.04

Abbreviations: COX, cyclooxygenase; NSAID, nonsteroidal anti-inflammatory drug.

* The ratio of the 50% inhibitory concentration (IC_{50}) of cyclooxygenase (COX)-2 to the IC_{50} of COX-1 in whole blood. A ratio <1 indicates selectivity for COX-2.

Feldman M, McMahon AT. *Ann Intern Med*. 2000;132:134-143.

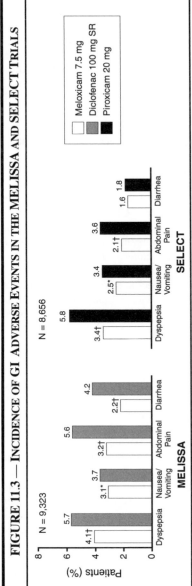

FIGURE 11.3 — INCIDENCE OF GI ADVERSE EVENTS IN THE MELISSA AND SELECT TRIALS

Abbreviations: GI, gastrointestinal; MELISSA, the Meloxicam Large-Scale International Study Safety Assessment [trial]; SELECT, Safety and Efficacy Large-Scale Evaluation of COX-Inhibiting Therapies [trial]; SR, slow release.

* P <0.05 vs comparator.
† P <0.001 vs comparator.

Hawkey C, et al. *Br J Rheumatol.* 1998;37:937-945; and Dequeker J, et al. *Br J Rheumatol.* 1998;37:946-951.

group, but only seven in the meloxicam group, incurred an upper GI perforation, ulceration, or bleed.

The results of the SELECT trial are consistent with those of another large-scale trial of similar design in which meloxicam 7.5 mg/d was compared with diclofenac slow release (SR) 100 mg/d. In this study (Meloxicam Large-Scale International Study Safety Assessment [MELISSA] trial),[72] more than 4600 patients per group were treated. Significantly fewer adverse events were reported by the meloxicam group, with fewer GI adverse events (13%, compared with diclofenac, 19%, $P < 0.001$). Dyspepsia, nausea, vomiting, abdominal pain, and diarrhea were all significantly less frequent with meloxicam than with diclofenac (**Figure 11.3**). Although it is unclear whether this reflects a reduction in underlying GI damage, the data also indicated a reduction in hospital admissions for GI complications in the meloxicam group. Three patients in the meloxicam group spent a total of 5 days in the hospital because of GI adverse events; 10 in the diclofenac group spent a total of 121 days in the hospital for GI adverse events.

Differences with respect to efficacy in the MELISSA trial consistently favored diclofenac but were small and, although statistically significant, did not exceed predetermined levels of clinical significance. Nonetheless, more patients discontinued meloxicam than diclofenac because of lack of efficacy ($P < 0.01$).[72]

In a double-blind study in normal subjects, meloxicam 7.5 mg/d was no different from placebo with respect to gastric mucosal damage.[73] However, consistent with the reduction of COX-2 selectivity seen with higher doses of this drug, a daily dose of 15 mg resulted in more gastric damage than placebo, although less than that with piroxicam 20 mg/d. In a 6-month, double-blind study in patients with hip or knee OA, the efficacy of meloxicam 15 mg/d was comparable to that of piroxicam 20 mg/d, and no significant difference was apparent between the two treatment groups with respect to the incidence of adverse events or patient withdrawals.[74] Lindén and colleagues[75] reported similar results in a 6-week study of patients with symptomatic hip OA.

Results of a placebo-controlled 12-week clinical trial[76] involving nearly 800 patients with hip or knee OA in the

United States who were randomized to treatment with meloxicam (3.75 mg, 7.5 mg, or 15 mg daily), placebo, or diclofenac (50 mg bid) permit a comparison with the MELISSA trial. However, it should be noted that although the total daily dose of diclofenac was identical in both studies, MELISSA employed a slow-release formulation of diclofenac, whereas the American study did not.

With respect to the incidence of GI adverse events and withdrawals because of GI adverse events or lack of efficacy, there were essentially no differences between the 7.5 mg/d and 15 mg/d doses of meloxicam in the American study. Pain scores showed a dose-response effect with significant superiority of both doses of meloxicam in comparison with placebo. Regardless of treatment group, withdrawals due to lack of efficacy were considerably higher in the American study (approximately 16% to 17% for meloxicam, 10.5% for diclofenac) than in the MELISSA trial (<2% in both treatment groups). After adjustment for the increased rate of dropouts due to lack of efficacy in the placebo group, however, the incidence of GI adverse events with each of the three doses of meloxicam was indistinguishable from that of placebo and lower than that of diclofenac ($P = 0.02$).

Rinder and colleagues,[77] in a placebo-controlled, double-blind trial involving 82 healthy volunteers randomized to treatment with meloxicam (7.5 mg, 15 mg, or 30 mg/d), placebo, or extended-release indomethacin 75 mg/d, found that meloxicam did not differ from placebo with respect to its effects on bleeding time and platelet aggregation over an 8-day course of treatment. Although a modest increase in bleeding time was observed with the highest dose of meloxicam, platelet aggregation responses to ADP and to arachidonic acid were preserved, whereas indomethacin significantly prolonged bleeding time and affected aggregation. These results are consistent with those of de Meijer and associates,[78] who found that meloxicam 15 mg inhibited TBX formation by 66% (in comparison with 95% inhibition by indomethacin) but did not inhibit platelet aggregation. It has been shown previously that the abolition of TBX-dependent platelet function does not occur until platelet TBX B_2 formation is inhibited by >95%.[79] The above study indicates that this high degree of TBX inhibition is not achieved with therapeutic or even supratherapeutic doses of meloxicam.

The clinical significance of the degree of COX-2 selectivity exhibited by meloxicam (**Table 11.1**) has not been tested in long-term GI safety studies analogous to the CLASS[55] or Vioxx Gastrointestinal Outcome Research (VIGOR)[80] trials of celecoxib and rofecoxib, respectively. However, Singh and Triadafilopoulos[81] presented an analysis of pooled data from 35 randomized trials in which meloxicam 7.5 mg/d or 15 mg/d was compared with diclofenac 100 to 150 mg/d, piroxicam 20 mg/d, naproxen 1000 mg/d, or placebo. Only trials in which the planned duration of treatment was at least 21 days were considered. Of the more than 24,000 patients analyzed, 42% received meloxicam in a dose of 7.5 mg/d and 12% received 15 mg/d.

Patients receiving meloxicam had a significantly lower rate of clinically significant upper GI events (ie, gastroduodenal perforation, gastric outlet obstruction, hemodynamically significant upper GI bleeding) than those receiving one of the other COX inhibitors (0.50 vs 2.16 events per 100 patient years, $P = 0.009$). Furthermore, no difference was noted between patients taking meloxicam and those taking one of the other NSAIDs with respect to thromboembolic cardiovascular complications, acute MI, congestive heart failure, or hypertension. No information was provided, however, with respect to the duration of treatment with meloxicam vs the comparator NSAIDs. Nor was information provided about the prevalence among the various treatment groups of risk factors for a serious NSAID-associated GI adverse event (in particular, use of low-dose aspirin). The latter point is particularly relevant in view of the results of the CLASS study,[55] in which low-dose aspirin appeared to mitigate the gastroprotective effect of celecoxib) (see Chapter 12, *NSAIDs That Are Selective Inhibitors of COX-2*).[55]

The authors drew a distinction between the above studies[81] and the CLASS[55] and VIGOR trials[80] in which patients who developed nonspecific GI symptoms and underwent endoscopy were discontinued from the study if endoscopy revealed an ulcer. In contrast, patients with a documented endoscopic ulcer or previous history of upper GI complication were not excluded from the clinical trials of meloxicam in the pooled analysis described. It has been suggested that some of the patients who were discontinued from the CLASS and VIGOR trials for the above reason would have developed clinically significant upper GI events (perforation, ulcer, bleeding) (**Table 11.2**) had they remained in the trial, so that the true incidence of clinically significant upper GI events among users of nonselective NSAIDs was systematically underestimated in the CLASS and VIGOR trials.

Results of a large-scale prospective 3-month observational cohort study of more than 13,000 patients in Germany who received meloxicam for a variety of rheumatic diseases further suggest its excellent tolerability.[82] In this study of patients with acute or chronic active rheumatic disease for whom NSAID therapy was indicated according to the prescribing information, a copy of which was distributed to each of some 4,000 medical practices throughout Germany shortly after the introduction of meloxicam, this agent was prescribed in a dose of 7.5 mg/d (65% of subjects) or 15 mg/d (33% of subjects). Sixty-one percent of the patients had OA, and 24%, rheumatoid arthritis; 12% had a previous history of a perforation, ulceration, or upper GI bleeding. Nearly 60% had received previous NSAID therapy that had been insufficiently effective (43%) or had been associated with an adverse drug reaction (21%).

In this study, only 0.8% reported GI adverse drug reactions and all cases of major GI toxicity (ulcer, perforation, bleeding) were associated with use of meloxicam in a dosing schedule that was not recommended. Tolerability of meloxicam was rated as good or very good by 94% of subjects, and effectiveness, as good or very good by 85%.

Recently, Singh and associates[83] reported the results of a nonblinded 6-month trial involving more than 1300 patients with OA of hand, hip, spine, or knee who were treated with meloxicam 7.5 mg/d or other NSAIDs that were on the formulary of the patient's managed care organization but had not been previously used by the patient. Treatment success was defined as completion of the study without switching to another NSAID. Based on the above definition, the meloxicam group experienced a 67% success rate and the "usual NSAID group" a 45% success rate

TABLE 11.2 — PERFORATIONS, OBSTRUCTIONS, AND BLEEDS IN PATIENTS ON THERAPEUTIC DOSES OF MELOXICAM OR OTHER NSAIDS

Treatment	Number of Patients	Exposure		Total Events		
		Mean (days)	Cumulative Person-Years	N	%	Rate Per 100 Person-Years Treatment
Meloxicam*	13,118	66	2379	12	0.1	0.50
Other NSAIDs[†]	11,078	40	1202	26	0.2	2.16

Abbreviation: NSAIDs, nonsteroidal anti-inflammatory drugs.

* 7.5 or 15 mg/d.

[†] Diclofenac 100 to 150 mg/d; piroxicam 20 mg/d; naproxen 1000 mg/d; or placebo.

Singh G, et al. *Am J Med*. Submitted for publication.

(P <0.0001). The meloxicam group showed significantly greater improvement in total Western Ontario and McMasters Universities Arthritis Index (WOMAC) score than the usual-care NSAID group (9.6 vs 6.1, P = 0.0001). Furthermore, a higher proportion of patients discontinued the usual NSAID prescribed at the onset of the study because of inefficacy or adverse events than discontinued meloxicam (**Figure 11.4**).

■ Other Adverse Effects of Nonselective NSAIDs on the GI Tract

In addition to their adverse effects on the gastric and duodenal mucosa, NSAIDs have been associated with deleterious effects on the small intestine, including:

- Inflammation associated with loss of blood and protein[84]
- Stricture[85]
- Ulceration
- Perforation
- Diarrhea.[86]

NSAIDs also cause large-bowel perforation and hemorrhage.[87] Clinical manifestations of the effects of NSAIDs on the small and large bowel, however, are much less frequent than upper GI tract problems.

■ Cardiovascular-Renal Effects of NSAIDs

Inhibition of prostaglandin biosynthesis by NSAIDs is also a well-recognized cause of other common, and occasionally severe, side effects, including:

- Hypertension
- Congestive heart failure
- Hyperkalemia
- Renal insufficiency.

Many classes of antihypertensive drugs exert their therapeutic effect, in part, through prostaglandin-mediated mechanisms (**Table 11.3**).[88] Although NSAIDs generally have little or no effect on blood pressure in normotensive individuals, they may increase blood pressure in hypertensive patients under treatment.[89,90] While the increase may be only some 4 to 5 mm Hg, it should be noted that an

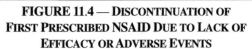

FIGURE 11.4 — DISCONTINUATION OF FIRST PRESCRIBED NSAID DUE TO LACK OF EFFICACY OR ADVERSE EVENTS

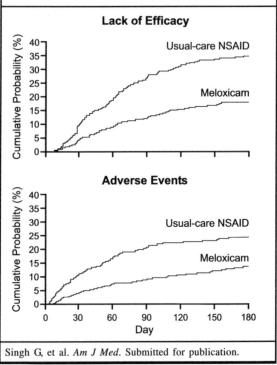

Singh G, et al. *Am J Med*. Submitted for publication.

increase in diastolic blood pressure as small as 5 to 6 mm Hg over a few years may increase the risk of cerebrovascular accident by 67% and of coronary artery disease by 15%,[91] while a decline in elevated diastolic blood pressure over a 3- to 5-year period may decrease the incidence of stroke and congestive heart failure by nearly 40% and 25%, respectively.[91]

Among elderly patients who were taking diuretics, concomitant use of an NSAID was associated with a 2-fold increase in the risk of hospitalization for congestive heart failure, with the majority of hospitalizations occurring within the first 30 days of NSAID use.[92]

It has been suggested that NSAID use is responsible for nearly 20% of all hospitalizations for congestive heart failure and that the burden of illness resulting from NSAID-related congestive failure may exceed that resulting from NSAID damage to the GI tract.[92]

Figure 11.5 depicts the consequences of inhibition of prostaglandin levels in the kidney, such as sodium and water retention, hyperkalemia, and renal failure.[93] Patients at greatest risk for renal complications from NSAIDs include those with preexisting renal disease, hypertension, congestive heart failure, cirrhosis, and volume depletion (as may occur with use of diuretics, hemorrhage, diarrhea, or profuse sweating) (**Table 11.4**). To treat patients with OA who have renal insufficiency, physicians have commonly prescribed sulindac, an NSAID promoted as having renal-sparing properties. This claim, however, is based primarily on studies in subjects with normal renal function.[94] Whelton and colleagues[95] noted a significant increase in serum creatinine concentration in patients with asymptomatic mild renal insufficiency treated with sulindac.

Among patients in whom acute deterioration of renal function occurred with a daily dose of ibuprofen 2400 mg, rechallenge with a daily dose of only 1200 mg also resulted in an acute decrease in renal function.[95] Therefore, even a dose of NSAID so low that it has minimal anti-inflammatory effects may lead to renal insufficiency.

While acute effects on renal blood flow are much more common than chronic renal changes in NSAID users, NSAIDs *can* cause chronic renal disease and, indeed, are much more likely to do so than ACET. The increased risk for chronic renal disease, which is largely confined to men >65 years of age, results in an odds ratio of 16:1 for daily NSAID use.[96]

Acute interstitial nephritis, with new-onset proteinuria usually in the nephrotic range, may occur at any time during NSAID therapy, although its prevalence is only 0.01% to 0.02%.[97] Histologic examination shows minimal-change glomerulonephritis and interstitial nephritis.[98] More recently, NSAID use has been associated with membranous glomerulonephritis and the nephrotic syndrome.[99] The problem usually remits within weeks after discontinuation of the NSAID, but resolution may take many months.

TABLE 11.3 — EFFECTS OF INHIBITION OF PROSTAGLANDIN SYNTHESIS IN THE PRESENCE OF VARIOUS ANTIHYPERTENSIVE DRUGS

Class of Antihypertensive	Primary Mode of Action	Effect of Blocking Prostaglandin Synthesis
Diuretic	↓ Extracellular volume and total peripheral resistance	↓ Loss of salt and water, exacerbated in presence of low plasma renin activity
β-Adrenergic blocker	Inhibits secretion of renin → ↓ in angiotensin and aldosterone	Inhibits renin release, may limit ability to reduce plasma renin activity; propranolol stimulates PGI_2 synthesis in patients with essential hypertension
ACE inhibitor	Inhibits formation of angiotensin II and aldosterone, inhibits inactivation of bradykinin	Interferes with release of bradykinin (which is mediated through local prostaglandin release)
Vasodilator	Unclear; thought to act through prostaglandin-mediated mechanisms	May interfere with prostaglandin-mediated mechanisms

Central α_2-agonist	↓ Sympathetic output from the CNS → ↓ in cardiac output and peripheral resistance	May ↑ total peripheral resistance
Peripheral α_1-adrenergic	Inhibits vasoconstriction induced by endogenous catecholamines. Prazosin stimulates formation of PGI_2 and PGE_2 *in vitro*	Potential attenuation of vasodilatory effect
Angiotensin II blocker	Blocks peripheral vasoconstriction and renal salt-sparing action of angiotensin II	In studies in animals, action of losartan was unaffected by inhibition of prostaglandin synthesis; in the same animal model, prostaglandin inhibition blocked angiotensin II-mediated ↑ in GFR

Abbreviations: ACE, angiotensin-converting enzyme; CNS, central nervous system; GFR, glomerular filtration rate; PGE, prostaglandin E; PGI, prostaglandin I.

Ruoff GE. *Clin Ther.* 1998;20:376-387; and Whelton A. *Am J Thers.* 2000;7:63-74.

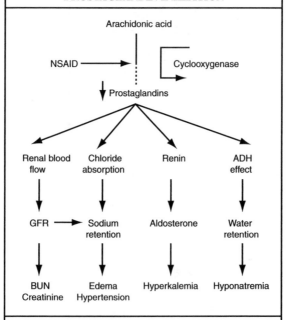

FIGURE 11.5 — RENAL EFFECTS ASSOCIATED WITH NSAID-INDUCED PROSTAGLANDIN INHIBITION

Arachidonic acid

NSAID → Cyclooxygenase

↓ Prostaglandins

Renal blood flow	Chloride absorption	Renin	ADH effect
↓	↓	↓	↓
GFR →	Sodium retention	Aldosterone	Water retention
↓	↓	↓	↓
BUN Creatinine	Edema Hypertension	Hyperkalemia	Hyponatremia

Abbreviations: ADH, antidiuretic hormone; BUN, blood urea nitrogen; GFR, glomerular filtration rate; NSAID, nonsteroidal anti-inflammatory drug.

Aronoff GR. *J Rheumatol.* 1992;19(suppl 36):25-31.

In every patient taking an NSAID chronically, blood pressure and renal and hepatic function should be monitored at regular intervals. If problems develop in any of these areas, therapy should be terminated. Chronic renal failure is a relative contraindication to use of an NSAID. Monitoring of renal function in NSAID users is important also if a complication develops that results in a decrease in renal perfusion, such as congestive heart failure or dehydration. Whelton has provided an excellent review of the renal effects of NSAIDs and analgesics.[100]

**TABLE 11.4 — RISK FACTORS FOR
NSAID-INDUCED RENAL DISEASE**

- Preexisting renal disease
- Diabetes mellitus
- Hypertension
- Congestive heart failure
- Cirrhosis
- Volume depletion (eg, due to diuretics, hemorrhage, diarrhea, profuse sweating)

Abbreviation: NSAID, nonsteroidal anti-inflammatory drug.

Inhibition by Ibuprofen of the Antiplatelet Effect of Aspirin

Evidence has been presented recently that the nonselective COX inhibitor ibuprofen may inhibit the antiplatelet effect of aspirin. Because patients with OA who have vascular disease may receive low-dose aspirin and NSAIDs concomitantly, potential interactions between aspirin and the latter drugs are highly relevant. A recent study by Catella-Lawson and colleagues[101] indicated that maximal inhibition of serum TBX B_2 levels (an index of COX-1 activity in the platelet) and of platelet aggregation produced by low-dose aspirin (81 mg) was blocked by a single daily dose of ibuprofen (400 mg) administered 2 hours prior to the dose of aspirin (**Color Plate 19**). Similar results were obtained with multiple daily doses of ibuprofen 400 mg tid, a dose commonly used in treatment of OA pain. In contrast, concomitant administration of rofecoxib, ACET, or diclofenac did not affect aspirin pharmacodynamics.

The inhibitory effects of multiple daily doses of ibuprofen were apparent even when subjects received aspirin *prior* to their morning dose of ibuprofen. The effect of multiple daily doses of ACET or of other NSAIDs was not tested. The results are consistent with antagonism of the irreversible effect of aspirin on the platelet by the multiple-dose regimen of ibuprofen. Theoretically, this could increase the risk of vascular thrombosis. These data would suggest that ACET is preferable to ibuprofen in patients taking low-dose aspirin for cardiovascular prophylaxis who require an analgesic.

A study was recently conducted of the records of more than 7000 patients who were discharged from the hospital after a first admission for cardiovascular disease. They were prescribed low-dose aspirin and survived for at least 1 month. In comparison with those who used aspirin alone, patients who were taking both aspirin and ibuprofen exhibited an increase risk of all-cause mortality (adjusted hazard ratio = 1.93, 95% CI = 1.30 – 2.87, P = 0.0011) and of cardiovascular mortality, in particular (adjusted hazard ratio = 1.73, 95 CI = 1.05 – 2.84, P = 0.03).[102]

These data support the possibility that ibuprofen interferes with the cardioprotective effects of aspirin, at least in patients with established cardiovascular disease. No such increased risk was apparent in those who used aspirin with diclofenac or with other nonselective NSAIDs. However, as pointed out by the authors, this study had several limitations: the number of subjects studied was relatively small, the effect of coxibs was not examined, and the severity of cardiovascular disease, the dose of individual NSAIDs and the presence of risk factors for cardiovascular mortality (eg, smoking, body mass index) were not taken into account.

Do NSAIDs Alter the Rate of Cartilage Breakdown in OA?

A number of reports suggest that NSAIDs may slow the progression of cartilage breakdown in OA, thus serving as disease-modifying OA drugs. Such claims, however, have been based largely on *in vitro* effects of the drug on cytokine production, release or activity of cartilage matrix-degrading proteases, inhibition of the production of toxic oxygen metabolites, etc.[103] There are *no* data from controlled, clinical trials in humans to indicate that any NSAID favorably influences progression of joint breakdown in OA.

Several NSAIDs inhibit proteoglycan (PG) synthesis by normal cartilage *in vitro*.[104-107] The augmented *in vitro* synthesis of PG in OA cartilage, which represents a repair effort by the chondrocytes,[108] is suppressed by salicylate to a much greater extent than that in normal cartilage.[109]

Because PGs are essential for the elasticity and compressive stiffness of the cartilage, suppression of their synthesis *in vivo* could have adverse consequences.

While the potential implications of the above studies are obvious, prediction of the *in vivo* effects of an NSAID based on its *in vitro* effects is naive. *In vitro* studies cannot predict the relative importance of:

- The effect of the NSAID on synovitis
- Its direct effect on chondrocyte metabolism
- Its analgesic action (perhaps resulting in overload of the damaged joint).

It is therefore notable that the *in vivo* effects of aspirin in the canine cruciate-deficiency model of OA are consistent with the *in vitro* data. Cartilage degeneration in the unstable knee of dogs fed aspirin in doses sufficient to maintain the serum salicylate concentration at 20 to 25 mg/dL was much more severe than that in the OA knee of dogs that did not receive the drug.[110] Aspirin also accelerated development of OA in C57 black mice.[111]

Several reports have implicated NSAIDs in the acceleration of joint damage in humans with OA,[112-115] but these suffer from the limitations inherent in retrospective studies. In a randomized prospective trial involving patients with hip OA, azapropazone, an analgesic with weak, prostaglandin synthase inhibitory action, was compared with indomethacin, a potent prostaglandin synthase inhibitor.[116] The indomethacin group showed more rapid radiographic deterioration of the OA joint than the group receiving azapropazone and took 50% less time to progress to arthroplasty. However, the technique used in that study for measurement of joint-space narrowing (a surrogate for loss of articular cartilage) has been criticized,[117] the surgeons who decided when arthroplasty was required were not blinded to the treatment the patients received, and pain scores were significantly higher in the azapropazone group than in those treated with indomethacin, raising the possibility of greater usage of the OA hip by subjects in the latter group and other between-group differences.

In another study, radiographic progression of knee OA was assessed in patients treated with indomethacin, tiaprofenic acid, or with a placebo matched to either the tiaprofenic acid capsules or the indomethacin tablets.[118] The rate of joint-space narrowing was significantly greater in the indomethacin group than in the placebo group, while no significant difference was found between tiaprofenic acid and placebo. Although the conclusions would support those of the study cited prior to this,[116] several concerns exist about the experimental design and interpretation of the results of this study.[119] Whether NSAIDs accelerate the progression of cartilage breakdown in humans with OA remains unclear. Better evidence is needed.

NSAID Withdrawal in Patients With OA

In general, the level of satisfaction of patients and physicians with NSAIDs is low. Patients with OA are typically switched from one NSAID to another because of lack of efficacy or adverse effects. Barring development of a serious adverse event, treatment with NSAIDs is rarely discontinued in patients with OA. Despite the tendency of physicians to maintain NSAID therapy in perpetuity for the patient with OA, it is important to recognize that it *is* possible to discontinue NSAIDs in many patients, to use NSAIDs only on an as-needed basis, or to decrease the dose. Because the risk of NSAID-associated adverse effects is dose-dependent, such measures are highly desirable.

The results of an NSAID-withdrawal study[120] (**Table 11.5**) in elderly subjects who were admitted acutely to geriatric hospitals for a variety of indications unrelated to OA or its treatment are illuminating. Ninety-one patients were identified who were taking a prescription NSAID at the time of admission. (Among the elderly, prescription of an NSAID is essentially tantamount to a diagnosis of OA, whereas in younger individuals NSAIDs may be prescribed for a multitude of reasons, eg, migraine, dysmenorrhea, sprains, strains, etc.) The study protocol involved withdrawal of the NSAID and replacement, as needed, by a simple analgesic, by hot or cold packs, massage, or a muscle relaxant, following which the patient's pain was monitored. If the above measures were ineffective, NSAID treatment was reinstituted. More than 50% of these elderly subjects did not require reinstitution of NSAID treatment over the ensuing 6-month follow-up period. The point is this: Many

TABLE 11.5 — SUCCESS OF NSAID WITHDRAWAL IN THE ELDERLY

Patient Status	Patients
Admitted on NSAID	91
NSAID withdrawn	78 (86%)
Alive and off NSAID	
at 4 weeks	45/67 (67%)
at 6 months	36/67 (54%)
Abbreviation: NSAID, nonsteroidal anti-inflammatory drug.	
Black D, et al. *J Am Geriatr Soc.* 1991;39:A26.	

patients with OA improve symptomatically—ie, they *get better*—and it is possible to decrease their dose of NSAID or to discontinue the NSAID.

A more recent study of the effects of an education intervention directed at nursing home staff provides additional evidence that NSAID withdrawal is feasible.[121] In this study of elderly nursing home residents who were regular NSAID users, nursing home staff and the responsible physician were informed that such individuals are at high risk for NSAID-associated adverse effects. Pharmacologic and nonpharmacologic alternatives that could permit discontinuation of the NSAID or reduction in dose were provided. In lieu of the patient's NSAID, ACET 650 mg tid and at bedtime as needed was prescribed. Throughout the study, the nurse reevaluated the patients to assure they did not experience an increase in pain as a result of the intervention. If that occurred, low-dose ibuprofen was added on an as-needed basis. If that was unsuccessful, a higher dose of ibuprofen was prescribed on a regular basis. If the latter was not successful, treatment with the original NSAID was reinstituted.

Analysis of the data indicated that the nursing home subjects had a considerable level of chronic pain at baseline. The intervention resulted in reduction of NSAID use from an average of 7 days per week to about 2 days per week in the experimental group (**Figure 11.6**). In many subjects, it was possible to discontinue the NSAID. Whereas little increase in ACET use was noted in the control nursing homes,

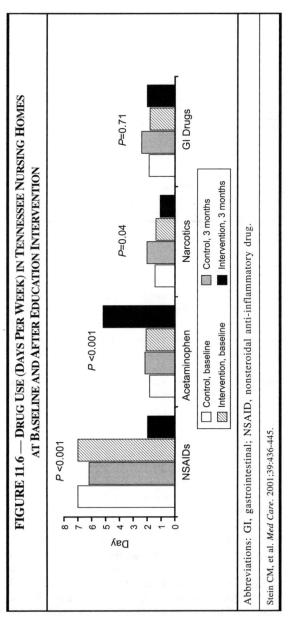

FIGURE 11.6 — DRUG USE (DAYS PER WEEK) IN TENNESSEE NURSING HOMES AT BASELINE AND AFTER EDUCATION INTERVENTION

Abbreviations: GI, gastrointestinal; NSAID, nonsteroidal anti-inflammatory drug.

Stein CM, et al. *Med Care*. 2001;39:436-445.

in the intervention nursing homes ACET use increased, on average, from 2 days per week to 5 days per week. Concurrently, opioid use decreased significantly in the intervention homes but increased in the control nursing homes. Pain scores showed little change from baseline in either treatment group, ie, the intervention did not exacerbate pain or disability. Thus in a controlled nursing home setting, with the cooperation of nursing home staff and physicians, the intervention resulted in a significant reduction in NSAID dose with no adverse effects on pain or function.

Notably, however, when a similar intervention was attempted by targeting primary care physicians in the community, only 10% of patients under the care of physicians in the intervention group were given a trial of ACET (vs 1% of patients in the practices of physicians in the control group).[122] No difference was noted between the two groups with respect to use of other pain medications or gastroprotective drugs or general health status.

Why the education intervention was so successful in reducing NSAID use among nursing home patients but failed to alter prescribing behaviors of community physicians is unclear. However, elderly patients with OA pain who visit the office of a community physician often also have a number of other problems related to comorbidities (eg, diabetes, heart disease, neurologic problems) that must be addressed in the course of a relatively brief follow-up visit, and these take precedence over management of the patient's joint pain. Blumenthal and associates[123] found recently that the mean duration of an office visit to a primary care physician was about 17 minutes.

REFERENCES

1. Day RO, Graham GG, Furst DE, Lee E. Ibuprofen, fenoprofen, ketoprofen. In: Paulus HE, Furst DE, Dromgoole SH, eds. *Drugs for Rheumatic Disease.* New York, NY: Churchill Livingstone; 1987: 315-345.

2. Giansiracusa JE, Donaldson MS, Koonce ML, Lefton TE, Ruoff GE, Brooks CD. Ibuprofen in osteoarthritis. *Curr Med Res Opin.* 1975; 3:481-484.

3. Levinson DJ, Rubinstein HM. Doubleblind comparison of fenoprofen calcium and ibuprofen in osteoarthritis of large joints. *Curr Ther Res.* 1983;34:280-284.

4. Owen-Smith BD, Burry HC. Ibuprofen in the management of osteoarthritis of the hip. *Rheumatol Phys Med.* 1972;11:281-286.

5. Petrick TJ, Bovenkerk WE. Multicenter studies in the United States and Canada of meclofenamate sodium in osteoarthritis of the hip and knee. Double blind comparison with placebo and long-term experience. *Arzneimittelforschung.* 1983;33:644-648.

6. Tyson VC, Glynne A. A comparative study of benoxaprofen and ibuprofen in osteoarthritis in general practice. *J Rheumatol.* 1980; 6(suppl):132-138.

7. Lister BJ, Poland M, DeLapp RE. Efficacy of nabumetone versus diclofenac, naproxen, ibuprofen, and piroxicam in osteoarthritis and rheumatoid arthritis. *Am J Med.* 1993;95:2S-9S.

8. Kvien TK, Brörs O, Staff PH, Rognstad S, Nordby J. Improved cost-effectiveness ratio with a patient self-adjusted naproxen dosing regimen in osteoarthritis treatment. *Scand J Rheumatol.* 1991;20:280-287.

9. McKenna F, Borenstein D, Wendt H, Wallemark C, Lefkowith JB, Geis GS. Celecoxib versus diclofenac in the management of osteoarthritis of the knee. *Scand J Rheumatol.* 2001;30:11-18.

10. Ehrich EW, Schnitzer TJ, McIlwain H, et al, for the Rofecoxib Osteoarthritis Pilot Study Group. Effect of specific COX-2 inhibition in osteoarthritis of the knee: a 6 week double blind, placebo controlled pilot study of rofecoxib. *J Rheumatol.* 1999;26:2438-2447.

11. Cannon GW, Cladwell JR, Holt P, et al, for the Rofecoxib Phase III Protocol 035 Study Group. Rofecoxib, a specific inhibitor of cyclooxygenase 2, with clinical efficacy comparable with that of diclofenac sodium: results of a one-year, randomized, clinical trial in patients with osteoarthritis of the knee and hip. *Arthritis Rheum.* 2000;43:978-987.

12. Dieppe P, Cushnaghan J, Jasani MK, McCrae F, Watt I. A two-year, placebo controlled trial of nonsteroidal anti-inflammatory therapy in osteoarthritis of the knee joint. *Br J Rheumatol*. 1993;32:595-600.

13. Williams HJ, Ward JR, Egger MJ, et al. Comparison of naproxen and acetaminophen in a two-year study of treatment of osteoarthritis of the knee. *Arthritis Rheum*. 1993;36:1196-1206.

14. Bradley JD, Brandt KD, Katz BP, Kalasinski LA, Ryan SI. Comparison of an anti-inflammatory dose of ibuprofen, an analgesic dose of ibuprofen, and acetaminophen in the treatment of patients with osteoarthritis of the knee. *N Engl J Med*. 1991;325:87-91.

15. Scholes D, Stergachis A, Penna PM, Normand EH, Hansten PD. Nonsteroidal antiinflammatory drug discontinuation in patients with osteoarthritis. *J Rheumatol*. 1995;22:708-712.

16. Fordyce WE. Evaluating and managing chronic pain. *Geriatrics*. 1978;33:59-62.

17. Seideman P, Samuelson P, Neander G. Naproxen and paracetamol compared with naproxen only in coxarthrosis. Increased effect of the combination in 18 patients. *Acta Orthop Scand*. 1993;64:285-288.

18. Armstrong CP, Blower AL. Non-steroidal anti-inflammatory drugs and life threatening complications of peptic ulceration. *Gut*. 1987; 28:527-532.

19. Duggan JM, Dobson AJ, Johnson H, Fahey P. Peptic ulcer and nonsteroidal anti-inflammatory agents. *Gut*. 1986;27:929-933.

20. Beard K, Walker AM, Perera DR, Jick H. Nonsteroidal anti-inflammatory drugs and hospitalization for gastroesophageal bleeding in the elderly. *Arch Intern Med*. 1987;147:1621-1623.

21. Carson JL, Strom BL, Soper KA, West SL, Morse ML. The association of nonsteroidal anti-inflammatory drugs with upper gastrointestinal tract bleeding. *Arch Intern Med*. 1987;147:85-88.

22. Somerville K, Faulkner G, Langman M. Non-steroidal anti-inflammatory drugs and bleeding peptic ulcer. *Lancet*. 1986;1:462-464.

23. Fries JF, Miller SR, Spitz PW, Williams CA, Hubert HB, Bloch DA. Toward an epidemiology of gastropathy associated with nonsteroidal antiinflammatory drug use. *Gastroenterology*. 1989;96(suppl 2):647-655.

24. Guess HA, West R, Strand LM, et al. Fatal upper gastrointestinal hemorrhage or perforation among users and nonusers of nonsteroidal anti-inflammatory drugs in Saskatchewan, Canada 1983. *J Clin Epidemiol*. 1988;41:35-45.

11

25. Griffin MR, Piper JM, Daughtery JR, Snowden M, Ray WA. Nonsteroidal anti-inflammatory drug use and increased risk for peptic ulcer disease in elderly persons. *Ann Intern Med.* 1991;114:257-263.

26. Wolfe MM, Lichtenstein DR, Singh G. Gastrointestinal toxicity of nonsteroidal antiinflammatory drugs. *N Engl J Med.* 1999;340: 1888-1899.

27. Singh G, Triadafilopoulos G. Epidemiology of NSAID induced gastrointestinal complications. *J Rheumatol.* 1999;56(suppl 26):18-24.

28. Smalley WE, Ray WA, Daugherty JR, Griffin MR. Nonsteroidal anti-inflammatory drugs and the incidence of hospitalizations for peptic ulcer disease in elderly persons. *Am J Epidemiol.* 1995;141:539-545.

29. Griffin MR, Ray WA, Schaffner W. Nonsteroidal anti-inflammatory drug use and death from peptic ulcer in elderly persons. *Ann Intern Med.* 1988;109:359-363.

30. Singh G, Ramey DR, Terry R, Triadafilopoulus G. NSAID-related effects on the GI tract: an ever widening spectrum. *Arthritis Rheum.* 1997;40(suppl):S93. Abstract.

31. Brooks PM, Day RO. Nonsteroidal antiinflammatory drugs – differences and similarities. *N Engl J Med.* 1991;324:1716-1725.

32. Singh G, Ramey DR, Morfeld D, Shi H, Hatoum HT, Fries JF. Gastrointestinal tract complications of nonsteroidal anti-inflammatory drug treatment in rheumatoid arthritis. A prospective observational cohort study. *Arch Intern Med.* 1996;156:1530-1536.

33. Gutthann SP, Garciá Rodriquez LA, Raiford DS. Individual nonsteroidal antiinflammatory drugs and other risk factors for upper gastrointestinal bleeding and perforation. *Epidemiology.* 1997;8:18-24.

34. Garciá Rodríguez LA, Jick H. Risk of upper gastrointestinal bleeding and perforation associated with individual non-steroidal anti-inflammatory drugs. *Lancet.* 1994;343:769-772.

35. Silverstein FE, Graham DY, Senior JR, et al. Misoprostol reduces serious gastrointestinal complications in patients with rheumatoid arthritis receiving nonsteroidal anti-inflammatory drugs. A randomized, double-blind, placebo-controlled trial. *Ann Intern Med.* 1995;123:241-249.

36. Fries JF, Williams CA, Bloch DA, Michel BA. Nonsteroidal anti-inflammatory drug-associated gastropathy: incidence and risk factor models. *Am J Med.* 1991;91:213-222.

37. Piper JM, Ray WA, Daugherty JR, Griffin MR. Corticosteroid use and peptic ulcer disease: role of nonsteroidal anti-inflammatory drugs. *Ann Intern Med.* 1991;114:735-740.

38. Huskisson EC, Hart FD, Shenfield GM, Taylor RT. Ibuprofen. A review. *Practitioner.* 1971;207:639-643.

39. Shorr RI, Ray WA, Daugherty JR, Griffin MR. Concurrent use of non-steroidal anti-inflammatory drugs and oral anticoagulants places elderly persons at high risk for hemorrhagic peptic ulcer disease. *Arch Intern Med.* 1993;153:1665-1670.

40. Langman MJ. Treating ulcers in patients receiving anti-arthritic drugs. *Q J Med.* 1989;73:1089-1091.

41. Henry D, Dobson A, Turner C. Variability in the risk of major gastrointestinal complications from nonaspirin nonsteroidal anti-inflammatory drugs. *Gastroenterology.* 1993;105:1078-1088.

42. Kim JG, Graham DY. *Helicobacter pylori* infection and development of gastric or duodenal ulcer in arthritic patients receiving chronic NSAID therapy. The Misoprostol Study Group. *Am J Gastroenterol.* 1994;89:203-207.

43. Graham DY, Lidsky MD, Cox AM, et al. Long-term nonsteroidal antiinflammatory drug use and *Helicobacter pylori* infection. *Gastroenterology.* 1991;100:1653-1657.

44. Laine L, Marin-Sorenson M, Weinstein WM. Nonsteroidal antiinflammatory drug-associated gastric ulcers do not require *Helicobacter pylori* for their development. *Am J Gastroenterol.* 1992;87:1398-1402.

45. Taha AS, Sturrock RD, Russell RI. Mucosal erosions in longterm nonsteroidal anti-inflammatory drug users: predisposition to ulceration and relation to *Helicobacter pylori. Gut.* 1995;36:334-336.

46. Chan FK, Sung JJ, Chung SC, et al. Randomised trial of eradication of *Helicobactor pylori* before non-steroidal anti-inflammatory drug therapy to prevent peptic ulcers. *Lancet.* 1997;350:975-979.

47. Hawkey CJ, Tulassay Z, Szczepanski L, et al. Randomised controlled trial of Helicobactor pylori eradication in patients on non-steroidal anti-inflammatory drugs: HELP NSAIDs study. Helicobacter Eradication for Lesions Prevention. *Lancet.* 1998;352:1016-1021.

48. Laine L. Approaches to nonsteroidal anti-inflammatory drug use in the high-risk patient. *Gastroenterology.* 2001;120:594-606.

49. Laine L, Bombardier C, Hawkey CJ, et al. Stratifying the risk of NSAID-related upper gastrointestinal clinical events: results of a double-blind outcomes study in patients with rheumatoid arthritis. *Gastroenterology.* 2002;123:1006-1012.

50. Larkai EN, Smith JL, Lidsky MD, Graham DY. Gastroduodenal mucosa and dyspeptic symptoms in arthritic patients during chronic nonsteroidal anti-inflammatory drug use. *Am J Gastroenterol.* 1987;82:1153-1158.

51. Weil J, Colin-Jones D, Langman M, et al. Prophylactic aspirin and risk of peptic ulcer bleeding. *BMJ.* 1995;310:827-830.

11

52. Kurata JH, Abbey DE. The effect of chronic aspirin use on duodenal and gastric ulcer hospitalizations. *J Clin Gastroenterol*. 1990; 12:260-266.

53. Roderick PJ, Wilkes HC, Meade TW. The gastrointestinal toxicity of aspirin: an overview of randomised controlled trials. *Br J Clin Pharmacol*. 1993;35:219-226.

54. Sorensen HT, Mellemkjaer L, Blot WJ, et al. Risk of upper gastrointestinal bleeding associated with use of low-dose aspirin. *Am J Gastroenterol*. 2000;95:2218-2224.

55. Silverstein FE, Faich G, Goldstein JL, et al. Gastrointestinal toxicity with celecoxib vs. nonsteroidal anti-inflammatory drugs for osteoarthritis and rheumatoid arthritis: the CLASS study: A randomized controlled trial. Celecoxib Long-term Arthritis Safety Study. *JAMA*. 2000;284;1247-1255.

56. Cryer B, Feldman M. Effects of very low dose daily, long-term aspirin therapy on gastric, duodenal, and rectal prostaglandin levels and on mucosal injury in healthy humans. *Gastroenterology*. 1999; 117:17-25.

57. Lai KC, Lam SK, Chu KM, et al. Lansoprazole for the prevention of recurrences of ulcer complications from long-term low-dose aspirin use. *N Engl J Med*. 2002;346:2033-2038.

58. Graham DY, Agrawal NM, Roth SH. Prevention of NSAID-induced gastric ulcer with misoprostol: multicentre, double-blind, placebo-controlled trial. *Lancet*. 1988;2:1277-1280.

59. Roth SH, Tindall EA, Jain AK, et al. A controlled study comparing the effects of nabumetone, ibuprofen, and ibuprofen plus misoprostol on the upper gastrointestinal tract mucosa. *Arch Intern Med*. 1993;153:2565-2571.

60. Barradell LB, Whittington R, Benfield P. Misoprostol: pharmacoeconomics of its use as prophylaxis against gastroduodenal damage induced by nonsteroidal anti-inflammatory drugs. *Pharmacoeconomics*. 1993;3:140-170.

61. Raskin JB, White RH, Jackson JE, et al. Misoprostol dosage in the prevention of nonsteroidal anti-inflammatory drug-induced gastric and duodenal ulcers: a comparison of three regimens. *Ann Intern Med*. 1995;123:344-350.

62. Taha AS, Hudson N, Hawkey CJ, et al. Famotidine for the prevention of gastric and duodenal ulcers caused by nonsteroidal antiinflammatory drugs. *N Engl J Med*. 1996;334:1435-1439.

63. Ekstrom P, Carling L, Wetterhus S, et al. Prevention of peptic ulcer and dyspeptic symptoms with omeprazole in patients receiving continuous non-steroidal anti-inflammatory drug therapy. A Nordic multicentre study. *Scand J Gastroenterol*. 1996;31:753-758.

64. Yeomans ND, Tulassay Z, Juhasz L, et al. A comparison of omeprazole with ranitidine for ulcers associated with nonsteroidal antiinflammatory drugs. Acid Suppression Trial: Ranitidine versus Omeprazole for NSAID-associated Ulcer Treatment (ASTRONAUT) Study Group. *N Engl J Med*. 1998;338:719-726.

65. Hawkey CJ, Karrasch JA, Szczepanski L, et al. Omeprazole compared with misoprostol for ulcers associated with nonsteroidal anti-inflammatory drugs. Omeprazole Versus Misoprostol for NSAID-induced Ulcer Management (OMNIUM) Study Group. *N Engl J Med*. 1998; 338:727-734.

66. Wilcox CM, Shalek KA, Cotsonis G. Striking prevalence of over-the counter nonsteroidal anti-inflammatory drug use in patients with upper gastrointestinal hemorrhage. *Arch Intern Med*. 1994;154:42-46.

67. Noble S, Balfour JA. Meloxicam. *Drugs*. 1996;51:424-432

68. Warner TD, Giuliano F, Vojnovic I, Bukasa A, Mitchell JA, Vane JR. Nonsteroid drug selectivities for cyclo-oxygenase-1 rather than cyclo-oxygenase-2 are associated with human gastrointestinal toxicity: a full *in vitro* analysis. *Proc Natl Acad Sci (USA)*. 1999;96:7563-7568.

69. Patrignani P, Panara MR, Sciulli MG, Santini G, Renda G, Patrono C. Differential inhibition of human prostaglandin endoperoxide synthase-1 and -2 by nonsteroidal anti-inflammatory drugs. *J Physiol Pharmacol*. 1997;48:623-631.

70. Gierse JK, McDonald JJ, Hauser SD, Rangwala SH, Koboldt CM, Seibert K. A single amino acid difference between cyclooxygenase-1 (COX-1) and -2 (COX-2) reverses the selectivity of COX-2 specific inhibitors. *J Biol Chem*. 1996;271:15810-15814.

71. Dequeker J, Hawkey C, Kahan A, et al. Improvement in gastrointestinal tolerability of the selective cyclooxygenase (COX)-2 inhibitor, meloxicam, compared with piroxicam: results of the Safety and Efficacy Large-scale Evaluation of COX-inhibiting Therapies (SELECT) trial in osteoarthritis. *Br J Rheumatol*. 1998;37:946-951.

72. Hawkey C, Kahan A, Steinbruck K, et al. Gastrointestinal tolerability of meloxicam compared to diclofenac in osteoarthritis patients. International MELISSA Study Group. Meloxicam Large-scale International Study Safety Assessment. *Br J Rheumatol*. 1998;37:937-945.

73. Patoia L, Santucci L, Furno P, et al. A 4-week, double-blind, parallel-group study to compare the gastrointestinal effects of meloxicam 7.5 mg, meloxicam 15 mg, piroxicam 20 mg and placebo by means of faecal blood loss, endoscopy and symptom evaluation in healthy volunteers. *Br J Rheumatol*. 1996;35:61-67.

74. Hosie J, Distel M, Bluhmki E. Efficacy and tolerability of meloxicam versus piroxicam in patients with osteoarthritis of the hip or knee: a six-month double-blind study. *Clin Drug Invest*. 1997;13:175-184.

75. Lindén B, Distel M, Bluhmki E. A double-blind study to compare the efficacy and safety of meloxicam 15 mg with piroxicam 20 mg in patients with osteoarthritis of the hip. *Br J Rheumatol.* 1996; 35(suppl 1):35-38.

76. Yocum D, Fleischmann R, Dalgin P, Caldwell J, Hall D, Roszko P. Safety and efficacy of meloxicam in the treatment of osteoarthritis: a 12-week, double-blind, multiple-dose, placebo-controlled trial. The Meloxicam Osteoarthritis Investigators. *Arch Intern Med.* 2000;160; 2947-2954.

77. Rinder HM, Tracey JB, Souhrada M, Wang, C, Gagnier RP, Wood CC. Effects of meloxicam on platelet function in healthy adults: a randomized, double-blind, placebo-controlled trial. *J Clin Pharmacol.* 2002;42:881-886.

78. de Meijer A, Vollaard H, de Metz M, Verbruggen B, Thomas C, Novakova I. Meloxicam, 15 mg/d, spares platelet function in healthy volunteers. *Clin Pharmacol Ther.* 1999;66:425-430.

79. Fitz Gerald GA, Oates JA, Hawiger J, et al. Endogenous biosynthesis of prostacyclin and thromboxane and platelet function during chronic administration of aspirin in man. *J Clin Invest.* 1983;71:676-688.

80. Bombardier C, Laine L, Reicin A, et al. Comparison of upper gastrointestinal toxicity of rofecoxib and naproxen in patients with rheumatoid arthritis. VIGOR Study Group. *N Engl J Med.* 2000;343: 1520-1528.

81. Singh G, Triadafilopoulos G. Risk of clinically significant upper gastrointestinal and cardiovascular thromboembolic complications with meloxicam. *Am J Med.* Submitted for publication.

82. Zeidler H, Kaltwasser JP, Leonard JP, et al. Prescription and tolerability of meloxicam in day-to-day practice. Postmarketing observational cohort study of 13,307 patients in Germany. *J Clin Rheumatol.* 2002;8:1-11.

83. Singh G, Tugwell P, Kobe M, et al. Meloxicam versus usual care NSAIDs for the treatment of osteoarthritis in a usual care setting. The results of the IMPROVE trial. *Am J Med.* Submitted for publication.

84. Bjarnason I, Zanelli G, Prouse P, et al. Blood and protein loss via small intestinal inflammation induced by nonsteroidal anti-inflammatory drugs. *Lancet.* 1987;2:711-714.

85. Matsuhashi N, Yamada A, Hiraishi M, et al. Multiple strictures of the small intestine after long-term nonsteroidal anti-inflammatory drug therapy. *Am J Gastroenterol.* 1992;87:1183-1186.

86. Kwo PY, Tremaine WJ. Nonsteroidal anti-inflammatory drug-induced enteropathy: case discussion and review of the literature. *Mayo Clin Proc.* 1995;70:55-61.

87. Langman MJ, Morgan L, Worrall A. Use of anti-inflammatory drugs by patients admitted with small or large bowel perforations and haemorrhage. *Br Med J*. 1985;290:347-349.

88. Ruoff GE. The impact of nonsteroidal anti-inflammatory drugs on hypertension: alternative analgesics for patients at risk. *Clin Ther*. 1998;20:376-387.

89. Pope JE, Anderson JJ, Felson DT. A meta-analysis of the effects of nonsteroidal anti-inflammatory drugs on blood pressure. *Arch Intern Med*. 1993;153:477-484.

90. Johnson AG, Nguyen TV, Day RO. Do nonsteroidal anti-inflammatory drugs affect blood pressure? A meta-analysis. *Ann Intern Med*. 1994;121:289-300.

91. Collins R, Peto R, MacMahon S, et al. Blood pressure, stroke, and coronary heart disease. Part 2, Short-term reductions in blood pressure: overview of randomised drug trials in their epidemiological context. *Lancet*. 1990;335:827-838.

92. Heerdink ER, Leufkens HG, Herings RM, Ottervanger JP, Stricker BH, Bakker A. NSAIDs associated with increased risk of congestive heart failure in elderly patients taking diuretics. *Arch Intern Med*. 1998;158:1108-1112.

11

93. Aronoff GR. Therapeutic implications associated with renal studies of nabumetone. *J Rheumatol*. 1992;19(suppl 36):25-31.

94. Brater DC, Anderson S, Baird B, Campbell WB. Effects of ibuprofen, naproxen and sulindac on prostaglandins in men. *Kidney Int*. 1985;27:66-73.

95. Whelton A, Stout RL, Spilman PS, Klassen DK. Renal effects of ibuprofen, piroxicam, and sulindac in patients with asymptomatic renal failure. A prospective, randomized, crossover comparison. *Ann Intern Med*. 1990;112:568-576.

96. Sandler DP, Burr FR, Weinberg CR. Nonsteroidal anti-inflammatory drugs and the risk for chronic renal disease. *Ann Intern Med*. 1991; 115:165-172.

97. Brater DC. Clinical aspects of renal prostaglandins and NSAID therapy. *Semin Arthritis Rheum*. 1987;17:17-22.

98. Bender WL, Whelton A, Beschorner WE, Darwish MO, Hall-Craggs M, Solez K. Interstitial nephritis, proteinuria, and renal failure caused by nonsteroidal anti-inflammatory drugs. Immunologic characterization of the inflammatory infiltrate. *Am J Med*. 1984;76:1006-1012.

99. Radford MG Jr, Holley KE, Grande JP, et al. Reversible membranous nephropathy associated with the use of nonsteroidal anti-inflammatory drugs. *JAMA*. 1996;276:466-469.

213

100. Whelton A. Renal and related cardiovascular effects of conventional and Cox-2 specific NSAIDs and non-NSAID analgesics. *Am J Ther*. 2000;7:63-74.

101. Catella-Lawson F, Reilly MP, Kapoor SC, et al. Cyclooxygenase inhibitors and the antiplatelet effects of aspirin. *N Engl J Med*. 2001;345:1809-1817.

102. MacDonald TM, Wei L. Effect of ibuprofen on cardioprotective effect of aspirin. *Lancet*. 2003;361:573-574.

103. Doherty M. "Chondroprotection" by non-steroidal anti-inflammatory drugs. *Ann Rheum Dis*. 1989;48:619-621.

104. McKenzie LS, Horsburgh BA, Ghosh P, Taylor TK. Effect of anti-inflammatory drugs on sulphated glycosaminoglycan synthesis in aged human articular cartilage. *Ann Rheum Dis*. 1976;35:487-497.

105. Herman JH, Hess EV. Nonsteroidal anti-inflammatory drugs and modulation of cartilaginous changes in osteoarthritis and rheumatoid arthritis. Clinical implications. *Am J Med*. 1984;77(suppl):16-25.

106. Brandt KD, Palmoski MJ. Effects of salicylates and other nonsteroidal anti-inflammatory drugs on articular cartilage. *Am J Med*. 1984;77:65-69.

107. de Vries BJ, van den Berg WB, Vitters E, van de Putte LB. Effects of NSAIDs on the metabolism of sulphated glycosaminoglycans in healthy and (post) arthritic murine articular cartilage. *Drugs*. 1988;35(suppl 1):24-32.

108. Adams ME, Brandt KD. Hypertrophic repair of canine articular cartilage in osteoarthritis after anterior cruciate ligament transection. *J Rheumatol*. 1991;18:428-435.

109. Palmoski MJ, Colyer RA, Brandt KD. Marked suppression by salicylate of the augmented proteoglycan synthesis in osteoarthritic cartilage. *Arthritis Rheum*. 1980;23:83-91.

110. Palmoski MJ, Brandt KD. *In vivo* effect of aspirin on canine osteoarthritic cartilage. *Arthritis Rheum*. 1983;26:994-1001.

111. Wilhelmi G. Fördende und hemmende einflüsse von tribenosid und acetylsalicylsäure auf die spontane arthrose der maus. *Arzheimittelforsch*. 1978;28:1724-1726.

112. Coke H. Longterm indomethacin therapy of coxarthrosis. *Ann Rheum Dis*. 1967;26:34.

113. Ronningen H, Langeland N. Indomethacin hips. *Acta Orthop Scand*. 1977;48:556.

114. Solomon L. Drug-induced arthropathy and necrosis of the femoral head. *J Bone Joint Surg Br*. 1973;55:246-261.

115. Newman NM, Ling RS. Acetabular bone destruction related to non-steroidal anti-inflammatory drugs. *Lancet*. 1985;2:11-14.

116. Rashad S, Revell P, Hemingway A, Low F, Rainsford K, Walker F. Effect of non-steroidal anti-inflammatory drugs on the course of osteoarthritis. *Lancet*. 1989;2:519-522.

117. Lequesne M, Lamotte L, Samson M. Conditions de d) stration radio cliniques d'un effet chondroprotecteur or chondroagresseur. In: Gaucher A, Netter P, Pourel J, Regent D, eds. *Pharmacologie Clinique Énantionmères/Microcristaux/Inflammation/Imagerie Ostéoarticulaire/Cartilage/Arthritis Experiméntales*. Paris, France: Masson; 1991:390.

118. Huskisson EC, Berry H, Gishen P, Jubb RW, Whitehead J. Effects of antiinflammatory drugs on the progression of osteoarthritis of the knee. LINK Study Group. Longitudinal Investigation of Nonsteroidal Anti-inflammatory Drugs in Knee Osteoarthritis. *J Rheumatol*. 1995;22:1941-1946.

119. Doherty M, Jones A. Indomethacin hastens large joint osteoarthritis in humans—how strong is the evidence? *J Rheumatol*. 1995;22:2013-2016.

120. Black D, Tuppen J, Heller A. NSAID withdrawal in elderly patients. *J Am Geriatr Soc*. 1991;39:A26.

121. Stein CM, Griffin MR, Taylor JA, Pichert JW, Brandt KD, Ray WA. Educational program for nursing home physicians and staff to reduce use of non-steroidal anti-inflammatory drugs among nursing home residents: a randomized controlled trial. *Med Care*. 2001;39:436-445.

122. Ray WA, Stein CM, Byrd V, et al. Educational program for physicians to reduce use of non-steroidal anti-inflammatory drugs among community-dwelling elderly persons. *Med Care*. 2001;39:425-435.

123. Blumenthal D, Causino N, Chang YC, et al. The duration of ambulatory visits to physicians. *J Fam Pract*. 1999;48:264-271.

11

NSAIDs That Are Selective Inhibitors of COX-2

The Molecular Basis for COX Inhibition

Recognition that inhibition of prostaglandin synthesis by aspirin and other nonsteroidal drugs (NSAIDs) resulted in analgesic, anti-inflammatory, and antipyretic effects was followed by recognition that inhibition of the enzyme cyclooxygenase (COX) was responsible also for the adverse effects of these drugs. As discussed below, it became apparent that two isoforms of COX existed and that it was possible pharmacologically to inhibit the inducible COX isoform, whose activity results in signs of inflammation, without inhibiting the constitutive isoform, the absence of whose activity can be associated with serious and even fatal adverse effects.

COX, which is also called prostaglandin (PG) H-synthase, catalyzes conversion of arachidonic acid to PGG_2 and then to PGH_2.[1-4] Activities of a variety of other specific enzymes then produce a spectrum of arachidonic acid metabolites, including platelet-derived thromboxane (TBX) A_2, endothelial cell-derived prostacyclin (PGI_2), and prostaglandins. Discovery in the late 1980s that COX expression in fibroblasts and monocytes could be markedly stimulated by interleukin-1 (IL-1) and inhibited by corticosteroids[5,6] was of singular importance insofar as it had been previously thought that the level of prostaglandin production was determined only by availability of the substrate, arachidonic acid. The above observations led to identification of two distinct COX isoforms, one constitutive and the other inducible.

Separate genes for the two enzymes have since been cloned and the regulation and expression of the two proteins clarified, providing insight into their distinct biologic roles.[5] The genes for the two isoforms are approximately 65% homologous in their coding regions.[7,8] Hence the proteins are similar with respect to their enzymatic activities and substrate specificities. However, crystallographic analysis has elucidated an important difference between COX-1 and COX-2 with respect to the configuration of the long hydrophobic channel that runs from the membrane-binding surface of the enzyme to its active site, deep in the interior of the molecule (**Color Plate 20**). In COX-2, the channel has a somewhat larger orifice than in COX-1 and a side pocket, pointing away from the catalytic site. Arachidonic acid released from damaged membranes adjacent to the opening of the channel is taken in and twisted around the hairpin bend of the channel, where two oxygens are inserted and a free radical extracted, generating a prostaglandin molecule.[9]

The difference between COX-1 and COX-2 is due to the existence of a single amino acid substitution at position 523, ie, at a site adjacent to arginine 120, which is present midway down the channel in both isoforms and is involved in the reversible hydrogen bonding of NSAIDs to COX.[8,10] Serine 530, the site of acetylation of the enzyme by aspirin, lies along the wall of the channel near tyrosine 385 (**Color Plate 20**), a residue implicated in COX catalytic activity. Acetylation of serine 530 by aspirin irreversibly inactivates the enzyme.[11-13]

The amino acid difference at position 523, with the isoleucine in COX-1 replaced by valine in COX-2, leaves a gap in the wall of the COX-2 channel, providing access to a side pocket, which in COX-1 is blocked by the bulkier isoleucine (**Color Plates 20 and 21**).[10] Structural modification of an NSAID by addition of a sulfonyl, sulfone, or sulfonamide group provides a rigid side extension that can enter the COX-2 side pocket but is too bulky to fit within the COX-1 channel. On this basis, inhibitors have been developed that block the activity of COX-2 at concentrations that have only minimal effect on COX-1 (**Table 11.1**). The degree of selectivity of COX inhibitors has generally been determined by analyzing the products of the reactions catalyzed by each of the two COX isoforms in the presence of the drug. For example, estimates of COX-2 inhibition may be made by examining the effect of the drug on PGE_2 production by monocytes exposed to bacterial lipopolysaccharide; estimates of the magnitude of COX-1 inhibition are based on inhibition of the generation of TBX B_2 (the degradation product of platelet TBX A_2) during the clotting of whole blood. COX-2 selectivity is reflected by a ratio of

COX-2 IC_{50} to COX-1 IC_{50} <1. New COX-2 inhibitors (eg, meloxicam, nimesulide, celecoxib, and rofecoxib), which have marked COX-2 selectivity, have IC_{50} ratios ≤0.1.[14-16]

Although, as indicated, NSAIDs *inhibit* COX-1 and COX-2 in clinically relevant concentrations, it was recently found that a very high (≥100 μm) concentration of diclofenac *induced* COX-2 protein production and COX activity in a transformed monocyte/macrophage cell line and that the enzyme activity was relatively insensitive to inhibition by diclofenac and other NSAIDs. Furthermore, in contrast to typical COX-2 activity, it could be inhibited by acetaminophen (ACET). These findings raise the question whether treatment with diclofenac and perhaps other NSAIDs could result in enzymatically distinct COX-2 populations (? COX-3).[17]

Although the two COX isoforms described have considerable structural homology, they differ with respect to the source of their arachidonic acid substrate: COX-2 utilizes intracellular arachidonic acid, and COX-1, extracellular substrate.[18,19] Phospholipase A_2, which is produced by a variety of cells, generates extracellular arachidonic acid substrate for COX-1. Therefore, to the extent that substrate concentration is an important determinant of the arachidonic acid metabolites produced by COX-1, regulation of phospholipase may modulate COX-1 activity.

As discussed in Chapter 11, *Nonselective NSAIDs*, concerns relative to the gastroenteropathy associated with nonselective NSAIDs are likely to be reduced considerably by the availability of selective COX-2 inhibitors such as celecoxib and rofecoxib,[20-29] both of which appear to be comparable in efficacy to—although not more effective than—nonselective NSAIDs (which themselves are COX-2 inhibitors) (see below). The advantage of selective COX-2 inhibitors resides not in their ability to inhibit COX-2 but in their lack of inhibition of COX-1 when they are used in clinically effective doses. Endoscopic studies have shown that the incidence of gastric and duodenal ulcers due to either of these drugs is lower than that due to comparator nonselective NSAIDs and no greater than that due to placebo.[22-25] Of additional advantage for the patient at risk for gastrointestinal (GI) bleeding, selective COX-2 inhibitors do not affect platelet aggregation or bleeding time.

12

It should be noted, however, that in many cases of GI hemorrhage in NSAID users, the bleeding site cannot be identified, and the correlation between endoscopically identified gastric and duodenal ulcers and clinically significant GI hemorrhage, perforation, or obstruction is unclear. Whether the striking reduction in endoscopically identifiable mucosal lesions in subjects taking selective COX-2 inhibitors is accompanied by a corresponding decrease in clinically important adverse events was addressed in large GI safety studies, the Celecoxib Long-term Arthritis Safety Study (CLASS)[30] and the Vioxx Gastrointestinal Outcome Research (VIGOR)[31] trial, as discussed below.

Homeostatic vs Proinflammatory Actions of COX-1 and COX-2

COX-1 is the only isoform expressed in normal gastric mucosa and in the platelet. In the gastric antrum, PGE_2 and PGI_2, synthesized as a result of the action of COX-1, promote vasodilatation, thereby maintaining mucosal integrity.[32] In the kidney, COX-1 generates vasodilatory prostaglandins that maintain renal blood flow and glomerular filtration rate, especially in the face of systemic vasoconstriction.[33,34] In platelets, COX-1 is essential for production of $TBX A_2$, which is required for platelet aggregation.[35]

Based on the above, the concept arose that the major (if not only) function of COX-1 was to maintain homeostasis and promote specific physiologic activities. In contrast, while COX-2 was undetectable in most normal tissues,[1-4,36] when cells, such as macrophages and endothelial cells, were challenged with inflammatory mediators, COX-2 expression was rapidly induced. In animal models, COX-2 messenger ribonucleic acid (mRNA) and COX-2 protein (but not COX-1) were up-regulated at sites of inflammation and detectable prior to the sharp increase in local prostaglandin production and clinical manifestations of inflammation.[37] This suggested that COX-2 was an inducible enzyme that accounted for a local increase in production of arachidonic acid metabolites, which produced vasodilatation, edema, and pain—the classic features of inflammation.

The situation is more complex, however. Studies in animals have shown that COX-2 is expressed constitutively in

220

kidney[38,39] and brain[40,41] and can be induced not only by inflammation but also by *physiologic* stimuli in kidney,[38] brain,[42] ovary,[43] uterus,[44,45] cartilage,[46] and bone,[47,48] while COX-1, which is constitutively present at many sites and plays a protective role, is also inducible, eg, in the crypt cells of the small intestine after radiation injury,[49] and may play a role in regeneration and contribute to inflammation.[50] It is clear that the initial paradigm (ie, "good" COX, "bad" COX) is an oversimplification and that targeted pharmacologic inhibition of a selective COX-1 isoform may result in unexpected outcomes. Consideration of the role of COX-1 in several organ systems serves to emphasize this point (see below).

■ Renal Function

In the kidney, COX-1 is expressed in the vasculature, glomeruli, and collecting ducts. It produces vasodilating prostaglandins that maintain renal plasma flow and glomerular filtration rate, especially during states of angiotensin-induced systemic vasoconstriction.[33,34] Nonselective NSAIDs impair this COX-1 protective response and may result in renal ischemia, tissue damage, or even papillary necrosis.

COX-2 may also be important in maintaining renal function. COX-2 knockout mice exhibit severe disruption of renal organogenesis.[51,52] COX-2 is expressed in the interstitial cells of the medulla of the normal rabbit kidney[39] and in the macula densa and thick ascending loop of Henle of the normal rat kidney.[38] In the human kidney, it is expressed in the podocytes of the glomerulus and endothelial cells of arteries and veins.[53,54] Chronic salt deprivation increases COX-2 expression in the rat kidney, suggesting that the prostaglandins it generates act to increase sodium absorption in response to volume depletion.[38] In the rat, renal COX-2 is also up-regulated by administration of angiotensin converting enzyme inhibitors or by angiotensin II receptor antagonist, suggesting that the renin-angiotensin system exerts feedback inhibition of COX-2 expression. Angiotensin II appears to down-regulate renal COX-2 expression, while COX-2 appears to be involved in the increased production of renin in response to inhibition of angiotensin II production.

In normal humans, selective COX-2 inhibitors induce sodium retention. This effect is associated with a marked decrease in renal PGI_2 production, presumably in the renal vasculature, and is independent of any effect on renal hemodynamics. As a consequence, selective COX-2 inhibitors may cause edema and an increase in blood pressure. They do not differ from nonselective NSAIDs in this respect. Although in normal individuals, even the elderly, the glomerular filtration rate does not appear to depend on renal COX-2 activity,[55] this may not be true in those with intrinsic renal disease, hypertension, or volume depletion.

■ Gastrointestinal Tract

COX-1 is the only COX isoform in the gastric mucosa and protects the stomach from erosions and ulceration.[32,56] GI bleeding caused by nonselective NSAIDs appears to relate to their inhibition of COX-1 activity both in the platelet, increasing the tendency to bleed,[57,58] and in the gastric mucosa, increasing the likelihood of ulceration (**Table 12.1**).[32,59]

Because COX-2 is not present in normal gastric mucosa or the platelet, it might be expected that inhibition would impose no risk of gastric ulceration or bleeding. However, COX-2 is expressed in animal models with acute gastric erosion and ulceration and may play a role in facilitating ulcer healing.[60] Similarly, in humans, COX-2 is induced with gastric injury and can be demonstrated at the rim of gastric ulcers.[60] Furthermore, COX-2 inhibitors retard ulcer healing in animals.[61] Whether healing of NSAID-induced ulcers will be impaired in patients who are switched from a nonselective NSAID to a selective COX-2 inhibitor is uncertain. It has been suggested that the latter will increase the risk of major GI adverse effects by retarding the healing of ulcers induced by other stimuli, eg, *Helicobacter pylori* or concomitant aspirin use.

Can selective COX-2 inhibitors *cause* ulcers in predisposed individuals? Patients with erosions or a history of ulcer are more likely to develop ulcers than those without erosions or ulcer history, probably because of reactivation of damage at the site of the ulcer scar.[62,63] Because it is likely that COX-2 is induced in both of these situations, it remains to be shown that selective COX-2 inhibitors will not increase ulcer risk in these subgroups.

TABLE 12.1 — GI BLEEDING FROM NSAID-INDUCED ULCERS

Mechanism*	COX Isoform Inhibited	Consequence
Prostaglandin inhibition in the GI tract	COX-1	Endoscopically apparent ulceration
Thromboxane inhibition in the platelet	COX-1	Increased bleeding tendency

Abbreviations: COX, cyclooxygenase; GI, gastrointestinal; NSAID, nonsteroidal anti-inflammatory drug.

* In patients with ulcer bleeding, both mechanisms are operative.

Cryer B. Personal communication.

COX-2 may also play an important physiologic role in other parts of the GI tract. It appears that invasion by pathogenic microorganisms leads to COX-2 production by intestinal cells, where it catalyzes production of PGE_2, which, in turn, stimulates the fluxes of chloride and fluid involved in expelling the pathogen.[64] Furthermore, COX-2 levels are increased in inflammatory bowel disease, such as ulcerative colitis,[65] and selective inhibition of COX-2 has been shown to exacerbate inflammation in an animal model of colitis.[66] It remains to be seen whether selective COX-2 inhibitors are safe in humans with ulcerative colitis.

■ The Effects of Coxibs on Colonic Neoplasms

Recent work has delineated a role for COX-2 in development of progression of adenomatous polyps and carcinoma of the colon.[67-70] It has been suggested that COX-2 inhibition may be beneficial in these conditions. The protective effect does not appear to be unique to coxibs, but may occur also as with nonselective NSAIDs.

Sandler and colleagues[71] found that daily use of aspirin 325 mg/d significantly reduced the incidence of colorectal adenomas in patients who had a previous diagnosis of colorectal cancer. Baron and associates[72] also reported a modest reduction in the incidence of colorectal adenomas in patients who had a recent history of histologically documented adenomas with use of aspirin 81 mg/d (but not of aspirin 325 mg/d). Notably, the protective effect of aspirin was greater for advanced neoplasms (adenomas 1 cm in diameter or with villous or tubulovillous features, dysplasia, or invasiveness; relative risk for 81 mg/d = 0.59; 95%, 0.38-4.92). It is not clear why protection appears to be conferred by low-dose aspirin but that a high dose of celecoxib (800 mg/d) was required for a protective effect in patients with familial adenomatous polyposis (FAP)[73] and a high dose of sulindac (300 mg/d) for a similar effect in patients with FAP and sporadic colonic polyps.

■ Thrombosis

Maintenance of normal blood flow and generation of an appropriate thrombogenic response to injury require a delicate balance between the activities of TBX A_2 produced by platelets and PGI_2 from vascular endothelial cells (**Table 12.2**).

TABLE 12.2 — CYCLOOXYGENASE ACTIVITY AND THROMBOSIS

Activity	Platelet	Endothelial Cell
COX isoform	COX-1	COX-2
Active arachidonic acid metabolite	Thromboxane A_2	Prostacyclin
Function of isoform	Activates fibrinogen receptors; induces vasoconstriction	Inhibits platelet function; stimulates smooth muscle relaxation and vasodilation

Abbreviation: COX, cyclooxygenase.

12

Activated platelets generate TBX A_2 via the action of COX-1.[27,53,54] Platelet aggregation results in the release of TBX A_2, which then provides a substrate and stimulus for production by vascular endothelial cells of PGI_2,[58] a potent vasodilator that counteracts the vasoconstrictive action of TBX A_2.[3] It has been shown that shear stress induces COX-2 expression in endothelial cells, leading to production of substantial amounts of PGI_2 by these cells.[74,75] A substantial proportion of systemic PGI_2 production is derived from the action of COX-2.

In humans, PGI_2 production can be inhibited by selective COX-2 inhibitors.[55,76] Because nonselective NSAIDs inhibit both COX-1 and COX-2, their effect on prothrombotic and antithrombotic activities is presumably in balance. However, selective COX-2 inhibitors may limit production of PGI_2 by endothelial cells, while having no effect on TBX A_2 production by platelets. This could theoretically result in an imbalance favoring platelet aggregation and vasoconstriction, with an increase in the frequency of vascular occlusion. Whether this is a clinically important effect of selective COX-2 inhibition, especially in patients at risk for ischemic events, remains to be determined. The question is important, since deaths from cardiovascular disease far outnumber those from NSAID-induced gastropathy.

■ Neural Function

The febrile response appears to involve COX-2. IL-1ß and perhaps other cytokines induce COX-2 production by endothelial cells of the brain vasculature,[77] generating prostaglandins, that act on temperature-regulating neurons. In experimental models, selective COX-2 inhibitors have been shown to block the febrile response.[78]

Although the data are relatively sparse, nonselective COX inhibitors appear to have negative effects on cognitive function in the elderly.[79] It is unclear whether selective COX-2 inhibitors will alter cognitive function or other neurophysiologic responses.

It has also been suggested that COX-2 may play a role in the progression of Alzheimer's disease (AD).[41,80,81] The benefit of selective COX-2 inhibition in this condition is under study.

With the premise that inflammation plays a significant role in the AD process[82], a recent one-year multicenter randomized double-blind, placebo-controlled, parallel group trial involving 351 subjects with mild-to-moderate AD was conducted in which patients were treated with rofecoxib 25 mg/d, naproxen 220 mg/bid, or placebo. Notably, neither NSAID slowed the progression of decline as assessed by the Alzheimer Disease Assessment Scale-cognitive (ADAS-Cog) subscale score. Nor was persistent benefit seen with either active treatment in several secondary outcome measures (eg, measures of activities of daily living, quality of life, and time to institutionalization). On the other hand, fatigue, dizziness, and hypertension were more common in the active treatment groups.[83]

As pointed out in an editorial by Launer[84], the generalizability of these results is uncertain. It is possible, for example, that drugs that are not effective in patients who already have full-blown AD might be effective in individuals who do not yet have clinical evidence of the disease but are at high risk, such as those with a family history of AD.

12

■ **Ovarian and Uterine Function**

COX-2–mediated prostaglandin production is associated with parturition[85] and implicated also in ovulation, fertilization, and implantation.[86,87] COX-2 induction occurs immediately following the surge of luteinizing hormone[88] and seems necessary for production of the proteolytic enzymes required for rupture of the ovarian follicle.[85] Inhibition of follicular rupture may explain the infertility associated with NSAID use.[89,90]

■ **Fracture Healing**

Two recent articles that report a delay in bone healing in animals in the absence of COX-2 activity have provoked controversy over the use of COX-2 selective NSAIDs during fracture repair.[91,92] Several previous studies had shown that administration of nonselective NSAIDs inhibited skeletal repair in various animal models of fracture healing.

The clinical implications of these studies are uncertain. As pointed out by Einhorn[93], the timing of administration of the COX-2 inhibitor may be important. In animal models, if drug administration was not continued throughout the first 3 weeks after the fracture, healing at 5 weeks was no different in rats that had been given a COX-2 inhibitor than in untreated controls, suggesting that the effects of inhibition are quickly reversed upon resumption of normal prostaglandin synthesis.

In humans, the data are sparse. However, in a single-center retrospective analysis of patients who had undergone spinal fusion, administration of the nonselective NSAID ketorolac increased the incidence of nonunion in a dose-dependent fashion.[94] On the other hand, analgesic doses of rofecoxib had no effect on the rate on nonunion in patients who underwent spinal fusion.[95] Although it has been known for years that NSAIDs inhibit heterotopic bone formation in patients undergoing total hip arthroplasty or in those with a pelvic fracture, they do not seem to interfere with the healing of pelvic fractures. It should be emphasized that the doses of NSAID (or coxib) used in animal studies such as those described are often much higher, on an mg/kg basis, than those used in humans and that randomized prospective controlled clinical trials do not exist to help answer the question. At present, if an NSAID is used for analgesia (eg, rather than an opioid) during a period in which bone healing is required, it may be reasonable to recommend that it be given for a relatively short period (<2 weeks) and perhaps not be administered to patients who have a condition that might impair fracture healing (eg, osteoporosis, glucocorticoid use).

The CLASS and VIGOR GI Safety Trials

Results of two major large-size GI safety studies, conducted by the manufacturers of celecoxib and rofecoxib, have been published—the CLASS trial[30] and the VIGOR study.[31] Both of these studies were designed to ascertain whether treatment with a coxib results in a lower incidence of clinically important NSAID-associated ulcers and ulcer complications than that seen with nonselective NSAIDs. It should be noted that the experimental designs of the CLASS and VIGOR studies differed in some important respects (**Table 12.3**).

In the VIGOR trial, a 50% to 60% reduction in the incidence of upper GI events was apparent in the rofecoxib treatment arm in comparison with the naproxen arm, providing clear evidence of a gastroprotective effect of rofecoxib (**Table 12.4**).

In the CLASS study, the difference between the annualized incidence rates of upper GI ulcer complications (the primary outcome measure) with celecoxib and comparator nonselective NSAIDs was not statistically significant. For ulcer complications combined with symptomatic ulcers, however, the difference was significant (2.08% vs 3.54%, respectively, $P = 0.02$). Among non-aspirin users, results over the first 6 months showed a significant reduction in ulcer complications with celecoxib, mimicking the results obtained with rofecoxib in the VIGOR trial (**Figure 12.1**). However, use of low-dose aspirin appeared to mitigate the gastroprotective effect of celecoxib. Furthermore, although only 22% of subjects in the CLASS study were taking low-dose aspirin, as many as 60% of OA patients over the age of 60 may do so in clinical practice.

It must be noted that the major publication describing the results of the CLASS trial[30] presented the data for only the first 6 months of treatment, although results were available for longer periods. In non-aspirin users, no significant difference between treatment groups was apparent with respect to the incidence of ulcer complications in patients treated for 12 months—ie, the superiority of celecoxib over the comparator NSAIDs observed during the first 6 months of treatment was not apparent in those who remained on treatment thereafter (**Figure 12.2**).

In addition, although the publication of the CLASS study reported the comparative incidence rates of two main outcome measures (upper GI ulcer complications and symptomatic ulcers) during the first 6 months of treatment in a three-arm trial comparing celecoxib with ibuprofen and diclofenac, the paper actually referred to a combined analysis of the results of two separate and longer trials, whose protocols differed from those in the published paper with respect to design, outcomes, duration of follow-up, and analysis. Specifically, two comparisons were originally planned: celecoxib vs ibuprofen and celecoxib vs diclofenac. Because the FDA was concerned that coxibs might interfere with ulcer healing, leading to a long-term increase in ulcer-related complications, the prespecified primary out-

12

TABLE 12.3 — COMPARISON OF STUDY DESIGNS FOR CELECOXIB (CLASS) AND ROFECOXIB (VIGOR) GI OUTCOMES TRIALS

Parameter	CLASS[30] Trial	VIGOR[31] Trial
Number of subjects	7982	8076
Mean age	~60 years; ~38% older than 65 years	~58 years
Underlying disease	Osteoarthritis 73%; rheumatoid arthritis 27%	Rheumatoid arthritis
Duration of follow-up	Median, 9 months; maximum, 13 months	Median, 9 months; maximum 13 months
Type of analysis	Excludes events on day 0-2 and >6 months	Intention to treat (includes events within 14 days of last dose of study drug)
Dose of coxib	Celecoxib 400 mg/d	Rofecoxib 50 mg/d
Comparator NSAID	Ibuprofen 2400 mg/d or diclofenac 150 mg/d	Naproxen 1000 mg/d
Low-dose aspirin	22%	Not permitted

Concurrent steroid use	30%	56%
Primary end point	Complicated ulcers	Clinical upper GI events
Secondary end point	Symptomatic + complicated ulcers	Complicated upper GI events

Abbreviations: CLASS, Celecoxib Long-term Arthritis Safety Study; GI, gastrointestinal; NSAID, nonsteroidal anti-inflammatory drug; VIGOR, Vioxx Gastrointestinal Outcome Research.

[30]Silverstein FE, et al. *JAMA.* 2000;284:1247-1255; [31]Bombardier C, et al. *N Engl J Med.* 2000;343:1520-1528.

TABLE 12.4 — SUMMARY OF GI EVENTS IN THE VIGOR TRIAL

End Points	Rofecoxib (%) (n = 4047)	Naproxen (%) (n = 4029)	Relative Risk	Risk Reduction (%)	P Value
Clinical upper GI events	2.1	4.5	.46	54	P <0.001
Complicated upper GI events	.6	1.4	.43	57	P = 0.005
Any GI bleeding	1.2	3.0	.38	62	P <0.001

Abbreviations: GI, gastrointestinal; VIGOR, Vioxx Gastrointestinal Outcome Research.

Bombardier C, et al. *N Engl J Med.* 2000;343:1520-1528.

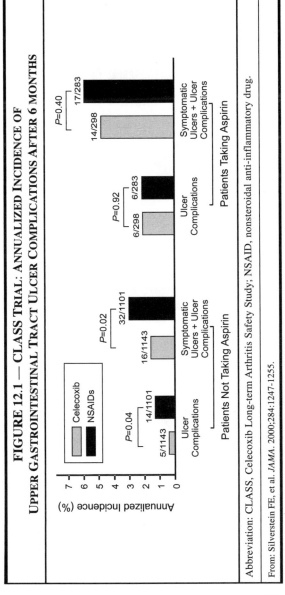

FIGURE 12.1 — CLASS TRIAL: ANNUALIZED INCIDENCE OF UPPER GASTROINTESTINAL TRACT ULCER COMPLICATIONS AFTER 6 MONTHS

Abbreviation: CLASS, Celecoxib Long-term Arthritis Safety Study; NSAID, nonsteroidal anti-inflammatory drug.

From: Silverstein FE, et al. *JAMA.* 2000;284:1247-1255.

12

233

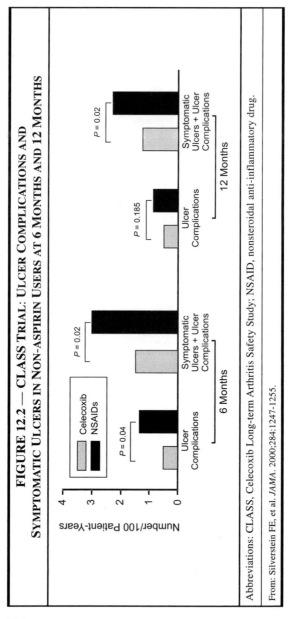

FIGURE 12.2 — CLASS TRIAL: ULCER COMPLICATIONS AND SYMPTOMATIC ULCERS IN NON-ASPIRIN USERS AT 6 MONTHS AND 12 MONTHS

Abbreviations: CLASS, Celecoxib Long-term Arthritis Safety Study; NSAID, nonsteroidal anti-inflammatory drug.

From: Silverstein FE, et al. *JAMA*. 2000;284:1247-1255.

come measure was ulcer complications (not symptomatic ulcers) in both of these trials, whose maximum duration of follow-up was 15 months and 12 months, respectively.

When the results of those studies were analyzed, the incidence of ulcer complications in all treatment groups was similar. Almost all of the ulcer complications that occurred during the second half of the trial (and were not reported in the publication) occurred in the celecoxib treatment group. These results, which were available when the manuscript was published but were not referred to in the article, contradict the published conclusions.[96]

Treatment With a Coxib vs Cotherapy With a Proton Pump Inhibitor and NSAID

Proton pump inhibitors (PPIs) have been shown to prevent NSAID-related gastroduodenal ulcers and to accelerate the healing of NSAID-induced gastric ulcers in the presence of continued NSAID use.[97,98] Furthermore, omeprazole has been shown to prevent the recurrence of gastroduodenal ulcers in arthritis patients and to permit the healing of ulcers in patients in whom NSAID therapy was continued.[63] When the efficacy of omeprazole 20 mg/d was compared with that of misoprostol 200 mg/bid for prevention of recurrent ulcers in patients with rheumatoid arthritis (RA) on NSAID therapy, only 3% of patients treated with omeprazole but 12% and 10%, respectively, of those treated with placebo or misoprostol developed a duodenal ulcer. Gastric ulcer recurred in 32%, 10%, and 13%, respectively, of patients receiving placebo, misoprostol, or omeprazole.[62]

How do coxibs compare with a PPI for prevention of recurrent ulcer bleeding? In a 6-month, double-blind trial in which patients with various types of arthritis who had ulcer bleeding and who tested negative for *H pylori* were randomized to treatment with celecoxib 200 mg/bid or with diclofenac 75 mg bid plus omeprazole 20 mg/d after healing of their ulcers, the annualized rate of recurrent bleeding was 9% with celecoxib and about 11% with the combination of diclofenac and PPI.[99] Although the number of patients in the above study was relatively small, increasing the possibility of a type 2 error (a false-negative result), and diclofenac appears to be a relatively safe nonselective

NSAID, these data indicate that *neither* treatment provided a very impressive level of protection from recurrent ulcer bleeding in these high-risk patients.

It is notable that the above study restricted enrollment to *H pylori*–negative patients. Because of the high likelihood of confounding ulcer disease and ulcer complications in *H pylori*–infected patients, Graham[100] has emphasized the importance of eradicating *H pylori* infection in studies of ulcers and ulcer complications associated with nonselective NSAIDs, coxibs, and aspirin. In any event, results from the Hong Kong group[99] raise questions about the magnitude of reduction of the risk of NSAID-associated ulcer complications with long-term use of coxibs or of a nonselective NSAID with PPI cotherapy.

Do COX-1–Sparing NSAIDs Increase the Risk of Thrombosis?

Analysis of the data from the VIGOR study revealed an unanticipated result: the incidence of myocardial infarction (MI) was four times greater among subjects treated with rofecoxib than among those treated with naproxen (**Table 12.5**). Although the total number of subjects who experienced an MI during the trial was low and the study was not powered to detect a significant difference in incidence of an MI between treatment groups, this observation raised significant concerns about possible detrimental cardiovascular effects of COX-1–sparing NSAIDs.

Nearly 40% of the MIs in the VIGOR study occurred in the 4% of subjects who had a cardiovascular indication for use of low-dose aspirin but were not taking aspirin. Dalen,[101] in a recent editorial accompanying three case-control studies,[102-106] supported the view that the increased incidence of MI in the rofecoxib treatment arm of the VIGOR trial, relative to the naproxen arm, may have been attributable to an antithrombotic effect of naproxen rather than to a detrimental effect of rofecoxib. However, in a large cohort study comparing more than 181,000 NSAIDs users and a comparable number of controls,[105] the incidence of coronary heart disease, acute MI, and death attributed to coronary heart disease in patients using NSAIDs was compa-

TABLE 12.5 — INCIDENCE OF MYOCARDIAL INFARCTION IN THE VIGOR TRIAL			
Event	Rofecoxib (%) (n = 4047)	Naproxen (%) (n = 4029)	Difference (95% CI)
All deaths	0.5	0.4	0.1 (-0.15–0.49)
Cardiovascular deaths	0.2	0.2	0.0 (-0.21–0.212)
Myocardial infarctions	0.4	0.1	0.3 (0.07–0.57)
Cerebrovascular accidents	0.2	0.2	0.0 (-0.17–0.27)

Abbreviation: CI, confidence interval; VIGOR, Vioxx Gastrointestinal Outcome Research.

Bombardier C. et al. *N Engl J Med.* 2000;343:1520-1528.

12

rable to that in age- and sex-matched controls who were not taking NSAIDs, and the incidence of coronary heart disease was the same in patients taking naproxen as in those not taking an NSAID. Although it has been contended that these results argue *against* a meaningful protective effect of naproxen, no information was available on the prevalence of over-the-counter aspirin use in this study.

In another recent retrospective cohort study involving more than 450,000 patients taking ibuprofen, naproxen, celecoxib, or rofecoxib (with the latter group broken down into those taking ≤ and ≥25 mg/day), the same group of investigators found that the incidence of hospital admission for MI or death from coronary heart disease was similar across each treatment group except for the high-dose rofecoxib group, in which the risk was increased by 70% ($P = 0.058$). Among new users of these drugs, the risk of serious coronary heart disease was nearly twice as great in the high-dose rofecoxib as in the other groups ($P = 0.02$). On this basis, the authors concluded that long-term use of rofecoxib in a dose ≥25 mg/day should be avoided.[107]

Indirectly supporting the possibility that COX-2 inhibition may have a prothrombotic effect by altering the balance between prostacyclin and thromboxane, Hennan and colleagues[106] showed that the aspirin-induced increase in time to occlusion in a canine coronary thrombosis model was abolished by administration of celecoxib. Furthermore, Cheng and associates[108] showed that transgenic knockout mice in which the prostaglandin receptor had been deleted— a model that presumably mimics the clinical effect of treatment with a COX-2 selective inhibitor—exhibited an enhanced proliferative response to injury and increase in synthesis of TBX A_2, suggesting that prostaglandin I_2 modulates the platelet-vessel wall interaction *in vivo* and has a beneficial effect by limiting the response of blood vessels to TBX A_2.

Jüni and colleagues[96] have also presented arguments against the likelihood that the increased incidence of MI in the rofecoxib arm of the VIGOR trial was due to a cardioprotective effect of naproxen. In a meta-analysis of the three case control studies cited,[102-104] they found that naproxen users were 0.81 times as likely to experience an MI as patients taking other agents (95% CI = 0.72 – 0.92), whereas patients in the naproxen arm of the VIGOR trial were only 0.20 times as likely to experience an MI as those receiving rofecoxib (95% CI = 0.07 – 0.58).[109] Any cardio-protective effect of naproxen suggested by the case-control studies, therefore, does not fully explain the increased risk of MI associated with rofecoxib in the VIGOR trial.

A recent meta-analysis of 23 clinical trials that compared rofecoxib with traditional NSAIDs or placebo revealed no increase of thrombotic events with rofecoxib relative to placebo (relative risk = 0.84; 95% CI = 0.51 – 1.38),[110] but was underpowered and most of the patients in these trials were at low risk for MI. This is in contrast to patients in the VIGOR trial, all of whom had RA, a disease that, as noted earlier, is associated with an increase in cardiovascular risk factors.[111]

Because the risk of MI is twice as great in RA as in osteoarthritis (OA), it is important to note that the VIGOR trial enrolled only patients with RA and, therefore, may have provided a more sensitive model for detection of thrombo-genic effects of selective COX-2 inhibition than clinical trials in patients with OA. However, because no information was provided with respect to the prevalence of risk factors for MI (**Table 12.6**) in the two treatment groups in the VIGOR trial, it is difficult to interpret the suggestion of an increased risk of thrombosis among patients with arthritis taking a COX-1–sparing NSAID. Also, the doses of coxibs employed in the CLASS and VIGOR studies were much higher than those used in treatment of OA, providing yet another basis for uncertainty about the relevance of the find-

---

TABLE 12.6 — RISK FACTORS FOR MYOCARDIAL INFARCTION

- Increased age
- Diabetes mellitus
- Hypercholesterolemia
- Prior thrombotic event
- Family history
- Hypertension
- Obesity
- Smoking

ings to treatment of patients in clinical practice. Nonetheless, the Food and Drug Administration has recently approved revision of the package insert for rofecoxib, which now recommends that caution be exercised when this drug is used in patients with a history of ischemic heart disease.

Other Adverse Effects of Coxibs

Coxibs are no less likely than nonselective NSAIDs to cause salt and water retention, hypertension, edema, and congestive heart failure, or to impair fracture healing. Nor are they free of nonspecific GI adverse effects, such as epigastric pain, dyspepsia, nausea, vomiting, and diarrhea, the incidence of which appears to be only slightly lower with coxibs than with nonselective COX inhibitors.[112]

In an analysis of eight published double-blind randomized trials (which varied among themselves with respect to treatment duration, comparator NSAIDs, and inclusion of a placebo group), the cumulative incidence of nonspecific GI adverse events (eg, dyspepsia) was modestly lower with rofecoxib than with nonselective NSAIDs over a 6-month treatment period (23.5% vs 25.5%, $P = 0.02$). However, the incidence thereafter was no better than that with nonselective NSAIDs.[113] Celecoxib and nonselective NSAIDs were both associated with more abdominal pain, dyspepsia, and diarrhea than placebo. However, use of celecoxib was accompanied by less abdominal pain than that with ibuprofen, diclofenac, or naproxen, and less dyspepsia than with naproxen. In general, nonspecific GI symptoms caused by rofecoxib did not differ from those caused by placebo or the comparator nonselective NSAID, except that diarrhea was more common with diclofenac than with rofecoxib.[112]

Although Geba and associates[114] reported recently that nonspecific GI adverse effects were as frequent in patients with knee OA who were treated with celecoxib or rofecoxib as in those treated with ACET, the significance of that observation is uncertain because of the lack of inclusion of a placebo control group.

An economic assessment of celecoxib and rofecoxib, sponsored by the Canadian Coordinating Office of Health Technology Assessment (CCOHTA) has recently been published.[115] Clinical benefits and cost-effectiveness of coxibs were compared with those of standard NSAIDs in patients with OA or RA who did not require treatment with low-dose aspirin. Data for GI risk and cardiovascular risk were obtained from the VIGOR and CLASS studies. The analysis considered patients at average risk and at high risk (ie, those with a history of a prior upper GI adverse event).

An attempt was made in the CCOHTA analysis to overcome the problems associated with the availability of only relatively short-term data from random controlled trials and to project cost utility over a 5-year period of treatment. The results, expressed as cost per quality-adjusted life year (QALY) gained relative to the age of the patient, are shown in **Figure 12.3**.

For subjects who had no risk factors (other than age), the cost per QALY gained did not fall below $50,000. The cost per QALY fell considerably, however, as additional risk factors were added into the analysis. Data for celecoxib were similar to those for rofecoxib.[116] The limitations of the CCOHTA study included the absence of an ACET comparator and of an analysis of indirect costs, eg, work disability. On the other hand, the CCOHTA analysis considered coxib-associated cardiovascular events, based on the data from the VIGOR study, that suggest a 4-fold increase in the risk of MI with rofecoxib in comparison with naproxen. However, it should be noted that the VIGOR study was conducted exclusively in patients with RA—in whom the risk of MI is approximately twice as great as in patients with OA—and employed a rofecoxib dose of 50 mg/d, ie, two to four times higher than the dose approved for treatment of OA.

The CCOHTA analysis concluded that rofecoxib and celecoxib were economically attractive in patients at high risk for an upper GI event if they use a nonselective NSAID and, specifically, in the elderly, but not in patients at average risk. Co-prescription of PPIs with nonselective NSAIDs was not economically attractive even among patients at high

241

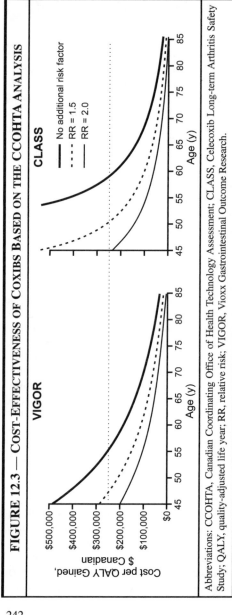

FIGURE 12.3 — COST-EFFECTIVENESS OF COXIBS BASED ON THE CCOHTA ANALYSIS

Abbreviations: CCOHTA, Canadian Coordinating Office of Health Technology Assessment; CLASS, Celecoxib Long-term Arthritis Safety Study; QALY, quality-adjusted life year; RR, relative risk; VIGOR, Vioxx Gastrointestinal Outcome Research.

Results of sensitivity analysis of the VIGOR Study (*left panel*) and CLASS study (*right panel*). (See text.)

Brandt KD, et al. *J Clin Rheum.* 2003;9(suppl):S1-S39; Silverstein FE, et al. *JAMA.* 2000;284:1247-1255; and Bombardier C, et al. *N Engl J Med.* 2000;343:1520-1528.

risk for a serious upper GI event and insufficient evidence existed to assess the economic advantages of a coxib in patients taking concomitant low-dose aspirin.

Until recently, none of the pharmacoeconomic studies have provided comparisons with ACET in patients with OA. Mandl and colleagues,[117] however, have reported a preliminary analysis of a variety of strategies for treatment of knee OA, based on guidelines of the American College of Rheumatology (ACR). Their results support the ACR recommendation that ACET should be the initial pharmacologic agent for treatment of OA and suggest that for patients in whom ACET is not effective, in the absence of a high risk for a GI bleed, a nonselective NSAID should be tried before adding a gastroprotective drug (specifically, misoprostol, in their analysis) or switching to a COX-2–selective NSAID.

REFERENCES

1. Dubois RN, Abramson SB, Crofford L, et al. Cyclooxygenase in biology and disease. *FASEB J.* 1998;12:1063-1073.

2. Vane JR. Inhibition of prostaglandin synthesis as a mechanism of action for the aspirin-like drugs. *Nat New Biol.* 1971;231:232-235.

3. Davies P, Bailey PJ, Goldenberg MM, Ford-Hutchinson AW. The role of arachidonic oxygenation products in pain and inflammation. *Annu Rev Immunol.* 1984;2:335-357.

4. Vane JR, Botting RM. Mechanism of action of aspirin-like drugs. *Semin Arthritis Rheum.* 1997;26:2-10.

5. Raz A, Wyche A, Needleman P. Temporal and pharmacological division of fibroblast cyclooxygenase expression into transcriptional and translational phases. *Proc Natl Acad Sci (USA).* 1989;86:1657-1661.

6. Fu YJ, Masferrer JL, Seibert K, Raz A, Needleman P. The induction and suppression of prostaglandin H_2 synthase (cyclooxygenase) in human monocytes. *J Biol Chem.* 1990;265:16737-16740.

7. Picot D, Loll PJ, Garavito M. The x-ray crystal structure of the membrane protein prostaglandin H2 synthase-1. *Nature.* 1994;367:243-249.

8. Luong C, Miller A, Barnett J, Chow J, Ramesha C, Browner MF. Flexibility of the NSAID binding site in the structure of human cyclooxygenase-2. *Nature Struct Biol.* 1996;3:927-933.

9. Hawkey CJ. Cox-2 inhibitors. *Lancet.* 1999;353:307-314.

12

10. Gierse JL, McDonald JJ, Hauser SO, Rangwala SH, Roboldt CM, Siebert K. A single amino acid difference between cyclooxygenase-1 (COX-1) and -2 (COX-2) reverses the selectivity of COX-2 specific inhibitors. *J Biol Chem.* 1996;271:15810-15814.

11. Smith WL, Eling TE, Kulmacz RJ, Marnett LJ, Tsai A. Tyrosyl radicals and their role in hydroperoxide-dependent activation and inactivation of prostaglandin endoperoxide synthase. *Biochemistry.* 1992; 31:3-7

12. Ruf HH, Raab-Brill U, Blau C. A model for the catalytic mechanism of prostaglandin endoperoxide synthase. *Biochem Soc Trans.* 1993; 21:739-744.

13. Shimokawa T, Smith WL. Prostaglandin endoperoxide synthase. The aspirin acetylation region. *J Biol Chem.* 1992;267:12387-12392.

14. Feldman M, McMahon AT. Do cyclooxygenase-2 inhibitors provide benefits similar to those of traditional nonsteroidal anti-inflammatory drugs, with less gastrointestinal toxicity? *Ann Intern Med.* 2000;132: 134-143.

15. Picot D, Loll PJ, Garavito RM. The x-ray crystal structure of the membrane protein prostaglandin H$_2$ synthase-1. *Nature. 1994;367:243-249.*

16. Kurumbail RG, Stevens Am, Gierse JK, et al. Structural basis for selective inhibition of cyclooxygenase-2 by antiinflammatory agents. *Nature.* 1996;384:644-648.

17. Simmons DL, Botting RM, Robertson PM, Madson ML, Vane JR. Induction of an acetaminophen-sensitive cyclooxygenase with reduced sensitivity to nonsteroid antiinflammatory drugs. *Proc Natl Acad Sci (USA).* 1999;96:3275-3280.

18. Murakami M, Matsumoto R, Austen KF, Arm JP. Prostaglandin endoperoxide synthase-1 and -2 couple to different transmembrane stimuli to generate prostaglandin D2 in mouse bone marrow-derived mast cells. *J Biol Chem.* 1994;269:22269-22275.

19. Kawata R, Reddy ST, Wolner B, Herschman HR. Prostaglandin synthase I and prostaglandin synthase 2 both participate in activation-induced prostaglandin D2 production in mast cell. *J Immunol.* 1995;155:818-825.

20. Silas S, Clegg DO. Selective COX-2 inhibition. *Bull Rheum Dis.* 1999;48:1-4.

21. Simon LS, Lanza FL, Lipsky PE, et al. Preliminary study of the safety and efficacy of SC-58635, a novel cyclooxygenase 2 inhibitor: efficacy and safety in two placebo-controlled trials in osteoarthritis and rheumatoid arthritis, and studies of gastrointestinal and platelet effects. *Arthritis Rheum.* 1998;41:1591-1602.

22. Lanza FL, Rack MF, Callison DA, et al. A pilot endoscopic study of the gastroduodenal effects of SC-58635, a novel COX-2-selective inhibitor. *Gastroenterology.* 1997;112(suppl 4):A194. Abstract

23. Geiss GS, Hubbard RC, Callison DA, Yu S, Zhao W. Safety and efficacy of celecoxib, a specific COX-2 inhibitor. *Rheumatol Eur.* 1998;27(suppl 1):118. Abstract.

24. Geiss GS, Stead H, Morant SV, Nandin R, Hubbard RC. Endoscopic and tolerability, results from a study of celecoxib, a specific COX-2 inhibitor, in patients with rheumatoid arthritis. *Rheumatol Eur.* 1998:27(suppl 1):118. Abstract

25. Smolen J. Clinical trials of COX-2 inhibitors. In: Vane J, ed. *The Promise of Specific COX-2 Inhibition by Novel Agents.* London: William Harvey Press; 1998:21.

26. Hubbard R, Geis GS, Woods E, Yu S, Zhao W. Efficacy, tolerability, and safety of celecoxib, a specific COX-2 inhibitor. *Arthritis Rheum.* 1998;41(suppl 9):S196. Abstract.

27. Celecoxib for arthritis. *Med Lett Drugs Ther.* 1999;41:11-12.

28. Cannon G, Caldwell J, Holt P, et al for the MK-0966 Phase III Protocol 035 Study Group. MK-0966, a specific COX-2 inhibitor, has clinical efficacy comparable to diclofenac in the treatment of knee and hip osteoarthritis in a 26-week controlled clinical trial. *Arthritis Rheum.* 1998;41(suppl 9):S196. Abstract.

29. Saag K, Fisher C, McKay J, et al for the MK-0966 Phase III Protocol 033 Study Group. MK-0966, a specific COX-2 inhibitor, has clinical efficacy comparable to ibuprofen in the treatment of knee and hip osteoarthritis in a 6-week controlled clinical trial. *Arthritis Rheum.* 1998;41(suppl 9):S196. Abstract.

30. Silverstein FE, Faich G, Goldstein JL, et al. Gastrointestinal toxicity with celecoxib vs nonsteroidal anti-inflammatory drugs for osteoarthritis and rheumatoid arthritis: the CLASS study: A randomized controlled trial. Celecoxib Long-term Arthritis Safety Study. *JAMA.* 2000;284:1247-1255.

31. Bombardier C, Laine L, Reicin A, et al. Comparison of upper gastrointestinal toxicity of rofecoxib and naproxen in patients with rheumatoid arthritis. VIGOR Study Group. *N Engl J Med.* 2000;343:1520-1528.

32. Scheiman JM. NSAIDs gastrointestinal injury, and cytoprotection. *Gastroenterol Clin North Am.* 1996;25:279-298.

33. Zambraski EJ. The effects of nonsteroidal anti-inflammatory drugs on renal function: experimental studies in animals. *Semin Nephrol.* 1995;15:205-213.

12

34. Breyer MD, Jacobson HR, Breyer RM. Functional and molecular aspects of renal prostaglandin receptors. *J Am Soc Nephrol.* 1996;7:8-17.

35. Burch JW, Stanford N, Majerus PW. Inhibition of platelet prostaglandin synthetase by oral aspirin. *J Clin Invest.* 1978;61:314-319.

36. Crofford LJ. COX-1 and COX-2 tissue expression: implications and predictions. *J Rheumatol.* 1997;24(suppl 49):15-19.

37. Anderson GD, Hauser SD, Bremer ME, McGarity KL, Isakson PC, Gregory SA. Selective inhibition of cyclo-oxygenase-2 reverses inflammation and expression of COX-2 and IL-6 in rat adjuvant arthritis. *J Clin Invest.* 1998;97:2672-2679.

38. Harris RC, McKanna JA, Akai Y, Jacobson HR, Dubois RN, Breyer MD. Cyclo-oxygenase-2 is associated with the macula densa of rat kidney and increases with salt restriction. *J Clin Invest.* 1994; 94:2504-2510.

39. Guan Y, Chang M, Cho W, et al. Cloning, expression, and regulation of rabbit cyclooxygenase-2 in renal medullary interstitial cells. *Am J Physiol.* 1997;273:F18-F26.

40. Kaufmann WE, Worley PF, Pegg J, Bremer M, Isakson P. COX-2, a synaptically induced enzyme, is expressed by excitatory neurons at postsynaptic sites in rat cerebral cortex. *Proc Natl Acad Sci (USA).* 1996;93:2317-2321.

41. Tocco G, Freire-Moar J, Schreiber SS, Sakhi SH, Aisen PS, Pasinetti GM. Maturational regulation and regional induction of cyclooxygenase-2 in rat brain: implications for Alzheimer's disease. *Exp Neurol.* 1997;144:339-349.

42. Miettinen S, Fusco FR, Yrjanheikki J, et al. Spreading depression and focal brain ischemia induce cyclooxygenase-2 in cortical neurons through N-methyl-D-aspartic acid-receptors and phospholipase A2. *Proc Natl Acad Sci.* (USA). 1997;94:6500-6505.

43. Narko K, Ritvos O, Ristimaki A. Induction of cyclooxygenase-2 and prostaglandin F2alpha receptor expression by interleukin-1 beta in cultured human granulosa-luteal cells. *Endocrinology.* 1997;138:3638-3644.

44. Chakraborty I, Das SK, Wang J, Dey SK. Developmental expression of the cyclo-oxygenase-1 and cyclo-oxygenase-2 genes in the peri-implantation mouse uterus and their differential regulation by the blastocyst and ovarian steroids. *J Mol Endocrinol.* 1996;16:107-122.

45. Yang ZM, Das SK, Wang J, Sugimoto Y, Ichikawa A, Dey SK. Potential sites of prostaglandin actions in the periimplantation mouse uterus: differential expression and regulation of prostaglandin receptor genes. *Biol Reprod.* 1997;56:368-379.

46. Amin AR, Attur M, Patel RN, et al. Superinduction of cyclooxygenase-2 activity in human osteoarthritis-affected cartilage. Influence of nitric oxide. *J Clin Invest.* 1997;99:1231-1237.

47. Tai H, Miyaura C, Pilbeam CC, et al. Transcriptional induction of cyclooxygenase-2 in osteoblasts is involved in interleukin-6-induced osteoclast formation. *Endocrinology.* 1997;138:2372-2379.

48. Onoe Y, Miyaura C, Kaminakayashiki T, et al. IL-13 and IL-4 inhibit bone resorption by suppressing cyclooxygenase-2-dependent prostaglandin synthesis in osteoblasts. *J Immunol.* 1996;156:758-764.

49. Cohn SM, Schloemann S, Tessner T, Seibert K, Stenson WF. Crypt stem cell survival in the mouse intestinal epithelium is regulated by prostaglandins synthesized through cyclooxygenase-1. *J Clin Invest.* 1997;99:1367-1379.

50. Langenbach R, Morham SG, Tirano HF, et al. Prostaglandin synthase 1 gene disruption in mice reduces arachidonic acid-induced inflammation and indomethacin-induced gastric ulceration. *Cell.* 1995; 83:483-492.

51. Dinchuk JE, Car BD, Focht RJ, et al. Renal abnormalities and an altered inflammatory response in mice lacking cyclooxygenase II. *Nature.* 1995;378:406-409.

52. Morham SG, Langenbach R, Loftin CD, et al. Prostaglandin synthase 2 gene disruption causes severe renal pathology in the mouse. *Cell.* 1995;83:473-482.

53. Komhoff M, Grone HJ, Klein T, Seyberth HW, Nusing RM. Localization of cyclooxygenase-1 and -2 in adult and fetal human kidney: Implication for renal function. *Am J Physiol.* 1997;272:F460-F468.

54. Khan KN, Venturini CM, Bunch RT, et al. Interspecies differences in renal localization of cyclooxygenase isoforms: implications in nonsteroidal antiinflammatory drug-related nephrotoxicity. *Toxicol Pathol.* 1998;26:612-620.

55. Catella-Lawson F, McAdam B, Morrison BW, et al. Effects of specific inhibition of cyclooxygenase 2 on sodium balance, hemodynamics, and vasoactive eicosanoids. *J Pharmacol Exp Ther.* 1999;289: 735-741.

56. Kargman S, Charleson S, Cartwright M, et al. Characterization of prostaglandin G/H Synthase 1 and 2 in rat, dog, monkey, and human gastrointestinal tracts. *Gastroenterology.* 1996;111:445-454.

57. Schafer AI. Effects of nonsteroidal antiinflammatory drugs on platelet function and systemic hemostasis. *J Clin Pharmacol.* 1995;35: 209-219.

58. Patrono C. Aspirin as an antiplatelet drug. *N Engl J Med.* 1994;330: 1287-1294.

12

59. Cryer B, Feldman M. Cyclooxygenase-1 and cyclooxygenase-2 selectivity of widely used nonsteroidal antiinflammatory drugs. *Am J Med*. 1998;104:413-421.

60. Mizuno H, Sakamoto C, Matsuda K, et al. Induction of cyclooxygenase 2 in gastric mucosal lesions and its inhibition by the specific antagonist delays healing in mice. *Gastroenterology*. 1997;112:387-397.

61. Schmassmann A, Peskar BM, Stettler C, et al. Effects of inhibition of prostaglandin endoperoxide synthase-2 in chronic gastro-intestinal ulcer models in rats. *Br J Pharmacol*. 1998;123:795-804.

62. Hawkey CJ, Karrasch JA, Szczepanski L, et al. Omeprazole compared with misoprostol for ulcers associated with nonsteroidal antiinflammatory drugs. Omeprazole versus Misoprostol for NSAID-induced Ulcer Management (OMNIUM) Study Group. *N Engl J Med*. 1998; 338:727-734.

63. Yeomans ND, Tulassay Z, Juhasz L, et al. A comparison of omeprazole with ranitidine for ulcers associated with nonsteroidal antiinflammatory drugs. Acid Suppression Trial: Ranitidine versus Omeprazole for NSAID-associated Ulcer Treatment (ASTRONAUT) Study Group. *N Engl J Med*. 1998;338:719-726.

64. Eckmann L, Stenson WF, Savidge TC, et al. Role of intestinal epithelial cells in the host secretory response to infection by invasive bacteria. Bacterial entry induces epithelial prostaglandin h synthase-2 expression and prostaglandin E2 and F2alpha production. *J Clin Invest*. 1997;100:296-309.

65. McLaughlin J, Seth R, Cole AT, Scott BB, Jenkins D, Hawkey CJ. Increased inducible cyclo-oxygenase associated with treatment failure in ulcerative colitis. *Gastroenterology*. 1966;110:A964.

66. Wallace JL, Keenan CM, Gale D, Shoupe TS. Exacerbation of experimental colitis by nonsteroidal anti-inflammatory drugs is not related to elevated leukotriene B4 synthesis. *Gastroenterology*. 1992; 102:18-27.

67. Oshima M, Dinchuk Je, Kargman SL, et al. Suppression of intestinal polyposis in Apc delta716 knockout mice by inhibition of cyclooxygenase 2 (COX-2). *Cell*. 1996;87:803-809.

68. Jacoby RF, Marshall DJ, Newton MA, et al. Chemoprevention of spontaneous intestinal adenomas in the Ape Min mouse model by the nonsteroidal anti-inflammatory drug piroxicam. *Cancer Res*. 1996;56:710-714.

69. Williams CS, Smalley W, DuBois RN. Aspirin use and potential mechanisms for colorectal cancer prevention. *J Clin Invest*. 1997; 100:1325-1329.

70. Sheng H, Shao J, Kirkland SC, et al. Inhibition of human colon cancer cell growth by selective inhibition of cyclooxygenase-2. *J Clin Invest*. 1997;99:2254-2259.

71. Sandler RS, Halabi S, Baron JA, et al. A randomized trial of aspirin to prevent colorectal adenomas in patients with previous colorectal cancer. *N Engl J Med*. 2003;348:883-890.

72. Baron JA, Cole BF, Sandler RS, et al. A randomized trial of aspirin to prevent colorectal adenomas. *N Engl J Med*. 2003;348:891-899.

73. Steinbach G, Lynch PM, Phillips RK, et al. The effect of celecoxib, a cyclooxygenase-2 inhibitor, in familial adenomatous polyposis. *N Engl J Med*. 2000;342:1946-1952.

74. Lim H, Dey SK. Prostaglandin E2 receptor subtype EP2 gene expression in the mouse uterus coincides with differentiation of the luminal epithelium for implantation. *Endocrinology*. 1997;138:4599-4606.

75. Topper JN, Cai J, Falb D, Gimbrone MA Jr. Identification of vascular endothelial genes differentially responsive to fluid mechanical stimuli: cyclooxygenases-2, manganese superoxide dismutase, and endothelial cell nitric oxide synthase are selectively up-regulated by steady laminar shear stress. *Proc Natl Acad Sci (USA)*. 1996; 93:10417-10422.

76. McAdam BF, Catella-Lawson F, Mardini FA, Kapoor S, Lawson JA, Fitzgerald GA. Systemic biosynthesis of prostacyclin by cyclooxygenase (COX)-2: the human pharmacology of a selective inhibitor of COX-2. *Proc Natl Acad Sci (USA)*. 1999;96:272-277.

77. Matsumura K, Cao C, Watanabe Y. Possible role of cyclooxygenase-2 in the brain vasculature in febrile response. *Ann NY Acad Sci*. 1997; 813:302-306.

78. Li S, Wang Y, Matsumura K, Ballou LR, Morham SG, Blatteis CM. The febrile response to lipopolysaccharide is blocked in cyclooxygenase-2$^{-/-}$ but not in cyclooxygenase-1$^{-/-}$ mice. *Brain Res*. 1999; 825:86-94.

79. Saag KG, Rubenstein LM, Chrischilles EA, Wallace RB. Nonsteroidal antiinflammatory drugs and cognitive decline in the elderly. *J Rheumatol*. 1995;22:2142-2147.

80. Stewart WF, Kawas C, Corrada M, Metter EJ. Risk of Alzheimer's disease and duration of NSAID use. *Neurology*. 1997;48:626-632.

81. McGeer PL, Schulzer M, McGeer EG. Arthritis and anti-inflammatory agents as possible protective factors for Alzheimer's disease: a review of 17 epidemiologic studies. *Neurology*. 1996;47:425-432.

82. McGeer PL, McGeer EG. Inflammation, autotoxicity and Alzheimer disease. *Neurobiol Aging*. 2001;22:799-809. Review.

83. Aisen PS, Schafer KA, Grundman M, et al. Effects of rofecoxib or naproxen vs placebo on Alzheimer disease progression: a randomized controlled trial. *JAMA*. 2003;289:2819-2826.

12

84.   Launer LJ. Nonsteroidal anti-inflammatory drugs and Alzheimer disease: what's next? *JAMA*. 2003;289:2865-2867.

85.   Sugimoto Y, Yamasaki A, Segi E, et al. Failure of parturition in mice lacking the prostaglandin F receptor. *Science*. 1997;277:681-683.

86.   Richards JS, Fitzpatrick SL, Clemens JW, Morris JK, Alliston T, Sirois J. Ovarian cell differentiation: a cascade of multiple hormones, cellular signals, and regulated genes. *Recent Prog Horm Res*. 1995;50:223-254.

87.   Lim H, Paria BC, Das SK, Dinchuk JE, et al. Multiple female reproductive failures in cyclooxygenase 2 deficient mice. *Cell*. 1997;91: 197-208.

88.   Tsafriri A. Ovulation as a tissue remodeling process. Proteolysis and cumulus expansion. *Adv Exp Med Biol*. 1995;377:121-140.

89.   Akil M, Amos RS, Stewart P. Infertility may sometimes be associated with NSAID consumption. *Br J Rheumatol*. 1996;35:76-78.

90.   Thylan S. NSAIDs and fertility. *Br J Rheumatol*. 1997;36:145-146.

91.   Simon AM, Manigrasso MB, O'Connor JP. Cyclo-oxygenase 2 function is essential for bone fracture healing. *J Bone Miner Res*. 2002; 17:963-976.

92.   Zhang X, Schwartz EM, Young DA, Puzas JE, Rosier RN, O'Keefe RJ. Cyclooxygenase-2 regulates mesenchymal cell differentiation into the osteoblast lineage and is critically involved in bone repair. *J Clin Invest*. 2002;109:1405-1414.

93.   Einhorn TA. Use of COX-2 inhibitors in patients with fractures. Is there a trade off between pain relief and healing? *Bull Am Acad Orthop Surg*. 2002;5:50.

94.   Glassman SD, Rose SM, Dimar JR, Puno RM, Campbell MJ, Johnson JR. The effect of postoperative nonsteroidal anti-inflammatory drug administration on spinal fusion. *Spine*. 1998;23:834-838.

95.   Matsumura J. Considerations in the use of COX-2 inhibitors in spinal fusion surgery. *Anesth Analg*. 2001;93:803-804.

96.   Jüni P, Dieppe P, Egger M. Risk of myocardial infarction associated with selective COX-2 inhibitors: questions remain. *Arch Intern Med*. 2002;162:2639-2640.

97.   Walan A, Bader JP, Classen M, et al. Effect of omeprazole and ranitidine on ulcer healing and relapse rates in patients with benign gastric ulcer. *N Engl J Med*. 1989;320:69-75.

98.   Agrawal NM, Campbell DR, Safdi MA, Lukasik NL, Huang B, Haber MM. Superiority of lansoprazole vs ranitidine in healing nonsteroidal anti- inflammatory drug-associated gastric ulcers: results of a double-blind, randomized, multicenter study. NSAID-Associated Gastric Ulcer Study Group. *Arch Intern Med*. 2000;160:1455-1461.

250

99. Chan FK, Hung LC, Suen BY, et al. Celecoxib versus diclofenac and omeprazole in reducing the risk of recurrent ulcer bleeding in patients with arthritis. *N Engl J Med*. 2002;347:2104-2110.

100. Graham DY. NSAIDs, Helicobacter pylori, and Pandora's Box. *N Engl J Med*. 2002;347:2162-2164.

101. Dalen JE. Selective COX-2 inhibitors, NSAIDs, aspirin, and myocardial infarction. *Arch Intern Med*. 2002;162:1091-1092.

102. Solomon DH, Glynn RJ, Levin R, Avorn J. Nonsteroidal anti-inflammatory drug use and acute myocardial infarction. *Arch Intern Med*. 2002;162:1099-1104.

103. Watson DJ, Rhodes T, Cai B, Guess HA. Lower risk of thromboembolic cardiovascular events with naproxen among patients with rheumatoid arthritis. *Arch Intern Med*. 2002;162:1105-1110.

104. Rahme E, Pilote L, LeLorier J. Association between naproxen use and protection against acute myocardial infarction. *Arch Intern Med*. 2002;162:1111-1115.

105. Ray WA, Stein CM, Hall K, Daugherty JR, Griffin MR. Non-steroidal anti-inflammatory drugs and risk of serious coronary heart disease: an observational cohort study. *Lancet*. 2002;359:118-123.

106. Hennan JK, Huang J, Barrett TD, et al. Effects of selective cyclooxygenase-2 inhibition on vascular responses and thrombosis in canine coronary arteries. *Circulation*. 2001;104:820-825.

107. Ray WA, Stein CM, Daugherty JR, Hall K, Arbogast PG, Griffin MR. COX-2 selective non-steroidal anti-inflammatory drugs and risk of serious coronary heart disease. *Lancet*. 2002;360:1071-1073.

108. Cheng Y, Austin SC, Rocca B, et al. Role of prostacyclin in the cardiovascular response to thromboxane A2. *Science*. 2002;296:539-541.

109. Targum SL. Cardiovascular safety review: rofecoxib, Food and Drug Administration Web site; February 1, 2001. Available at: http://www.fda.gov/ohrms/dockets/ac/01/briefing/3677b2_06_cardio.pdf. Accessed June 27, 2003.

110. Konstam MA, Weir MR, Reicin A, et al. Cardiovascular thrombotic events in controlled, clinical trials of rofecoxib. *Circulation*. 2001; 104:2280-2288.

111. Van Doornum S, McColl G, Wicks IP. Accelerated atherosclerosis: an extraarticular feature of rheumatoid arthritis? *Arthritis Rheum*. 2002; 46:862-873.

112. Feldman M, McMahon AT. Do cyclooxygenase-2 inhibitors provide benefit similar to those of traditional nonsteroidal anti-inflammatory drugs, with less gastrointestinal toxicity? *Ann Intern Med*. 2000;132:134-143.

12

113. Langmann MJ, Jensen DM, Watson DJ, et al. Adverse upper gastrointestinal effects of rofecoxib compared with NSAIDs. *JAMA*. 1999;282:1929-1933.

114. Geba GP, Weaver AL, Polis AB, et al. Efficacy of rofecoxib, celecoxib, and acetaminophen in osteoarthritis of the knee: a randomized trial. *JAMA*. 2002;287:64-71.

115. Rahme E, Marentette MA, Kong SX , LeLorier J. Does income affect the accessibility of COX-2 inhibitors: a drug utilization review study (abstract #39). Toronto: Canadian Association of Population Therapeutics, Annual Conference; 2002.

116. Brandt KD, Doherty M, Raffa RB, et al. Proceedings of symposium: controversies and practical issues in the management of osteoarthritis. *J Clin Rheum*. 2003;9(suppl):S1-S39.

117. Mandl LA, Liang MH, Fisman DN. Cost-effectiveness of competing strategies for management of knee osteoarthritis. *Arthritis Rheum*. 2002;46:S582.

13 Opioids

In general, chronic opioid therapy has had little place in the management of chronic osteoarthritis (OA) pain. Opioid side effects that may be especially problematic in the elderly include:

- Nausea
- Vomiting
- Constipation
- Urinary retention
- Mental confusion
- Drowsiness
- Respiratory depression.

Among patients who have chronic obstructive pulmonary disease or decreased respiratory reserve, depression of the respiratory drive may occur even with a low dose of an opioid. Furthermore, although the elderly patient without pulmonary disease who takes an opioid chronically is often tolerant to the respiratory depressant effect, the addition of a general anesthetic, sedative-hypnotic, or other central nervous system (CNS) depressant will increase the risk.

The CNS effects of opioids (eg, dizziness) may have particularly serious consequences in the elderly. Elderly persons for whom either codeine or propoxyphene were prescribed were found to have a relative risk of hip fracture of 1.6 (95% CI = 1.4 to 1.9).[1] Concurrent use of these opioids and a psychotropic drug (eg, sedative, antidepressant, antipsychotic) carried a fracture risk 2.6 times that in nonusers of drugs in either class.

In addition to their concerns about side effects, health professionals and patients hold concerns related to tolerance to opioids and physical and psychologic dependence. Many physicians are reluctant to prescribe opioids for patients with nonmalignant chronic pain because of their concerns about legal action by governmental regulatory agencies. More recent evidence, however, suggests that prohibition of opioids on these grounds may require reevaluation.[2] The desire to reduce illicit drug use in society may exaggerate fears of drug dependency and addiction. In fact, people aged ≥60 account for fewer than 1% of patients attending methadone maintenance programs, suggesting that the prevalence of narcotic abuse among older people is low.[3] **Table 13.1** provides a list of signs that are suggestive of opioid addiction.[4]

The dose of opioid analgesic needed to treat chronic nonmalignant pain, such as OA pain, is often lower than that needed for cancer-related pain. If opioid treatment is started with a low dose that is then increased gradually, se-

---

TABLE 13.1 — SIGNS SUGGESTIVE OF ADDICTION IN PATIENTS TAKING AN OPIOID FOR PAIN*

Loss of Control
- Compulsive overuse, unable to take medications as prescribed
- Frequently runs out of medication early despite dose agreement
- Frequently reports lost or stolen prescriptions
- Solicits multiple prescribers
- Uses multiple pharmacies to fill prescriptions

Preoccupation With Drug Use
- Noncompliant with other treatment recommendations
- Misses other appointments, always arrives for opioid prescriptions
- Uses street drugs, involved with street culture
- Preference for short-acting or bolus-dose medications
- Reports no relief with other medications or treatments
- Reports allergies to all other drugs

Adverse Consequences of Opioid Use
- Declining function despite apparent analgesia
- Observed to be frequently intoxicated or "high"
- Persistently oversedated

* Occasional occurrences may be understandable in the context of pain alone. However, a persistent pattern of behavior should raise concern regarding possible addiction.

Savage SR. *Med Clin North Am.* 1999;83:761-786.

---

rious side effects (eg, impaired consciousness, respiratory depression) are rare. With chronic use, tolerance to opioids is common; the patient first notices a shorter duration of analgesia and then a decrease in effectiveness of each dose. Tolerance can be delayed by using low doses and concomitantly administering a nonopioid analgesic. Notably, tolerance to most of the adverse effects of opioids develops as rapidly as, or more rapidly than, tolerance to their analgesic action so that adequate analgesia can be restored safely by increasing the dose.

What about the efficacy of commonly used opioids? Oral codeine, taken alone in a dose of 60 mg, is no more effective than 650 mg of aspirin or acetaminophen (ACET). Codeine, therefore, is usually used in combination with these drugs to treat moderate or moderately severe pain. Although the codeine congener, propoxyphene, which is available as 65 mg of the hydrochloride or 100 mg of the napsylate, is no more effective than aspirin, ACET, or 32 mg of codeine, formulations of propoxyphene in combination with ACET or aspirin are more effective than propoxyphene alone. In individuals who take propoxyphene in supratherapeutic doses, a toxic metabolite, norpropoxyphene, may lead to convulsions and cardiotoxicity.

Controlled clinical trials have demonstrated the efficacy of opioids in treatment of OA pain. A fixed-dose combination of codeine, ibuprofen, and ACET was more effective than ibuprofen alone,[5] and a controlled-release formulation of dihydrocodeine was as effective as a fixed-dose combination of dextropropoxyphene and ACET.[6] In an open-label trial of controlled-release oxycodone, pain control in patients with OA was maintained by a stable dose for as long as 18 months without evidence of tolerance or interference with daily activities; indeed, the incidence of common opioid side effects decreased during this period.[7]

In patients with OA who had moderate to severe joint pain despite regular use of nonsteroidal anti-inflammatory drugs (NSAIDs), oxycodone, or an immediate-release formulation of oxycodone/ACET, given on an around-the-clock basis, resulted in significant reduction in pain intensity and improved quality of sleep in comparison with placebo.[8] Furthermore, controlled-release oxycodone appeared to be associated with a lower incidence of nausea than the combination product.

It is probable that opioids are underutilized in treatment of chronic OA pain.[9] They deserve consideration for acute flares of joint pain when ACET or an NSAID does not produce adequate analgesia or when the patient is unable to tolerate NSAIDs. The effective dose varies widely. If an opioid is necessary for treatment of chronic OA pain, once the optimal dose needed to provide adequate analgesia (preferably for at least 4 hours) has been established by titration, the drug should generally be given on a fixed schedule, with the patient informed that he may omit a dose if not in pain. Around-the-clock administration is more effective than waiting for severe pain to return before administering the next dose and may decrease the total dose required. It should be emphasized, however, that in most OA patients for whom an opioid is prescribed, joint pain is not constant and nonopioid analgesics, NSAIDs, and non-pharmacologic measures will be effective in combating joint pain and permitting reduction in the opioid dose. Indeed, in most patients with OA, such measures obviate the need for opioid therapy.

Tramadol hydrochloride is a centrally acting analgesic with a dual mechanism of action:

- The molecule is a μ-opioid agonist
- It inhibits reuptake of norepinephrine and serotonin.

Affinity of binding to the μ-opioid regimen is some 6000 times lower than that of morphine. Because its opioid and nonopioid activities are synergistic,[10,11] the analgesic effect of tramadol is only partly antagonized by naloxone. Tramadol does not inhibit prostaglandin synthesis. Hence, in contrast to NSAIDs, it has no adverse effects on the kidney, platelet, or gastric mucosa.

Oral administration of tramadol may be useful in management of moderate to moderately severe pain. Tramadol 300 mg/d was more effective than dextropropoxyphene 300 mg/d.[12] A dose of tramadol 100 mg was more effective than codeine 60 mg and about as effective as combinations of codeine with aspirin or with ACET (which are considerably less expensive).[13,14] In a randomized double-blinded parallel study of subjects with chronic joint pain, tramadol 200

256

mg/d to 400 mg/d produced a level of improvement similar to that seen with ibuprofen 1200 mg/d to 2400 mg/d.[15,16] Tramadol was reported to be a useful adjunct in patients with OA whose symptoms were inadequately controlled with NSAIDs.[17] In a placebo-controlled trial in patients with knee OA who demonstrated an ability to tolerate tramadol in an initial "run-in" phase of the study and whose joint pain improved with naproxen 1000 mg/d, addition of tramadol permitted reduction in the dose of NSAID, ie, tramadol was NSAID-sparing.[18]

However, tramadol may have significant side effects. In a 4-week clinical trial comparing it with an ACET/codeine combination, nausea was significantly more common with tramadol (10.3% vs 4.5%, $P = 0.05$).[19] Central nervous system side effects (ie, dizziness, vertigo, somnolence) also were more common with tramadol, although the differences were not significant. Adverse events considered by the investigators as being probably related to treatment occurred in 17% of the tramadol group and 12.2% of the ACET/codeine group, but they led to discontinuation of treatment in twice as many patients taking tramadol as ACET/codeine (18.8%, 9.6%, respectively, $P < 0.05$).

The frequency and severity of side effects of tramadol may be reduced considerably if treatment is initiated at a very low dose (eg, 25 mg/d), which is then increased gradually every few days. (This "go-slow" approach, however, limits the usefulness of the drug in management of acute pain). Development of tolerance or dependence with long-term administration of tramadol appears to be uncommon.[20] Accordingly, tramadol has not been scheduled as a controlled substance. The rate of abuse/dependence among tramadol users was found to be 1.55 cases per 100,000 individuals exposed, and among those who abused tramadol, 97% had a prior history of substance abuse.[21]

Because it inhibits reuptake of serotonin and norepinephrine, tramadol should not generally be given to patients who are receiving a tricyclic antidepressant, selective serotonin reuptake inhibitor, or monoamine oxidase inhibitor. The combination has been reported to cause convulsions. Even in the absence of concomitant therapy with the aforementioned agents, seizures may occur in some patients taking tramadol;[22] the risk is greater in patients with previous seizures.

13

Tramadol may be particularly useful for treatment of OA pain in patients in whom ACET or a low-dose NSAID is ineffective or those in whom contraindications exist to use of an NSAID.

Recently, a tablet containing tramadol 37.5 mg/ ACET 325 mg (Ultracet) has become available. In a randomized placebo-controlled trial in patients with low back pain or hip and/or knee OA, its efficacy was comparable to that of codeine 30 mg/ACET 300 mg, with average total daily doses of 3.5 tablets for each of the two agents (ie, tramadol 131 mg/ACET 1.3 g; codeine 105 mg/ACET 1.05 g, respectively). Notably, constipation was much less common with tramadol/ACET than with codeine/ACET (11% vs 21%, respectively).[23]

The "start-low, go-slow" dosing regimen that is required to minimize the incidence of adverse effects with tramadol (eg, nausea, vomiting, dizziness) does not seem to be necessary with the tramadol/ACET combination, which may be dosed initially in amounts of 1 to 2 tablets up to four times daily. The cost of Ultracet is considerably greater than that of a combination of generic tramadol and over-the-counter ACET. The importance of the ratio of tramadol to ACET in Ultracet in determining its efficacy and adverse effects in comparison with those that might occur with ratios of the generic products taken separately has not been determined.

REFERENCES

1. Shorr RI, Griffin MR, Daugherty JR, Ray WA. Opioid analgesics and the risk of hip fracture in the elderly: codeine and propoxyphene. *J Gerontol.* 1992;47:M111-M115.

2. Foley KM. Changing concepts of tolerance to opioids. What the cancer patient has taught us. In: Chapman CR, Foley KM, eds. *Current and Emerging Issues in Cancer Pain: Research and Practice.* New York, NY: Lippincott Williams & Wilkins; 1993:331-350.

3. Schuckit MA. Geriatric alcoholism and drug abuse. *Gerontologist.* 1977;17:168-174.

4. Savage SR. Opioid use in the management of chronic pain. *Med Clin North Am.* 1999;83:761-786.

5. Vlok GJ,van Vuren JP. Comparison of a standard ibuprofen treatment regimen with a new ibuprofen/paracetamol/codeine combination in chronic osteo-arthritis. *S Afr Med J.* 1987;1(suppl):4-6.

6. Lloyd RS, Costello F, Eves MJ, James IG, Miller AJ. The efficacy and tolerability of controlled-release dihydrocodeine tablets and combination dextropropoxyphene/paracetamol tablets in patients with severe osteoarthritis of the hips. *Curr Med Res Opin.* 1992;13:37-48.

7. Roth S, Iwan T, Hou Y, Fitzmartin R, Kaiko R, Lacouture PG. Long term opioid administration: stable doses and pain control with reduction in side effects over time. Proceedings of the 8th World Congress on Pain of the International Association for the Study of Pain, August 17-22, 1996. Seattle, Wash: ISAP Press; 1996:53. Abstract.

8. Caldwell JR, Hale ME, Boyd RE, et al. Treatment of osteoarthritis pain with controlled release oxycodone or fixed combination oxycodone plus acetaminophen added to nonsteroidal antiinflammatory drugs: a double blind, randomized, multicenter, placebo controlled trial. *J Rheumatol.* 1999;26:862-869.

9. Popp B, Portenoy RK. Management of chronic pain in the elderly; pharmacology of opioids and other analgesic drugs. In: Ferrell BR, Ferrell BA, eds. *Pain in the Elderly.* Seattle, Wash: IASP Press; 1996:21-34.

10. Lee CR, McTavish D, Sorkin EM. Tramadol. A preliminary review of its pharmacodynamic and pharmacokinetic properties, and therapeutic potential in acute and chronic pain states. *Drugs.* 1993;46:313-340.

11. Raffa RB, Friderichs E, Reimann W, Shank RP, Codd EE, Vaught JL. Opioid and nonopioid components independently contribute to the mechanism of action of tramadol, an 'atypical' opioid analgesic. *J Pharmacol Exp Ther.* 1992;260:275-285.

13

12. Jensen EM, Ginsberg F. Tramadol vs dextropropoxyphene in the treatment of osteoarthritis: short-term, double-blind study. *Drug Invest.* 1994;8:211-218.

13. Sunshine A. New clinical experience with tramadol. *Drugs.* 1994; 47(suppl 1):8-18.

14. Barkin RL. Focus on tramadol: centrally acting analgesic for moderate to moderately severe pain. *Hospital Formulary.* 1995;30:321-325.

15. Dalgin P and the TPS-OA Study Group. Comparison of tramadol and ibuprofen for the chronic pain of osteoarthritis. *Arthritis Rheum.* 1997;40(suppl 9):S86. Abstract.

16. Katz WB. Progress with tramadol: US experience. *Clinical Courier.* 1997;14:1-12.

17. Roth SH. Efficacy and safety of tramadol HCl in breakthrough musculoskeletal pain attributed to osteoarthritis. *J Rheumatol.* 1998;25: 1358-1363.

18. Schnitzer TJ, Kamin M, Olson WH. Tramadol allows reduction of naproxen dose among patients with naproxen-responsive osteoarthritis pain: a randomized, double-blind, placebo-controlled study. *Arthritis Rheum.* 1999;42:1370-1377.

19. Rauck RL, Ruoff GE, McMillen JI. Comparison of tramadol and acetaminophen with codeine for long-term pain management in elderly patients. *Curr Ther Res.* 1994;55:1417-1431.

20. Budd K. Chronic pain—challenge and response. *Drugs.* 1994; 47(suppl 1):33-38.

21. Cicero TJ, Senay EC, Munoz A for the Independent Steering Committee. Proactive surveillance program to assess ultram (tramadol) abuse. *Pharmacoepidemiology and Drug Safety.* 1998;7:S79-S215.

22. Kahn LH, Alderfer RJ, Graham DJ. Seizures reported with tramadol. *JAMA.* 1997;278:1661.

23. Mullican WS, Lacy JR, TRAMAP-ANAG-066 Study Group. Tramadol/acetaminophen combination tablets and codeine/acetaminophen combination capsules for the management of chronic pain: a comparative trial. *Clin Ther.* 2001;23:1429-1445.

14   Glucosamine and Chondroitin Sulfate

Glucosamine and chondroitin sulfate have recently enjoyed striking popularity for treatment of osteoarthritis (OA).[1] They are sold widely in pharmacies, supermarkets, and health food stores, although not approved for use in OA by the Food and Drug Administration. Several studies have shown glucosamine to be superior to placebo and comparable to nonsteroidal anti-inflammatory drugs (NSAIDs) with respect to efficacy in patients with knee OA, and with a better safety profile than NSAIDs.[2] However, the efficacy of neither glucosamine nor chondroitin sulfate has been examined in large well-designed placebo-controlled trials. In a meta-analysis of six randomized, double-blind, placebo-controlled studies of glucosamine and nine of chondroitin sulfate, McAlindon and colleagues[3] concluded that moderate symptomatic benefit was demonstrated for both of these agents relative to placebo. In studies of chondroitin sulfate, symptomatic improvement was apparent as long as 12 months after the onset of treatment. However, when only high-quality or large-size trials were considered, the effect sizes for glucosamine and chondroitin sulfate were diminished, ie, the better the study design, the smaller the therapeutic benefit.

Because company sponsorship has been shown to affect the likelihood of positive results,[4] it is notable that most of the published clinical trials of glucosamine have been supported by the manufacturer. Among 12 trials in which the manufacturer was clearly involved, all gave positive results.[5] (In nine other trials that reported positive findings, the funding source was not identified.) In contrast, in three recent randomized double-blind trials in which the manufacturer was not involved with acquisition of the data or data analysis, glucosamine was no more effective than placebo.[6-8]

The question of whether glucosamine and chondroitin sulfate have disease-modifying OA effects, ie, slow the progression of structural damage in the OA joint, is discussed in Chapter 19, *Disease-Modifying Drugs for OA.*

REFERENCES

1. Lozada CJ, Altman RD. New and investigational therapies for osteoarthritis. In: Moskowitz RW, Howell DS, Altman RD, Buckwalter JA, Goldberg VM, eds. *Osteoarthritis. Diagnosis and Medical/Surgical Management.* 3rd Ed. Philadelphia: WB Saunders; 2001:447-456.

2. Brandt KD, Doherty MA, Raffa RB, et al. Symposium proceedings: controversies and practical issues in the management of osteoarthritis. *J Clin Rheum.* 2003;9(suppl):S1-S39.

3. McAlindon TE, LaValley MP, Gulin JP, Felson DT. Glucosamine and chondroitin for treatment of osteoarthritis: a systematic quality assessment and meta-analysis. *JAMA.* 2000;283:1469-1475.

4. Rochon PA, Gurwitz JH, Simms RW, et al. A study of manufacturer-supported trials of nonsteroidal anti-inflammatory drugs in the treatment of arthritis. *Arch Intern Med.* 1994;154:157-163.

5. Chard J, Dieppe P. Glucosamine for osteoarthritis: magic, hype, or confusion? It's probably safe – but there's no good evidence that it works. *BMJ.* 2001;322:1439-1440.

6. Hughes R, Carr A. A randomized, double-blind, placebo-controlled trial of glucosamine sulphate as an analgesic in osteoarthritis of the knee. *Rheumatology.* 2002;41:279-284.

7. Rindone JP, Hiller D, Collacott E, Nordhaugen N, Arriola G. Randomized, controlled trial of glucosamine for treating osteoarthritis of the knee. *West J Med.* 2000;172:91-94.

8. Houpt JB, McMillan R, Wein C, Paget-Dellio SD. Effect of glucosamine hydrochloride in the treatment of osteoarthritis of the knee. *J Rheumatol.* 1999;26:2423-2430.

15 Rubefacients and Capsaicin Cream

Although nonsteroidal anti-inflammatory drugs (NSAIDs) and analgesics, such as acetaminophen, are the agents most commonly used to control the pain of osteoarthritis (OA), they often produce no more than a moderate reduction in joint pain and their use, especially in the elderly, is often attended by side effects, such as dyspepsia, gastrointestinal bleeding, and renal dysfunction. Furthermore, older individuals with OA often require systemic medication for comorbid conditions (eg, hypertension, heart disease, diabetes mellitus), increasing the risk of serious drug interactions with NSAIDs and compounding the problem of compliance with prescribed dosing. For this reason, management of OA pain by topical therapy holds considerable appeal.

Application of topical irritants to painful joints and muscles and the local heat provided by rubefacients may be beneficial. However, although topical medications are widely used in the United States as over-the-counter preparations, physicians in this country do not often prescribe them for OA, chiefly because evidence of their efficacy is limited. Topical NSAIDs, in particular, enjoy considerable popularity in Europe but have not been approved for use in the United States. It is unclear whether the benefit attributed to their use is mediated through a pharmacologic action, through placebo effect, or through their action as a rubefacient. On the other hand, in contrast to the uncertainties surrounding the use of topical NSAIDs, controlled clinical trials indicate that topically applied capsaicin cream may relieve joint pain in patients with OA of the hand or knee.

Capsaicin (trans-8-methyl-N-vanillyl-6-nonenamide) is an alkaloid derived from the seeds and membranes of the Solanaceae (nightshade) family of plants, which includes the common pepper plant.[1,2] It is the active ingredient in Tabasco sauce. Initially, it was believed that capsaicin worked via a "counterirritant" mechanism, but it was sub-

263

sequently shown that when applied topically, capsaicin stimulates release of substance P from peripheral nerves and prevents reaccumulation of substance P from cell bodies and nerve terminals in both the central and peripheral nervous systems.[3] This action is relevant because substance P is an important neuropeptide mediator responsible for transmission of pain from the periphery to the central nervous system. Capsaicin has been used successfully in treatment of a variety of painful disorders, including postherpetic neuralgia, cluster headaches, diabetic neuropathy, phantom limb pain, and postmastectomy pain.[4-7] Because local application of capsaicin results in depletion of substance P from the entire neuron, branches from the peripheral nerves to deeper structures, such as the joint, are effectively depleted.[3,8] Initially, external transport of substance P is blocked; with continued treatment, the synthesis of substance P is reduced.

Although articular cartilage is not innervated and therefore cannot be a source of pain, histologic studies have shown that the joint capsule, tendons, ligaments, and periosteum are extensively innervated.[9,10] Nerve fibers are present also in the subchondral bone. Small-diameter nerve fibers in the synovium have been shown to localize antiserum to substance P[11] and synovial fluid concentrations of substance P are increased in patients with OA.[12,13]

In addition to modulating pain, substance P may mediate inflammation within the joint. For example, intra-articular infusion of substance P in rats with adjuvant arthritis increased the severity of joint inflammation.[14] Intra-articular injection of substance P increases blood flow to the joint, transudation of plasma proteins, and release of lysosomal enzymes.[15] Substance P is a chemoattractant for neutrophils and monocytes[15] and stimulates synovial cells to produce prostaglandins and collagenase, mediators associated with joint damage.[14,16] Although the importance of substance P in the pathogenesis of joint inflammation in OA is not clear, it plays a significant role in mediating joint pain in OA, and its pharmacologic inhibition may be useful in palliation of joint pain in this disease.

Several placebo-controlled studies[17-20] have demonstrated the efficacy of capsaicin cream in treatment of OA pain. While patients in most of these clinical trials have generally been permitted to continue their usual treatment with

264

NSAIDs or analgesics, capsaicin cream has been shown to be effective even when employed as monotherapy for OA.[19] Improvement in pain scores under such conditions has been shown to persist for as long as 12 weeks and to be as great as that which can be achieved with NSAIDs.

A local burning sensation is common in patients who use capsaicin preparations but diminishes with continued treatment and seldom results in discontinuation of treatment. Intolerance may also be managed by temporarily switching to a lower-strength preparation (if the 0.025% formulation is not the initial choice). A higher-potency cream may then be used, if necessary, after tolerance to the skin-irritating effect of the lower-strength preparation has developed. Because burning at the application site affects blinding in clinical trials and could favor a positive response to capsaicin, it is notable that the therapeutic response among subjects who have experienced burning after treatment with capsaicin was comparable to that in those who did not incur this side effect.

Topical capsaicin therapy appears to be safe and effective and warrants initial consideration in management of OA pain. Patients should apply the cream in a thin film to all sides of the involved joint and should be instructed to wash their hands immediately after application of the cream and to avoid contact with broken or inflamed skin, eyes, and mucous membranes.

REFERENCES

15

1. Bunny S. *The Illustrated Book of Herbs. Their Medicinal and Culinary Uses*. New York, NY: Gallery Books; 1985:96.

2. Brandt KD, Bradley JD. Topical capsaicin cream. In: Brandt KD, Doherty M, Lohmander LS, eds. *Osteoarthritis*. 2nd ed. Oxford, UK: Oxford University Press. In press.

3. Virus RM, Gebhart GF. Pharmacologic actions of capsaicin: apparent involvement of substance P and serotonin. *Life Sci.* 1979;25:1273-1283.

4. Bernstein JE, Korman NJ, Bickers DR, Dahl MV, Millikan LE. Topical capsaicin treatment of chronic postherpetic neuralgia. *J Am Acad Dermatol.* 1989;21:265-270.

5. Sicuteri F, Fusco BM, Marabini S, Fanciullacci M. Capsaicin as a potential medication for cluster headache. *Med Sci Res.* 1988;16:1079-1080.

6. Ross Dr, Varipapa RJ. Treatment of painful diabetic neuropathy with topical capsaicin. *N Engl J Med.* 1989;321:474-475.

7. Rayner HC, Atkins RC, Westerman RA. Relief of local stump pain by capsaicin cream. *Lancet.* 1989;2:1276-1277.

8. Fitzgerald M. Capsaicin and sensory neurones—a review. *Pain.* 1983; 15:109-130.

9. Samuel EP. The autonomic and somatic innervation of the articular capsule. *Anat Rec.* 1952;113:84-93.

10. Ralston HJ, Miller MR, Kasahara M. Nerve ending in human fasciae, tendons, ligaments, periosteum and joint synovial membrane. *Anat Rec.* 1960;1136:137-147.

11. Kidd BL, Mapp PI, Blake DR, Gibson SJ, Polak JM. Neurogenic influences in arthritis. *Ann Rheum Dis.* 1990;49:649-652.

12. Menkes CJ, Mauborgne A, Loussadi S, Renoux M. Bruxelle J, Cesselin F. Substance P (SP) levels in synovial tissue and synovial fluid from rheumatoid arthritis (RA) and osteoarthritis (OA) patients. *Arthritis Rheum.* 1990;33(suppl 9):S112.

13. Marshall KW, Chiu B, Inman RD. Substance P and arthritis: analysis of plasma and synovial fluid levels. *Arthritis Rheum.* 1990;33:87-90.

14. Levine JD, Clark R, Devor M, Helms C, Moskowitz MA, Basbaum AI. Intraneuronal substance P contributes to the severity of experimental arthritis. *Science.* 1984;226:547-549.

15. Kimball ES. Substance P, cytokines, and arthritis. *Ann NY Acad Sci.* 1990;594:293-308.

16. Lotz M, Carson DA, Vaughan JH. Substance P activation of rheumatoid synoviocytes: neural pathway in pathogenesis of arthritis. *Science.* 1987;235:893-895.

17. Deal CL, Schnitzer, TJ, Lipstein E, et al. Treatment of arthritis with topical capsaicin: a double-blind trial. *Clin Ther.* 1991;13:383-395.

18. McCarthy GM, McCarty DJ. Effect of topical capsaicin in the therapy of painful osteoarthritis of the hands. *J Rheumatol.* 1992;19:604-607.

19. Altman RD, Aven A, Holmburg, CE, et al. Capsaicin cream 0.025% as monotherapy for osteoarthritis: a double-blind study. *Semin Arthritis Rheum.* 1994;23:25-33.

20. Schnitzer T, Posner M, Lawrence I. High strength capsaicin cream for osteoarthritis pain: rapid onset of action and improved efficacy with twice daily dosing. *J Clin Rheumatol.* 1995;1:268-273.

16 Intra-articular Injection of Corticosteroid

Systemic treatment with a corticosteroid or administration of an adrenocorticotropic hormone has no place in the treatment of osteoarthritis (OA). The benefits are equivocal and the side effects associated with prolonged use of these agents, especially in the elderly, outweigh any possible efficacy. On the other hand, intra-articular (IA) injection of corticosteroids may be of benefit in OA. Hollander reported marked to complete relief of symptoms in 87% of 231 patients who received repeated injections over a 20-year period.[1] Similar results were noted in a review of nearly 1000 patients with knee OA who received IA steroid injections as needed over a 9-year period: Nearly 60% no longer had enough pain to require further injections, about 20% were still receiving injections, and about 20% had not benefited from the procedure or had been lost to follow-up.[2] These data, however, must be viewed along with the results of studies that have shown similar benefit after a single injection of 1% procaine,[3] isotonic saline,[3] or the suspending vehicle.[4]

Symptomatic improvement after IA steroid injection is likely to be only temporary (**Table 16**.1).[5-10] **Figure 16**.1 presents the results of several placebo-controlled trials of IA steroid injection in patients with knee OA and depicts the limited duration of benefit in each case. It shows the magnitude and duration of improvement in joint pain relative to the baseline pain scores of subjects who received IA corticoid injection in several studies analyzed by Kirwan and Rankin[11] and, for comparison, changes in these outcome measures after IA injection of placebo. To a considerable extent, joint aspiration alone may improve knee pain in patients with OA through a placebo response or as a result of regression to the mean (ie, patients selected for IA injection have more severe symptoms than those who are not selected and who, given the variability and severity of OA symptoms over time, would tend to regress toward the mean level of pain severity independent of the procedure). The

TABLE 16.1 — PLACEBO-CONTROLLED TRIALS OF INTRA-ARTICULAR GLUCOCORTICOID INJECTION IN PATIENTS WITH OA

Author	Intervention	Number of Patients Randomized (Completing)	Design	Duration (wk)	Efficacy
Cederlof[5]	Prednisolone 25 mg vs PL	44 (44)	Parallel	8	Equal
Friedman[6]	TH 20 mg vs PL	34 (34)	Parallel	8	TH > PL at 1 wk only
Dieppe[7]	TH 20 mg vs PL	12 + 16 (12 + 16)	Parallel/crossover	6/2	TH > PL at 2 wk only
Gaffney[8]	TH 20 mg vs PL	84 (84)	Parallel	6	TH > PL at 1 wk only
Jones[9]	MP 40 mg vs PL	59 (47)	Crossover	8	MP > PL at 3 wk only

Abbreviations: MP, methylprednisolone; PL, placebo; TH, triamcinolone hexacetonide.

[5]Cederlof S, Jonson G. *Acta Chir Scand.* 1966;132:532-537; [6]Friedman DM, Moore ME. *J Rheumatol.* 1980;7:850-856; [7]Dieppe PA, et al. *Rheumatol Rehabil.* 1980;19:212-217; [8]Valtonen EI. *Scand J Rheumatol.* 1981;41(suppl):1-7; [9]Jones A, Doherty M. *Ann Rheum Dis.* 1996;55:829-832.

Adapted from: Creamer P. *Curr Opin Rheumatol.* 1999;11:417-421.

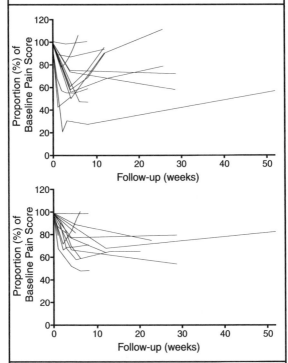

FIGURE 16.1 — IMPROVEMENT IN PAIN SCORE AFTER INTRA-ARTICULAR INJECTION OF GLUCOCORTICOID

Improvement in pain score as a percentage of baseline pain score after intra-articular injection of placebo (top) or glucocorticoid (bottom). Combined results of several studies analyzed by Kirwan JR and Rankin E.

Kirwan JR, Rankin E. *Baillières Clin Rheumatol.* 1997;11:769-794.

16

data indicate that, on average, IA injection of glucocorticoid may produce greater symptomatic benefit than placebo for a couple of weeks but does not afford benefit of longer duration.

With respect to the question of whether the benefits of intra-articular steroid injection are sustained, Raynauld and associates[12] recently reported the results of a randomized double-blind trial in which 68 patients with knee OA received intra-articular injections of triamcinolone acetonide or saline every 3 months for as long as 2 years. Based on values for the WOMAC pain subscale and severity of nocturnal pain and values for range of motion, steroid-injected knees showed a trend toward greater symptomatic improvement, especially at 1 year ($P = 0.05$), than saline-injected knees. Area-under-the-curve analysis showed significant improvement throughout the study with repeated injections of steroids, but not of saline ($P < 0.05$).

The adverse effects of corticosteroid injections are generally relatively minor but some, such as skin atrophy (**Color Plate 22**), may result in litigation. The incidence of corticosteroid-induced atrophy of subcutaneous fat and skin is unclear. This complication results in a depressed, atrophic area that is often made more obvious by associated hypopigmentation. Factors associated with development of atrophy include poor localization of the injection and use of potent fluorinated steroids. It is prudent to warn patients of the possibility of cutaneous or subcutaneous atrophy before injecting superficial sites, such as the acromioclavicular joint or small joints of the hands, and to document this discussion in the medical record. Injection of fluorinated steroids should be avoided at these sites. In addition to the risk of cutaneous atrophy, hyperglucocorticoidism has been implicated as an etiologic factor in osteonecrosis. Rarely, osteonecrosis may develop after IA injection of a long-acting depot glucocorticoid preparation.[13]

Although temporary deterioration in diabetes control might be expected due to systemic absorption of corticosteroid, it is not common.[14] Nonetheless, it is best to warn patients of the possibility. In some patients, facial flushing occurs after an IA corticosteroid injection. The incidence of flushing is unclear, but one prospective study has suggested that it may be as high as 40% and may be severe in

12% of patients.[15] Changing to a different corticosteroid may reduce the frequency of subsequent flushing. Anaphylaxis has been reported after corticosteroid injection but is rare.[16]

Sepsis is the most worrisome complication of IA steroid injection and may result in severe morbidity and even mortality. Infection may be a complication of any IA puncture, but many consider that the risk is greater in the presence of corticosteroids. The true risk of joint infection following corticosteroid injection is unknown. Most estimates are derived from retrospective records and are on the order of 1 per 15,000 to 1 per 50,000 injections. Clearly, the risk of joint infection with steroid injection is low.

Although clinical experience with IA steroid therapy supports its safety, rapidly progressive joint failure has been observed after frequent, repeated injections in large doses into the same joint.[17-20] The masking of pain by IA steroid injections may lead to overuse, with subsequent breakdown and instability of the joint (analgesic arthropathy).[21,22] Steroid injection may also damage articular cartilage directly. Weekly injections into rabbit joints resulted in degeneration of the articular cartilage, with fissures and cyst formation, associated with inhibition of synthesis of collagen and proteoglycans by the chondrocytes.[23] Because of these concerns, IA steroid injections are generally given at intervals not shorter than 3 to 4 months.

Some clinicians recommend weeks of joint rest (eg, crutch walking) after an IA steroid injection, while others permit the patient to return promptly to usual daily activities.[24] The deleterious effects of IA steroids on cartilage seen in a rabbit model of OA were potentiated by exercise,[23] arguing in favor of a period of postinjection joint rest. Patients who were hospitalized and placed at rest after an IA injection of steroids have been found to have had a longer duration of response than ambulatory patients.[25] Many physicians caution the patient to minimize joint loading for a period of time following the injection, even though controlled data to support this recommendation are not available.

Counterbalancing the possibility that excessive doses of IA steroids and/or too-frequent injection of steroid into the same joint may lead to joint damage is the observation that IA steroid injection ameliorates some of the pathologic changes of OA in animal models,[23,26] raising the possibility that this therapy may be disease-modifying, in addition to any effect it may have on palliation of joint pain. Experimental evidence suggests that IA steroids may exert a chondroprotective effect by suppressing synthesis of matrix metalloproteinases, such as stromelysin,[27] that have been implicated in the breakdown of OA cartilage. No evidence exists, however, that steroids favorably influence either the pathologic changes in articular cartilage or osteophytosis in humans with OA.

How important is accuracy in the placement of a joint injection? It would appear that injections are often inaccurate. In a study of patients receiving IA steroid injections in a variety of joints, injections were shown by contrast radiography to be extra-articular in as many as 30% of cases.[28] Aspiration of joint fluid was associated with improved accuracy. Inaccuracy of the injection would not matter if it did not affect efficacy, but unfortunately the same study suggested that inaccurate injections produced less improvement than those delivered into the joint space. Thus if an injection is ineffective, this may be due to inaccuracy of placement and therefore consideration should be given to repeating the procedure.

Which patient with OA is a candidate for IA steroid injection? Several studies have failed to demonstrate any clear-cut predictors of response to corticosteroids other than possibly the presence of an effusion.[10] (As indicated above, effusion may simply be a surrogate for the accuracy of the injection.[28]) Although many authors suggest that IA steroid injections in patients with OA should be reserved for those with acute synovitis, there are no data to support this view. It is reasonable to consider using a corticosteroid injection in patients who fail to respond to other conservative therapy and in those unwilling or unable to undergo surgery.

Finally, it should be recognized that OA pain may arise from para-articular structures. In those cases, injection of steroid into painful pericapsular sites and ligaments might produce symptomatic relief.[29,30]

REFERENCES

1. Hollander JL. Intra-articular hydrocortisone in arthritis and allied conditions. *J Bone Joint Surg*. 1953;35A:983-990.

2. Hollander JL. Treatment of osteoarthritis of the knees. *Arthritis Rheum*. 1960;3:564-566.

3. Traut EF. Procaine and procainamide hydrochloride in skeletal pain. *JAMA*. 1952;150:785-789.

4. Wright V, Chandler G, Morison RAH, Hartfall SJ. Intra-articular therapy in osteoarthritis: comparison of hydrocortisone acetate and hydrocortisone tertiary butylacetate. *Ann Rheum Dis*. 1960;19:257-261.

5. Cederlof S, Jonson G. Intraarticular prednisolone injection for osteoarthritis of the knee. A double bind test with placebo. *Acta Chir Scand*. 1966;132:532-537.

6. Friedman DM, Moore ME. The efficacy of intraarticular steroids in osteoarthritis: a double-blind study. *J Rheumatol*. 1980;7:850-856.

7. Dieppe PA, Sathapatayavongs B, Jones HE, Bacon PA, Ring EF. Intra-articular steroids in osteoarthritis. *Rheumatol Rehabil*. 1980; 19:212-217.

8. Valtonen EJ. Clinical comparison of triamcinolonehexacetonide and betamethasone in the treatment of osteoarthritis of the knee joint. *Scand J Rheumatol*. 1981;41(suppl):1-7.

9. Jones A, Doherty M. Intra-articular corticosteroids are effective in osteoarthritis but there are no clinical predictors of response. *Ann Rheum Dis*. 1996;55:829-832.

10. Gaffney K, Ledingham J, Perry JD. Intra-articular triamcinolone hexacetonide in knee osteoarthritis: factors influencing the clinical response. *Ann Rheum Dis*. 1995;54:379-381.

11. Kirwan JR, Rankin E. Intra-articular therapy in osteoarthritis. *Baillières Clin Rheumatol*. 1997;11:769-794.

12. Raynauld JP, Buckland-Wright C, Ward R, et al. Safety and efficacy of long-term intraarticular steroid injections in osteoarthritis of the knee: a randomized, double-blind placebo-controlled trial. *Arthritis Rheum*. 2003;48:370-377.

13. Laroche M, Arlet J, Mazieres B. Osteonecrosis of the femoral and humeral heads after intraarticular corticosteroid injections. *J Rheumatol*. 1990;17:549-551.

14. Clemmesen S. Triamcinolone hexacetonide for intraarticular and intramuscular therapy. *Acta Rheumatol Scand*. 1971;17:273-278.

15. Pattrick M, Doherty M. Facial flushing after intra-articular injection of steroid. *Br Med J*. 1987;295:1380.

16. Hopper JM, Carter SR. Anaphylaxis after intra-articular injection of bupivicaine and methylprednisolone. *J Bone Joint Surg Br*. 1993;75: 505-506.

16

17. Zachariae L. Deleterious effects of corticosteroids administered topically, in particular intra-articularly. *Acta Orthop Scand.* 1965;36:127-136.

18. Keagy RD, Keim HA. Intra-articular steroid therapy: repeated use in patients with chronic arthritis. *Am J Med Sci.* 1967;253:45-51.

19. Balch HW, Gibson JM, El-Ghobarey AF, Bain LS, Lynch MP. Repeated corticosteroid injections into knee joints. *Rheumatol Rehabil.* 1977;16:137-140.

20. Gray RG, Gottlieb NL. Intra-articular corticosteroids. An updated assessment. *Clin Orthop.* 1983;177:235-263.

21. Alarcón-Segovia D, Ward LE. Marked destructive changes occurring in osteoarthritic finger joints after intra-articular injection of corticosteroids. *Arthritis Rheum.* 1966;9:443-463.

22. Miller WT, Restifo RA. Steroid arthropathy. *Radiology.* 1966; 86:652-657.

23. Moskowitz RW, Goldberg VM, Schwab W, Berman L. Effects of intra-articular corticosteroids and exercise in experimental models of inflammatory and degenerative arthritis. *Arthritis Rheum.* 1975;18:417. Abstract.

24. McCarty DJ. Intrasynovial therapy with adreno-corticosteroid esters. *Wis Med J.* 1978;77:S75-S76.

25. Neustadt DH. Intra-articular steroid therapy. In: Moskowitz RW, Howell DS, Godberg VM, Mankin HF, eds. *Osteoarthritis: Diagnosis and Medical/Surgical Management.* Philadelphia, PA: WB Saunders Co; 1984:493-510.

26. Colombo C, Butler M, Hickman L, Selwyn M, Chart J, Steinetz B. A new model of osteoarthrosis in rabbits. II. Evaluation of anti-osteoarthritic effects of selected antirheumatic drugs administered systemically. *Arthritis Rheum.* 1983;26:1132-1139.

27. Pelletier JP, Mineau F, Raynauld JP, Woessner JF Jr, Gunja-Smith Z, Martell-Pelletier J. Intraarticular injections with methylprednisolone acetate reduce osteoarthritic lesions in parallel with chondrocyte stromelysin synthesis in experimental osteoarthritis. *Arthritis Rheum.* 1994;37:414-423.

28. Jones A, Regan M, Ledingham J, Pattrick M, Manhire A, Doherty M. Importance of placement of intra-articular steroid injections. *BMJ.* 1993;307:1329-1330.

29. Sambrook PN, Champion GD, Browne CD, et al. Corticosteroid injection for osteoarthritis of the knee: peripatellar compared to intra-articular route. *Clin Exp Rheumatol.* 1989;7:609-613.

30. Creamer P. Intra-articular corticosteroid treatment in osteoarthritis. *Curr Opin Rheumatol.* 1999;11:417-421.

17 Intra-articular Injection of Hyaluronic Acid

Hyaluronan (HA) is a large, polydisperse linear glycosaminoglycan composed of repeating disaccharides of glucuronic acid and N-acetylglucosamine. Synoviocytes, fibroblasts, and chondrocytes all synthesize HA, which is present in all mammalian connective tissues at concentrations of 0.05% to 5%, with an average molecular weight (MW) of 6×10^4 to 12×10^6 d.[1] Synovial fluid is a plasma ultrafiltrate modified by addition of a high concentration of HA, which is synthesized and secreted into the joint cavity by the type B cells of the synovial lining.[2-5] In normal human synovial fluid, the MW of HA is 6 to 7×10^6 d, and the concentration, 2 mg/mL to 4 mg/mL.[2]

In osteoarthritis (OA), the concentration and MW of synovial fluid HA are reduced and the viscoelastic properties of the fluid compromised.[6,7] Injection of exogenous HA into the joint presumably supplements the endogenous HA and has been reported to relieve joint pain in patients with OA, sometimes for many months (despite evidence that the injected HA is cleared from the joint in no more than a few days), and to increase the MW and the quantity of HA synthesized by the synovium.[8-10]

HA preparations marketed for intra-articular (IA) injection range from 0.25 to 2×10^6 d and have been purified from rooster comb or human umbilical cord or have been produced by bacteria. To increase the average MW, prolong its half-life within the joint, and—it has been claimed—improve its clinical efficacy, HA has been modified to form hylans, chemically cross-linked HA molecules with an average MW as high as 23×10^6 d. One HA preparation, Hyalgan (MW = 5 to 7.5×10^5 d), and one hylan, Synvisc (hylan G-F20), have been approved by the Food and Drug Administration for use in humans with knee OA whose joint pain has not responded to nonmedicinal measures and analgesic drugs. Synvisc is a highly purified formulation of rooster comb HA, the major portion of which

17

is cross-linked with formaldehyde and the remainder with vinylsulfone to form a highly viscous gel, whose MW is 6 to 7×10^6 d.[11] As indicated, injected HA has a short residence time in the joint. For Hyalgan, the half-life is 17 hours[12]; the smaller component of Synvisc (90% of the preparation) has a half-life of 1.5 days, and the larger component, 8.8 days.[13] Insufficient information is available to establish the optimal number of injections or the dose necessary for a successful therapeutic outcome or to permit direct comparison of the efficacy and adverse effects of the two HA preparations currently approved by the FDA for use in humans.

Possible Mechanisms of Action

Hyaluronan molecules in solution form an extensive network. High-MW HA is viscoelastic, ie, it behaves as a viscous liquid at low shear rates and an elastic solid at high shear rates. Because of its HA content, joint fluid acts as a viscous lubricant during slow movement of the joint, as in walking, and as an elastic shock absorber during rapid movement, as in running. Various functions have been attributed to synovial fluid HA, including lubrication of the soft tissues (eg, adjacent fronds of synovial villi) and formation of a surface layer or the articular cartilage. Hyaluronan has a variety of effects on cells *in vitro* that may relate to its reported effects in joint disease. For example, it inhibits prostaglandin E_2 synthesis induced by interleukin (IL)-1[14,15]; protects against proteoglycan depletion and cytotoxicity induced by IL-1, mononuclear cell-conditioned medium, and oxygen-derived free radicals[16,17]; and affects leukocyte adherence, proliferation, migration, and phagocytosis.[3] Reduction of cellular damage by reactive oxygen species in the presence of HA has been attributed to two mechanisms: the first, competition between HA and cells for free radicals, is independent of the MW of the HA, while the second, prevention of contact between the target cell and enzymes that produce reactive oxygen, is proportional to the MW of the HA.[16,17] In addition, during degradation of HA by free radicals, the latter are consumed in the reaction, reducing their concentration in the synovial fluid.[18,19] Hyaluronan has been shown to have a direct effect on control mechanisms of monocyte activation, eg, it increases messenger ribonucleic acid (mRNA) expression for IL-1ß, tumor necrosis factor (TNF)-α, and insulinlike growth factor-1 (IGF-1).[20] Monoclonal antibodies to the HA receptor, CD44, block the effect of HA on expression of IL-1ß, TNF-α, and IGF-1, indicating a direct interaction of HA with the cell.[20] In cartilage, HA has been shown to suppress extracellular matrix degradation by fibronectin fragments.[21,22]

It is not clear whether any of the effects of HA on cultured cells are relevant to clinical outcomes after intra-articular (IA) injection. Furthermore, it should be noted that the effects of exogenous HA on cellular activity *in vivo* are generally compared with activities in control cultures in which the medium contains little or no HA, although even in a diseased joint, the concentration of endogenous HA is 0.5 mg/mL to 1 mg/mL[6,7] and the average MW 5×10^6 d.[7]

It has also been suggested that HA may modify fluid flow through the joint. A constant flow of HA occurs through the normal joint, with a half-life of 0.5 to 1.0 days in rabbit and sheep, respectively.[23,24] Although it has been reported that synovial fluid flow is diminished in OA,[2] most measurements indicate more rapid clearance of both HA and protein from inflamed joints, even when synovitis is mild, as in OA.[25,26] Others have suggested that HA acts as a chemical sponge, binding or entangling both macromolecules and particulate debris in the diseased joint and that the rapid clearance of injected HA results in removal of these deleterious substances from the joint space.[27] However, experimental manipulation of the MW and concentration of HA in canine knee joints by injection of exogenous HA had no effect on the rate of clearance of radiolabeled albumin.[28] There is little evidence that injection of HA promotes clearance of metabolites and debris or significantly augments the fluid flow through the joint.

17

The original rationale proposed for IA HA treatment of OA was to increase the viscosity of the synovial fluid.[29] According to Balazs and others,[2,30] injection of an OA joint with HA or hylan restores the viscoelasticity of the synovial fluid, augments the flow of joint fluid, normalizes endogenous HA synthesis and/or inhibits HA degradation, and reduces joint pain. These investigators have contended that altered properties of synovial fluid contribute importantly to progression of joint destruction in OA and that transient supplementation of joint fluid leads to long-lasting increases in the MW and concentration of endogenous HA, resulting in improved joint function.[2] However, although the concept that viscosupplementation by IA injection of HA is useful in treatment of OA has been proposed, few data exist to support this mechanism of action. Data from humans, in particular, are scarce. While the MW of synovial fluid HA may increase temporarily after injection of exogenous HA, no evidence exists that this treatment returns either the concentration or the MW of synovial fluid HA to a level approximating that in normal synovial fluid (**Table 17.1**). Indeed, there is no evidence that *any* abnormality in synovial fluid HA leads to OA or progression of established joint damage.

Effects of HA Injection on OA Pain

Intra-articular injections of HA have been employed with some enthusiasm in the past few years for treatment of OA pain that has not responded to a program of ACET and nonpharmacologic measures.[31] Although IA HA therapy is expensive (approximately $500 for a series of injections, in addition to the physician's fees for the 3 to 5 weekly visits required), it has been argued that it is cost-effective, insofar as it is not associated with systemic effects and permits reduction in the patient's nonsteroidal anti-inflammatory dose (NSAID) dose, thereby reducing the risk of NSAID-associated gastrointestinal ulcers and ulcer complications and the cost of the periodic laboratory studies needed to monitor chronic NSAID therapy. However, there is no evidence that reduction in NSAID dose or withdrawal of NSAIDs occurs with any greater frequency in patients treated with IA HA than in those who are not and, as discussed below, recent studies have failed to demonstrate superiority of IA HA therapy to IA injections of saline or of enzymatically degraded HA (in which the viscoelasticity has been drastically reduced) (**Figure 17.1**).[32-34]

In 1997, Kirwan and Rankin[35] reviewed published studies of the effects of IA HA therapy and compared outcomes with those obtained after IA injection of placebo or corticosteroid. The data indicate that joint aspiration alone improves knee pain in patients with OA. HA injections appear to result in improvement that is similar in magnitude

TABLE 17.1 — EFFECTS OF INTRA-ARTICULAR INJECTION OF HEALON ON LIMITING VISCOSITY AND HA CONCENTRATION OF SYNOVIAL FLUID FROM HUMAN SUBJECTS

Sample	Limiting Viscosity (cc/g)		HA Concentration (mg/mL)	
	Mean ± SD	Range	Mean ± SD	Range
Healon	—	2000-2500	10	10
Normal synovial fluid*	5230 ± 140	4500-6000	2.26 ± 0.13	1.45-2.94
OA synovial fluid				
Pretreatment	3325 ± 650[†]	3000-4300[†]	1.56 ± 0.36[‡]	1.14-1.99[‡]
Post-treatment	3825 ± 512[†]	3300-4500[†]	1.73 ± 0.29[‡]	1.38-2.14[‡]
Increase after	500 ± 316[†]	200-900[†]	0.17 ± 0.27[‡]	-0.39-0.42[‡]

Abbreviations: HA, hyaluronic acid; OA, osteoarthritis; SD, standard deviation.

* Values obtained on samples from 71 joints of 42 donors, collected as 10 pooled samples and 3 individual samples.[6]
† Values for samples from 4 of 7 patients[6] in whom intrinsic viscosity was measured 1 week after injection of Healon; note that post-treatment values remain ~25% lower than those for normal human synovial fluid.
‡ Values from 7 patients.[9]

[6]Balazs EA, et al. *Arthritis Rheum.* 1967;10:357-376; [9]Peyron JG, Balazs EA. *Pathol Biol.* 1974;22:731-736.

17

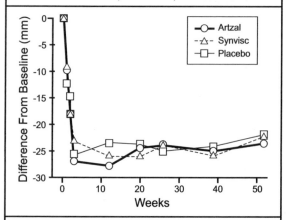

FIGURE 17.1 — KNEE PAIN IMPROVEMENT RELATIVE TO BASELINE IN PATIENTS TREATED WITH ARTZAL, SYNVISC, OR PLACEBO

Improvement in knee pain, relative to baseline, in patients treated with the chemically cross-linked high molecular weight hylan, Synvisc; the lower molecular weight hyaluronan, Artzal; or placebo (a series of 3 weekly intra-articular injections of saline). No significant difference was noted between the 3 treatment groups.

From: Karlsson, et al. *Rheumatology.* 2002;41:1240-1248.

to that of arthrocentesis or placebo but of somewhat greater duration. The magnitude of improvement after a series of IA HA injections appears comparable to that after an injection of steroid (**Figure 17.2**).[36] However, although the latter produces improvement more rapidly, the benefit appears to be more short-lived than after IA HA. Whether improvement after HA injection is due to a placebo effect or regression to the mean (ie, selection of patients for IA injection whose symptoms are more severe than average and whose pain would improve even without treatment) is unclear.

Considerable caution is required in interpreting the results of clinical trials of IA HA treatment. In particular, the magnitude and duration of the placebo response to IA injections is large and may be sustained for 6 months or longer (**Figure 17.2**), making evaluation of any IA therapy diffi-

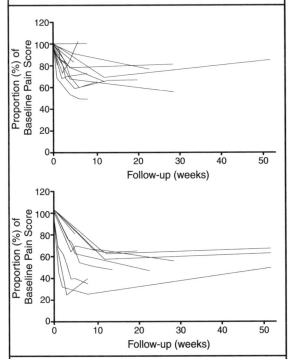

FIGURE 17.2 — IMPROVEMENT IN PAIN SCORE AFTER INTRA-ARTICULAR INJECTION OF HYALURONIC ACID

Improvement in pain score as a percentage of baseline pain score after intra-articular injection of placebo (top) or hyaluronic acid (bottom). Combined results of several studies analyzed by Kirwan JR and Rankin E.

Kirwan JR, Rankin E. *Baillières Clin Rheumatol.* 1997;11:769-794.

cult. It is not clear that the difference between HA and placebo, even if statistically significant, is *clinically* significant.

As illustration, a recently reported study in which patients were treated with 5 weekly IA injections of HA or saline or with naproxen 500 mg bid serves to emphasize the vigor of the placebo response to IA injections.[37] Subjects who received IA injections were given dummy tablets, as a control for the naproxen, while subjects in the naproxen arm received 5 weekly subcutaneous injections of lidocaine as a blind for the IA injections. Among patients who completed the study (approximately 67%), a decrease in knee pain after a 50-foot walk of 20 mm (on a 100-mm visual analog scale) was seen in 56% of those who received HA and in 41% of the placebo group. Twenty-six weeks after initiation of treatment, 47.6% of patients in the HA group, but only 33.1% of those in the saline group, were pain-free or reported only mild pain ($P = 0.039$). Results in the HA group were similar to those in the naproxen group. The authors concluded that treatment with HA was as effective as naproxen for patients with knee OA and had fewer side effects.

However, an intention-to-treat analysis of all subjects randomized to treatment (rather than of only the completers) showed that a series of IA saline injections were as effective as the positive control, naproxen (**Table 17.2**). The failure to demonstrate superiority of naproxen over placebo in this study stands in sharp contrast to the results of virtually every published placebo-controlled trial of an NSAID, in which the NSAID produces greater relief of OA pain than placebo. However, a distinction must be made; in the typical NSAID study, the placebo is a dummy tablet or capsule that mirrors the active NSAID in color, size, shape, and odor. In studies of HA, the placebo is a series of IA injections of saline or the vehicle.

Furthermore, the large placebo response is by no means the only important limitation of the clinical trials that have reported a positive effect from IA HA therapy.[38] For example, in some studies[39,40] the person who performed the patient evaluations was not blinded with respect to treatment group, raising the possibility that bias was introduced because the HA and saline control solutions are so readily distinguished from each other by the marked differences in their viscosity.

In a study in which the authors concluded that HA treatment was superior to placebo, a decrease in synovial effusion was the major outcome measure.[39] However, the severity of joint pain and mean volume of synovial effusion at baseline were both significantly greater in the HA group than in the placebo group, and synovial effusion volumes in both treatment groups were substantial (18.5 ± 14.0

TABLE 17.2 — LEVEL OF PAIN ON A 100-MM VISUAL ANALOG SCALE AFTER A 50-FOOT WALK*

Study Group	Week of Study						Improvement in Pain Compared With Baseline (%)		
	Baseline	12	16	26	Last Observation		Week 12	Week 26	Last Observation
HA, n Mean (SD)	163 54 (29)	115 23 (25)	109 21 (24)	105 18 (21)	160 27 (27)		57	67	50
Placebo, n Mean (SD)	167 55 (29)	129 24 (26)	123 22 (25)	113 24 (27)	163 28 (30)		56	56	49
Naproxen, n Mean (SD)	162 54 (28)	125 21 (25)	119 24 (28)	111 21 (25)	160 25 (28)		61	61	54

Abbreviations: HA, hyaluronic acid; SD, standard deviation.

* Results for all patients randomized.

Altman RD, et al. *J Rheumatol.* 1998;25:2203-2212.

17

cc, 13.9 ± 9.6 cc)—much larger than is characteristic of OA. Synovial fluid analyses were not reported, but these relatively large effusion volumes raise the possibility that, at least in some cases, the arthropathy was due to some cause other than OA (eg, gout, calcium pyrophosphate dihydrate, crystal deposition disease). Furthermore, effusion volume has not been validated as an outcome measure in OA clinical trials. Because of the difficulty in completely aspirating a knee effusion, it is not well suited to this purpose.

Although the above discussion emphasizes the large placebo response in clinical trials of IA HA, it should be noted that several preclinical studies suggest an analgesic effect that cannot readily be attributed to a placebo response, although they provide no insight into possible underlying mechanisms. However, relief of joint pain for months after the injected material has been cleared from the joint, as has been reported in some clinical trials in humans, is difficult to explain by *any* mechanism, whether it is biochemical, physicochemical, or mechanical.

Disease-Modifying Effects of Intra-articular Hyaluronan Injection

Whether IA HA injections may modify the progression of structural damage in OA is discussed in Chapter 19, *Disease-Modifying Drugs for OA*.

Safety

Is IA HA therapy safe? Certainly, it carries none of the concerns associated with systemic inhibition of prostaglandin synthesis by NSAIDs. Local reactions at the injection site, with pain, tenderness, and erythema, are generally transient and require little more than reassurance of the patient and an ice pack. However, some reports have suggested a relatively high incidence of local reactions following treatment with hylan G-F 20. In a study of 22 patients who received a total of 88 injections in 28 knees, postinjection "flares" occurred in 27% of patients and after 11% of injections.[41] In some cases, acute synovitis was associated with joint swelling lasting up to 3 weeks and the synovial fluid leukocyte count exceeded 50,000 cells per mm^3, raising concern about the presence of acute bacterial infection, although bacterial cultures of the synovial fluid and crystal analysis were negative. In a few cases, however, IA injection of HA has been followed promptly by an acute attack of pseudogout, confirmed by the identification of weakly positively birefringent crystals in the synovial fluid.[42,43] No direct comparisons are available of the incidence of local reactions after IA injection of hylan G-F 20 and those after injection of other HA preparations, arthrocentesis alone, or corticosteroid.

Although, in the short run, IA HA therapy seems safe (except perhaps for the occasional "pseudoseptic" reaction as indicated above), force-plate studies in animals suggest that overloading of the damaged joint may occur after this treatment, which may lead to depletion of proteoglycans in articular cartilage and could, in the long run, increase structural damage of the joint. Given the increasing use of HA in humans, this is an important area for further study.

REFERENCES

1. Balazs EA. The physical properties of synovial fluid and the special role of hyaluronic acid. In: Helfet A, ed. *Disorders of the Knee*. 2nd ed. Philadelphia, Pa: JB Lippincott; 1982:61-74.

2. Balazs EA, Denlinger JL. Viscosupplementation: a new concept in the treatment of osteoarthritis. *J Rheumatol*. 1993;39(suppl):3-9.

3. Ghosh P. The role of hyaluronic acid (hyaluronan) in health and disease: interactions with cells, cartilage and components of the synovial fluid. *Clin Exp Rheumatol*. 1994;12:75-82.

4. Abatangelo G, O'Regan M. Hyaluronan: biological role and function in articular joints. *Eur J Rheum Inflammation*. 1995;15:9-16.

5. Laurent TC, Laurent UB, Fraser JR. The structure and function of hyaluronan. An overview. *Immunol Cell Biol*. 1996;74:A1-A7.

6. Balazs EA, Watson D, Duff IF, Roseman S. Hyaluronic acid in synovial fluid. I. Molecular parameters of hyaluronic acid in normal and arthritis human fluids. *Arthritis Rheum*. 1967;10:357-376.

7. Dahl LB, Dahl IM, Engstrom-Laurent A, Granath K. Concentration and molecular weight of sodium hyaluronate in synovial fluid from patients with rheumatoid arthritis and other arthropathies. *Ann Rheum Dis*. 1985;44:817-822.

17

285

8. Iwata H. Pharmacologic and clinical aspects of intraarticular injection of hyaluronate. *Clin Orthop.* 1993;289:285-291.

9. Peyron JG, Balazs EA. Preliminary clinical assessment of Na-hyaluronate injection into human arthritic joints. *Pathol Biol.* 1974;22:731-736.

10. Mensiteri M, Ambrosio L, Innace S, Perbellini A, Nicolais L. Viscoelastic evaluation of different knee osteoarthritis therapies. *J Mat Sci: Mat Med.* 1995;6:130-137.

11. Wobig M, Dickhut A, Maier R, Vetter G. Viscosupplementation with hylan G-F20: a 26-week controlled trial of efficacy and safety in the osteoarthritic knee. *Clin Ther.* 1998;20:410-423.

12. Fiorentini R. Proceedings of the United States Food and Drug Administration Advisory Panel on Orthopaedic and Rehabilitation Devices Panel, 11/21/96. Fairfax, Va: CASET Associates, Ltd; 1996:8.

13. Berkowitz D. Proceedings of the United States Food and Drug Administration Advisory Panel on Orthopaedic and Rehabilitation Devices Panel, 11/20/96. Fairfax, Va: CASET Associates, Ltd; 1996:87.

14. Yasui T, Akatsuka M, Tobetto K, Hayaishi M, Ando T. The effect of hyaluronan on interleukin-1 alpha-induced prostaglandin-E_2 production in human osteoarthritic synovial cells. *Agents Actions.* 1992;37:155-156.

15. Tobetto K, Yasui T, Ando T, et al. Inhibitory effects of hyaluronan on (^{14}C) arachidonic acid release from labeled human synovial fibroblasts. *Jpn J Pharmacol.* 1992;60:79-84.

16. Larsen NE, Lombard KM, Parent EG, Balazs EA. Effect of hylan on cartilage and chondrocyte cultures. *J Orthop Res.* 1992;10:23-32.

17. Presti D, Scott JE. Hyaluronan-mediated protective effect against cell damage caused by enzymatically produced hydroxyl (OH) radicals is dependent on hyaluronan molecular mass. *Cell Biochem Funct.* 1994; 12:281-288.

18. McNeil JD, Wiebkin OW, Betts WH, Cleland LG. Depolymerisation products of hyaluronic acid after exposure to oxygen-derived free radicals. *Ann Rheum Dis.* 1985;44:780-789.

19. Greenwald RA, Moy WW. Effect of oxygen-derived free radicals on hyaluronic acid. *Arthritis Rheum.* 1980;23:455-463.

20. Noble PW, Lake FR, Henson PM, Riches DW. Hyaluronate activation of CD44 induces insulin-like growth factor-1 expression by a tumor necrosis factor-alpha-dependent mechanism in murine macrophages. *J Clin Invest.* 1993;91:2368-2377.

21. Homandberg GA, Hui F, Wen C, Kuettner KE, Williams JM. Hyaluronic acid suppresses fibronectin fragment mediated cartilage chondrolysis: I. In vitro. *Osteoarthritis Cartilage.* 1997;5:309-319.

22. Williams JM, Plaza V, Hui F, Wen C, Kuettner KE, Homandberg GA. Hyaluronic acid suppresses fibronectin fragment mediated cartilage chondrolysis: II. In vitro. *Osteoarthritis Cartilage.* 1997;5:235-240.

23. Brown TJ, Laurent UB, Fraser JR. Turnover of hyaluronan in synovial joints: elimination of labelled hyaluronan from the knee joint of the rabbit. *Exp Physiol.* 1991;76:125-134.

24. Fraser JR, Kimpton WG, Pierscionek BK, Cahill RN. The kinetics of hyaluronan in normal and acutely inflamed synovial joints: observations with experimental arthritis in sheep. *Semin Arthritis Rheum.* 1993;22(suppl 1):9-17.

25. Myers SL. Effect of synovial fluid hyaluronan on the clearance of albumin from the canine knee. *Ann Rheum Dis.* 1995;54:433-434.

26. Myers SL, Brandt KD, Eilam O. Even low-grade synovitis significantly accelerates the clearance of protein from the canine knee. Implications for measurement of synovial fluid "markers" of osteoarthritis. *Arthritis Rheum.* 1995;38:1085-1091.

27. Engstrom-Laurent A. Hyaluronan in joint disease. *J Intern Med.* 1997; 242:57-60.

28. Myers SL, Brandt KD. Effects of synovial fluid hyaluronan concentration and molecular size on clearance of protein from the canine knee. *J Rheumatol.* 1995;22:1732-1739.

29. Peyron JG. Intraarticular hyaluronan injections in the treatment of osteoarthritis: state-of-the-art review. *J Rheumatol.* 1993;39(suppl):10-15.

30. Rydell N, Balazs EA. Effect of intra-articular injection of hyaluronic acid on the clinical symptoms of osteoarthritis and on granulation tissue formation. *Clin Orthop.* 1971;80:25-32.

31. Altman RD, Hochberg MC, Moskowitz RW, Schnitzer TJ. Recommendations for the medical management of osteoarthritis of the hip and knee: 2000 update. *Arthritis Rheum.* 2000;9:1905-1915.

32. Brandt KD, Block JA, Michalski JP, Moreland LW, Caldwell JR, Lavin PT. Efficacy and safety of intraarticular sodium hyaluronate in knee osteoarthritis. ORTHOVISC Study Group. *Clin Orthop.* 2001; 385:130-143.

33. Allard S and O'Regan M. The role of elastoviscosity in the efficacy of viscosupplementation for osteoarthritis of the knee: a comparison of hylan G-F 20 and lower-molecular-weight hyaluronan. *Clin Ther.* 2000;22:792-793.

34. Karlsson J, Sjögren LS, Lohmander LS. Comparison of two hyaluronan drugs and placebo in patients with knee osteoarthritis. A controlled, randomized, double-blind, parallel-design multicentre study. *Rheumatology.* 2002;41:1240-1248.

17

35. Kirwan JR, Rankin E. Intra-articular therapy in osteoarthritis. *Baillières Clin Rheumatol.* 1997;11:769-794.

36. Jones AC, Pattrick M, Doherty S, Doherty M. Intra-articular hyaluronic acid compared to intra-articular triamcinolone hexacetonide in inflammatory knee osteoarthritis. *Osteoarthritis Cartilage.* 1995;3: 269-273.

37. Altman RD, Moskowitz R. Intraarticular sodium hyaluronate (Hyalgan) in the treatment of patients with osteoarthritis of the knee: a randomized clinical trial. Hyalgan Study Group. *J Rheumatol.* 1998;25: 2203-2212.

38. Brandt KD, Smith GN Jr, Simon LS. Intraarticular injection of hyaluronan as treatment for knee osteoarthritis: what is the evidence? *Arthritis Rheum.* 2000;43:1192-1203.

39. Dougados M, Nguyen M, Listrat V, Amor B. High molecular weight sodium hyaluronate (hyalectin) in osteoarthritis of the knee: a 1 year placebo-controlled trial. *Osteoarthritis Cartilage.* 1993;1:97-103.

40. Adams ME, Atkinson MH, Lussier AJ, et al. The role of viscosupplementation with hylan G-F 20 (Synvisc) in the treatment of osteoarthritis of the knee: a Canadian multicenter trial comparing hylan G-F 20 alone, hylan G-F 20 with non-steroidal anti-inflammatory drugs (NSAIDs) and NSAIDs alone. *Osteoarthritis Cartilage.* 1995;3:213-225.

41. Puttick MP, Wade JP, Chalmers A, Connell DG, Rangno KK. Acute local reactions after intraarticular hylan for osteoarthritis of the knee. *J Rheumatol.* 1995;22:1311-1314.

42. Luzar MJ, Altawil B. Pseudogout following intraarticular injection of sodium hyaluronate. *Arthritis Rheum.* 1998;41:939-940.

43. Maillefert JF, Hirschhorn P, Pascaud F, Piroth C, Tavernier C. Acute attack of chondrocalcinosis after an intraarticular injection of hyaluronan. *Rev Rheum Engl Ed.* 1997;64:593-594.

18 A Rational Strategy for Therapy for OA Pain

Although most physicians initiate treatment for osteoarthritis (OA) pain with a nonsteroidal anti-inflammatory drug (NSAID), *the data argue persuasively for a change in this strategy* and support the recommendation that acetaminophen (ACET) should be prescribed initially, in a dose up to 4000 mg/d, in parallel with implementation of nonpharmacologic measures appropriate for the individual patient.[1,2] Although some contend that the presence of clinical signs of inflammation (eg, warmth or erythema over the joint, synovial effusion) warrants initial treatment with an NSAID rather than an analgesic, there is no evidence to support that view. ACET may be as effective as an NSAID in OA patients with clinical signs of joint inflammation (eg, joint swelling and tenderness)[3] or histologic evidence of synovitis[4] as in those in whom these are absent.

Given their potential adverse effects and cost (**Table 18**.1) and the fact that no drug has been shown unequivocally to prevent, delay progression of, or reverse the pathologic changes of OA in humans, drugs should serve an *adjunctive or complementary, rather than primary,* role in management of OA pain. Nonpharmacologic measures are as important—and often more important—than drug treatment and may include:

- Instruction of the patient in principles of joint protection
- Thermal modalities
- Isometric exercises to strengthen periarticular muscles in patients with knee OA
- Weight reduction, if the patient is obese
- Avoidance of excessive loading of the arthritic hip or knee by use of a cane or walker

18

TABLE 18.1 — APPROXIMATE RETAIL COST IN DOLLARS FOR 30 DAYS OF TREATMENT OF OA PAIN WITH VARIOUS REGIMENS*†

Drug (Generic/Trade)	Dose	Average Cost ($)		% Change May 2001–March 2003
		May 2001	March 2003	
Acetaminophen (generic)				
Tablets	3 g/d	8.30	8.92	+ 7.5
Caplets	3 g/d	8.30	9.42	+ 13.5
Gelcaps	3 g/d	8.76	10.62	+ 11.4
Celecoxib (Celebrex)	200 mg/d	81.64	87.10	+ 6.7
Rofecoxib (Vioxx)	12.5 mg/d	81.82	94.37	+ 15.3
	25 mg/d	83.89	87.45	+ 4.2

Naproxen (generic)	750 mg/d	20.52	24.13	+ 17.5
	1000 mg/d	24.87	23.41	− 5.9
Naproxen (generic), 1000 mg/d				
+ Misoprostol	800 µg/d	164.50[†]	151.09	− 8.2
+ Omeprazole	20 mg/d[†]	151.33[‡]	139.40	− 7.9
+ Esomeprazole (Nexium)	20 mg/d	—	160.71	—

* Average for four randomly chosen Indianapolis pharmacies for which retail prices were obtained in the months indicated.
† Generic misoprostol was not available in May 2001. The figure shown for that date represents cost of the branded product Cytotec.
‡ Generic omeprazole was not available in May 2001. The figure shown represents the cost of the branded product Prilosec.

18

- Shoes with well-cushioned soles
- Orthotics for the patient with varus or valgus knee deformity
- Patellar taping (for patellofemoral OA).

A health-education program designed to assist patients with self-management can reduce pain and decrease health care costs. Furthermore, the benefits may persist for years.

The above notwithstanding, it is clear that some patients experience greater relief of knee pain with an NSAID than with ACET. However, there is no way to predict which OA patient will obtain greater benefit from an NSAID than from an analgesic. The evidence suggests that ACET is at least as effective as an NSAID in relieving joint pain in *nearly 50%* of patients with OA. In a survey of 668 patients with OA of hip or knee who were asked to compare the effectiveness of, and their overall satisfaction with, ACET in comparison with NSAIDs that they had received, approximately 45% reported that ACET was about the same as or more effective than their NSAID.[5] A comparable proportion of patients reported that they were as satisfied, or more satisfied with ACET as with the NSAIDs that they had received (**Table 18.2**). Similarly, in a double-blind crossover study comparing a diclofenac/misoprostol formulation (Arthrotec) with ACET in patients with OA of the hip or knee, even though the magnitude of improvement in joint pain, function, and quality of life was greater with NSAID treatment than with ACET, 22% of patients reported no difference between the two drugs and an additional 20% reported ACET to be "better" or "much better" than diclofenac/misoprostol.[6] Ratings of overall efficacy by the physician were similar to those of the patients.

The use of ACET in a dose up to 4000 mg/d as the initial drug of choice for systemic treatment of OA pain is consistent with the 1995 American College of Rheumatology Guidelines for Management of OA,[1,2] which state: "Toxicity is the major reason for not recommending the use of NSAIDs as first-line therapy for patients with OA." The serious adverse events associated with NSAIDs (especially those related to inhibition of cyclooxygenase [COX]-1, such as gastric or duodenal ulcers, gastrointestinal [GI] bleed-

TABLE 18.2 — EFFECTIVENESS OF AND OVERALL SATISFACTION WITH ACETAMINOPHEN VS NSAIDS AS REPORTED BY PATIENTS WITH HIP OR KNEE OA

Patient's Judgment of Acetaminophen, Relative to NSAID(s)	Patients in Each Category (%)		
	Much Less/Somewhat Less	Same/More/Much More	Total
Effectiveness	56	45	101*
Satisfaction	52	48	100

Abbreviations: NSAID, nonsteroidal anti-inflammatory drug; OA, osteoarthritis.

* Total exceeds 100% due to rounding off.

Wolfe F, et al. *Arthritis Rheum*. 2000;43:378-385.

18

ing, renal insufficiency, inhibition of platelet aggregation) are not seen with ACET.

The Vioxx Gastrointestinal Outcome Research (VIGOR) study[7] has confirmed that the striking reduction in the incidence of endoscopically evident gastroduodenal ulceration seen with a coxib is accompanied by a corresponding decrease in clinically important adverse GI events, such as bleeding, ulceration, and perforation. The Celecoxib Long-term Arthritis Safety Study (CLASS)[8] showed a similar effect after the first 6 months of treatment, but the gastroprotective effect appeared to be mitigated by concomitant use of low-dose aspirin for cardiovascular prophylaxis and the statistically significant benefit seen at 6 months in non-aspirin users was no longer apparent at 12 months.

Furthermore, even if coxibs do have clinically significant gastroprotective effects they—like nonselective NSAIDs—are associated with other adverse effects, such as renal insufficiency edema, and congestive heart failure.[9] Furthermore, as indicated in Chapter 10, *Acetaminophen,* Chapter 11, *Nonselective NSAIDs,* and Chapter 12, *NSAIDs That Are Selective Inhibitors of COX-2*, the incidence of nonspecific GI side effects (eg, dyspepsia, abdominal pain) with coxibs is higher than that associated with placebo and may not be appreciably different from that seen with nonselective NSAIDs.[10,11]

It is clear that the safety profiles of the new selective COX-2 inhibitors are less favorable than that of ACET. Furthermore, COX-2 inhibitors are much more expensive than ACET. Hence, there is no basis for a recommendation that a coxib is an acceptable alternative to ACET as a first-line drug for OA pain.

However, if sufficient improvement in symptoms does not result within a few weeks after initiation of treatment with ACET and appropriate nonpharmacologic measures, it is reasonable to add a low (analgesic) dose of NSAID. If risk factors for serious adverse GI side effects of NSAIDs are present (see Chapter 10, *Acetaminophen,* Chapter 11, *Nonselective NSAIDs,* and Chapter 12, *NSAIDs That Are Selective Inhibitors of COX-2*) and a nonselective NSAID is used, even in a low dose, it is reasonable to coadminister a gastroprotective agent, such as misoprostol or a proton pump inhibitor (PPI). As an alternative, codeine/ACET or tramadol/ACET may be considered. If this approach does not produce sufficient symptomatic relief, nonmedicinal measures should be continued and the NSAID prescribed in a higher (anti-inflammatory) dose. Selective COX-2 inhibitors are no more effective in relieving OA pain than nonselective NSAIDs.[12-16] However, in patients at high risk for an NSAID-associated GI catastrophe, a coxib may be preferable to even a low dose of a nonselective COX inhibitor.

Whether a coxib is preferable to a low dose of a nonselective NSAID in the patient who is at low risk of incurring a serious NSAID-related adverse event has not been established. The recent cost-effectiveness analysis provided by the Canadian government[17] (see Chapter 12, *NSAIDs That Are Selective Inhibitors of COX-2*) would suggest that except in the elderly, coxibs are not cost-effective in this setting. Although the CLASS[8] and VIGOR[7] studies were designed as GI safety studies, they point out the importance of considering *overall* patient safety when considering prescription of an NSAID.

The evidence needed to fully inform the physician with respect to which patient with OA might benefit most from a coxib and in which patient a coxib might be contraindicated is lacking. Are the gastroprotective effects of coxibs negated by concomitant use of low-dose aspirin? Should COX-1–sparing NSAIDs not be used in patients at risk for coronary thrombosis or stroke? Only large-scale randomized clinical trials of sufficient duration to answer these questions will illuminate these issues.

Meanwhile, however, physicians are faced with treatment choices for patients with OA pain, which they must make without the benefit of such data. It would seem reasonable to consider each OA patient individually in prescribing pharmacologic therapy. Therapeutic recommendations for patients with risk factors for cardiovascular disease and a paucity of risk factors for an NSAID-associated peptic ulcer may differ from those for patients with obvious risk factors for a GI catastrophe if they are treated with a nonselective NSAID but who have no (or minimal) risk factors for MI (**Figure 18.1**).

As an alternative to the above strategy, a nonacetylated salicylate (eg, salsalate, choline magnesium trisalicylate) may be prescribed. Because these drugs have minimal ef-

18

FIGURE 18.1 — RATIONAL APPROACH TO TREATMENT OF OA PAIN WITH NSAIDS

Patient Characteristics	Treatment Recommendation
↑ CV risk factors* + ↓ UGI risk factors †	Nonselective NSAID ± gastroprotection with misoprostol or PPI
↑ GI risk factors* + ↓ CV risk factors*	Coxib

Abbreviations: CV, cardiovascular; GI, gastrointestinal; NSAID, nonsteroidal anti-inflammatory drug; PPI, proton pump inhibitor; UGI, upper gastrointestinal.

* Increased age, diabetes mellitus, hypercholesterolemia, prior thrombotic event, family history, hypertension, obesity, smoking.
† Increased age, cormobidity (poor or fair general health), oral glucocorticoids, history of peptic ulcer disease, history of UGI bleeding, anticoagulation, combination NSAID therapy, increasing NSAID dose, smoking, alcohol use.

fects on systemic prostaglandin synthesis, they do not cause the renal toxicity or inhibition of platelet aggregation associated with other NSAIDs. Furthermore, while the incidence of serious GI side effects with nonacetylated salicylates is lower than that with nonselective COX-2 inhibitors, they are as effective as the latter in relieving OA pain. However, ototoxicity and central nervous system toxicity may limit the utility of salicylates in the older patient.

Because the risk of an NSAID-associated GI catastrophe is dose-dependent, when nonselective NSAIDs are used, the lowest effective dose should be employed. Increases in dose are not necessarily accompanied by increases in efficacy. In general, higher doses should be avoided in most patients with OA. The analgesia produced by ACET and that achieved with an NSAID may be additive, so that concomitant use of ACET may permit a reduction in the daily dose of NSAID. As noted, addition of ACET (4000 mg/d) to a low dose of naproxen (500 mg/day) was as effective as a 1500 mg/d dose of naproxen alone in patients with hip OA.[18]

As indicated in Chapter 12, *NSAIDs That Are Selective Inhibitors of COX-2*, although the VIGOR study[7] and other evidence have raised a concern that treatment with a coxib may increase the risk of a cardiovascular complication (eg, myocardial infarction), the issue remains unclear.

On the other hand, there is no question that patients who are at risk for cardiovascular disease are frequently treated with low-dose aspirin for primary and secondary prophylaxis and that this increases the risk for GI damage.[19-21] Because OA affects primarily the elderly (ie, a segment of the population at risk for cardiovascular events such as myocardial infarction [MI] and stroke) in whom low-dose aspirin prophylaxis for primary and secondary prevention is being utilized with increasing frequency, it is important to recognize that the combination of aspirin and an NSAID is particularly damaging to the gastric mucosa.

In a study from Denmark[21] in which the incidence rate ratio of GI bleeding with low-dose aspirin was 2.6, the rate was twice as high among patients who were also taking an NSAID. Notably, in the CLASS trial,[8] the incidence of upper GI complications, with or without symptomatic ulcers, in aspirin users was no lower in those receiving celecoxib than in those receiving diclofenac or ibuprofen (see Chapter 12, *NSAIDs That Are Selective Inhibitors of COX-2*).

In the patient with OA in whom ACET is not efficacious, prescription of an NSAID as an alternative or supplement to ACET should be based on the patient's prior GI history and current use of aspirin. In addition, because a large number of patients with OA take a PPI for gastroesophageal reflux disease (GERD) or for nonspecific GI complaints, NSAID selection must also take that into account.

Table 18.3 provides an approach to NSAID treatment for the patient with OA, based on these issues:

- In patients who are not taking low-dose aspirin and have no history of ulcer disease and can be considered to be at low risk for an NSAID-associated serious GI adverse event, it is reasonable to prescribe a nonselective NSAID.
- If the patient is not taking aspirin but is at significant risk for a serious GI adverse event, in choosing an NSAID, one should consider whether the patient is taking a PPI or misoprostol: if not, based on

18

TABLE 18.3 — APPROACH TO NSAID TREATMENT OF OA PAIN BASED ON CONCOMITANT USE OF LOW-DOSE ASPIRIN FOR CARDIOVASCULAR PROPHYLAXIS*

Aspirin Use	Low Risk of GI Adverse Event[†]	High Risk of GI Adverse Event[†]	Comment
No	Nonselective NSAID	Coxib	If patient is already taking a PPI (eg, for GERD), a nonselective NSAID may be considered rather than a coxib. However, if patient has a history of prior ulcer or GI bleeding, a coxib may be preferable to a nonselective NSAID
Yes	Nonselective NSAID + PPI or misoprostol	Coxib[‡] or nonselective NSAID + mandatory PPI or misoprostol	If patient has a history of ulcer or GI bleeding, coxib may be preferable to a nonselective NSAID

Abbreviations: GERD, gastroesophageal reflux disease; GI, gastrointestinal; NSAID, nonsteroidal anti-inflammatory drug; OA, osteoarthritis; PPI, proton pump inhibitor.

* Recommendations are independent of the presence of nonspecific GI symptoms, eg, dyspepsia, epigastric pain, nausea, and diarrhea. Only 20% of patients who develop a complicated ulcer with NSAID use have antecedent symptoms.

† See Chapter 11, *Nonselective NSAIDs*, for discussion of risk factors.

‡ Results of the CLASS study (Silverstein FE, et al. *JAMA*. 2000;284:1247-1255) suggest the gastroprotective effect of a coxib is mitigated by concomitant use of low-dose aspirin.

current evidence, a COX-1–sparing NSAID might be considered the drug of choice. If the patient is receiving a PPI or misoprostol (eg, for GERD), a nonselective NSAID would be a reasonable alternative unless the patient has a history of ulcer or an ulcer complication (eg, hemorrhage), in which case a coxib may be preferable.

- For the OA patient taking low-dose aspirin, if an NSAID is prescribed, a gastroprotective agent is indicated, especially if the patient has a history of ulcers. It is worth noting that histamine (H_2) receptor antagonists have not been shown to prevent NSAID-induced upper GI ulceration,[22] and that a recent comparison of the PPI lansoprazole with misoprostol showed greater symptomatic benefit with better tolerability and greater compliance with the PPI.[23]

- For the aspirin user, in the absence of a significant apparent risk for an NSAID-associated GI adverse event, a nonselective NSAID may be recommended in conjunction with a PPI or misoprostol. However, in the patient taking low-dose aspirin who is judged to have significant risk for a GI adverse event and, especially in the patient with a history of ulcer or ulcer complication, a coxib may be preferable to a nonselective NSAID. It should be recognized, however, that the results of the CLASS[8] trial strongly suggest that the gastroprotective effect by coxib is mitigated by concomitant use of low-dose aspirin.

- In the patient at high risk for a serious GI adverse event who requires an NSAID and is taking low-dose aspirin, concomitant gastroprotective therapy should be considered mandatory. In these circumstances, despite the added cost, it is reasonable to consider the combination of a coxib and a PPI.

18

In any case, regardless of whether the patient is taking concomitant low-dose aspirin and regardless of whether the physician recommends a nonselective NSAID or COX-1–sparing NSAID, the NSAID should be used in the lowest effective dose and for the shortest period of time. Nonpharmacologic measures (see Chapter 9, *Nonmedicinal Therapy for OA Pain*) and supplementary analgesia (eg,

ACET, codeine/ACET, or tramadol/ACET), are effective NSAID-sparing interventions.

Finally, the patient and physician should understand that for most patients with OA, the goals of decreasing joint pain, increasing mobility, and achieving a better quality of life are *realistic and attainable.*

Optimization of Drug Therapy for the Patient With OA Already Under Treatment

In patients with OA who are already taking an NSAID but who have not incorporated relevant nonpharmacologic measures, these should be instituted. It will often be possible to then reduce the dose of NSAID or to replace the NSAID with ACET, which may be used on an as-needed basis. There is no reason that once an NSAID is prescribed for palliation of OA pain, it must be continued in perpetuity. When NSAIDs are required, they, too, may be employed as needed, rather than in a fixed daily dose; pain control has been shown to be comparable under these circumstances and the risk of toxicity will be reduced.

In the patient who is taking a nonselective NSAID and doing well, should an attempt be made to switch to a COX-2–selective agent? Certainly if the patient is at risk for a GI adverse event, that approach is reasonable. As pointed out by Peterson and Cryer,[24] if we consider a patient with a 5% risk of developing a complicated ulcer while taking an NSAID (eg, an elderly person 75 years of age or older, with a prior history of ulcer and GI bleeding) and we assume that a COX-1–sparing NSAID would reduce that risk by approximately 50%, in order to prevent a single ulcer complication, 40 patients would require treatment with the COX-1–sparing agent instead of a nonselective NSAID. The yearly incremental cost of this approach to prevention of a complicated ulcer would be approximately $30,000—low enough to justify switching such patients to a COX-1–sparing drug. This strategy would be approximately 40% less expensive than prescribing a generic NSAID and cotherapy with misoprostol or a PPI (**Table 18.1**), although a direct comparison of the incidence rates for complicated ulcers with these two strategies is not available.

REFERENCES

1. Hochberg MC, Altman RD, Brandt KD, et al. Guidelines for the medical management of osteoarthritis. Part I. Osteoarthritis of the hip. American College of Rheumatology. *Arthritis Rheum*. 1995;38:1535-1540.

2. Hochberg MC, Altman RD, Brandt KD, et al. Guidelines for the medical management of osteoarthritis. Part II. Osteoarthritis of the knee. American College of Rheumatology. *Arthritis Rheum*. 1995;38:1541-1546.

3. Bradley JD, Brandt KD, Katz BP, Kalasinski LA, Ryan SI. Treatment of knee osteoarthritis: relationship of clinical features of joint inflammation to the response to a nonsteroidal antiinflammatory drug or pure analgesic. *J Rheumatol*. 1992;19:1950-1954.

4. Hugenberg ST, Myers SL, Brandt KD, Ryan S. Synovitis does not predict response to nonsteroidal anti-inflammatory drug therapy in knee osteoarthritis. *Arthritis Rheum*. 1991;34:S84.

5. Wolfe F, Zhao S, Lane N. Preference for nonsteroidal antiinflammatory drugs over acetaminophen by rheumatic disease patients: a survey of 1799 patients with osteoarthritis, rheumatoid arthritis and fibromyalgia. *Arthritis Rheum*. 2000;43:378-385.

6. Pincus T, Koch GG, Sokka T, et al. A randomized, double-blind, crossover clinical trial of diclofenac plus misoprostol versus acetaminophen in patients with osteoarthritis of the hip or knee. *Arthritis Rheum*. 2001;44:1587-1598.

7. Bombardier C, Laine L, Reicin A, et al. Comparison of upper gastrointestinal toxicity of rofecoxib and naproxen in patients with rheumatoid arthritis. VIGOR Study Group. *N Engl J Med*. 2000;343:1520-1528.

8. Silverstein FE, Faich G, Goldstein JL, et al. Gastrointestinal toxicity with celecoxib vs nonsteroidal anti-inflammatory drugs for osteoarthritis and rheumatoid arthritis: the CLASS study: A randomized controlled trial. Celecoxib Long-term Arthritis Safety Study. *JAMA*. 2000;284:1247-1255.

9. Heerdink ER, Leufkens HG, Herings RM, Ottervanger JP, Stricker BH, Bakker A. NSAIDs associated with increased risk of congestive heart failure in elderly patients taking diuretics. *Arch Intern Med*. 1998; 158:1108-1112.

10. Langmann MJ, Jensen DM, Watson DJ, et al. Adverse upper gastrointestinal effects of rofecoxib compared with NSAIDs. *JAMA*. 1999;282:1929-1933.

11. Feldman M, McMahon AT. Do cyclooxygenase-2 inhibitors provide benefits similar to those of traditional nonsteroidal anti-inflammatory drugs, with less gastrointestinal toxicity? *Ann Intern Med*. 2000;132: 134-143.

12. Simon LS, Lanza FL, Lipsky PE, et al. Preliminary study of the safety and efficacy of SC-58365, a novel cyclooxygenase 2 inhibitor: efficacy and safety in two placebo-controlled trials in osteoarthritis and rheumatoid arthritis, and studies of gastrointestinal and platelet effects. *Arthritis Rheum*. 1998;41:1591-1602.

18

13. Hubbard R, Geis GS, Woods E, Yu S, Zhao W. Efficacy, intolerability, and safety of celecoxib, a specific COX-2 inhibitor. *Arthritis Rheum.* 1998;41(suppl 9):S196.

14. Celecoxib for arthritis. *Med Lett Drugs Ther.* 1999;41:11-12.

15. Cannon G, Caldwell J, Holt P, et al for the MK-0966 Phase III Protocol 035 Study Group. MK-0966, a specific Cox-2 inhibitor, has clinical efficacy comparable to diclofenac in the treatment of knee and hip osteoarthritis in a 26-week controlled clinical trial. *Arthritis Rheum.* 1998;41(suppl 9):S196.

16. Saag K, Fisher C, McKay J, et al for the MK-0966 Phase III Protocol 033 Study Group. MK-0966, a specific Cox-2 inhibitor, has clinical efficacy comparable to ibuprofen in the treatment of knee and hip osteoarthritis in a 6-week controlled clinical trial. *Arthritis Rheum.* 1998;41(suppl 9):S196.

17. Maetzel A, Krahn M, Naglie G. The cost-effectiveness of celecoxib and rofecoxib in patients with osteoarthritis or rheumatoid arthritis. Ottawa: Canadian Coordinating Office for Health Technology Assessment (CCOHTA); 2001. Technology report no 23.

18. Seideman P, Samuelson P, Neander G. Naproxen and paracetamol compared with naproxen only in coxarthrosis. Increased effect of the combination in 18 patients. *Acta Orthop Scand.* 1993;64:285-288.

19. Weil J, Colin-Jones D, Langman M, et al. Prophylactic aspirin and risk of peptic ulcer bleeding. *BMJ.* 1995;310:827-830.

20. Lai KC, Lam SK, Chu KM, et al. Lansoprazole for the prevention of recurrences of ulcer complications from long-term low-dose aspirin use. *N Engl J Med.* 2002;346:2033-2038.

21. Sorensen HT, Mellemkjaer L, Blot WJ, et al. Risk of upper gastrointestinal bleeding associated with use of low-dose aspirin. *Am J Gastroenterol.* 2000;95:2218-2224.

22. Koch M, Dezi A, Ferrario F, Capurso I. Prevention of nonsteroidal anti-inflammatory drug-induced gastrointestinal mucosal injury. A meta-analysis of randomized controlled clinical trials. *Arch Intern Med.* 1996;156:2321-2332.

23. Graham DY, Agrawal NM, Campbell DR, et al. Ulcer prevention in long-term users of nonsteroidal anti-inflammatory drugs: results of a double-blind, randomized, multicenter, active- and placebo-controlled study of misoprostol vs lansoprazole. *Arch Intern Med.* 2002;162:169-175.

24. Peterson WL, Cryer B. COX-1–sparing NSAIDs—is the enthusiasm justified? *JAMA.* 1999;282:1961-1963.

19

Disease-Modifying Drugs for OA

As discussed earlier, for many patients with osteoarthritis (OA), symptomatic treatment with a nonsteroidal antiinflammatory drug (NSAID) or analgesic may achieve some reduction in joint pain, but because of limitations in efficacy, cost, and/or side effects, it is by no means satisfactory. Interest has arisen, therefore, in the possibility of pharmacologically *modifying the disease process*. Drugs that may prevent or retard progression of articular cartilage breakdown in OA are now receiving increasing attention. A number of pharmacologic agents have been shown to reduce proteolytic breakdown of articular cartilage and/or to stimulate matrix repair in animal models of OA in which morphologic, biochemical, and metabolic changes in the OA cartilage mimic, more or less closely, those in human OA cartilage. Such agents have been called "chondroprotective" drugs. However, because not only the cartilage but also all of the tissues of the joint are involved in this disease, it has been suggested recently that the preferable label is Disease-Modifying OA Drug (DMOAD).[1]

DMOADs range from empiric compounds, eg, tissue extracts,[2] to site-specific metalloproteinase inhibitors, designed by structural analysis to fit precisely into the catalytic site of the enzyme.[3] Excellent reviews of the subject by Altman and Howell[4] and by Di Pasquale[5] have been published. Some of the agents reported to exhibit a DMOAD effect include:

- Tamoxifen
- Diacerhein
- Hyaluronic acid
- Glucocorticoids
- Heparinoids (eg, glycosaminoglycan polysulfate [GAGPS], pentosan polysulfate [PPS], and glycosaminoglycan peptide-complex [GP-C])
- NSAIDs
- Doxycycline.

19

Several of the agents receiving current attention are discussed below. (See Chapter 17, *Intra-articular Injection of Hyaluronic Acid*, for discussion of the data relative to a possible DMOAD effect of hyaluronic acid.)

Nonsteroidal Anti-inflammatory Drugs

Claims that NSAIDs have DMOAD activity are based almost exclusively on *in vitro* evidence that the drug may modify proteoglycan (PG) or collagen metabolism, cytokine-mediated matrix degeneration, release or activity of matrix metalloproteinases (MMP), and/or the actions of toxic oxygen metabolites.[6] The number of *in vivo* studies of NSAIDs in experimental models of OA is remarkably limited, because all of the animal species that are commonly employed as models (eg, the dog, the mouse, the rabbit, the guinea pig) are markedly sensitive to the gastrointestinal (GI) side effects of NSAIDs and develop GI hemorrhage or perforation before the joint pathology is well established.

On the other hand, some NSAIDs inhibit the synthesis of PGs by chondrocytes *in vitro*[7] and some, such as salicylate, rather than exhibiting a protective effect, have been shown to *accelerate* progression of cartilage degeneration *in vivo* in animal models of OA.[8]

In humans, *in vivo* evidence that NSAIDs exhibit DMOAD activity is no less adequate than that in animal models. Although in an uncontrolled study, aspirin administration was reported to reduce the prevalence of degenerative changes in articular cartilage in humans recurrent after dislocation of the patella,[9] in a prospective controlled study of patients with chondromalacia patellae in whom arthroscopy was performed before and after treatment, aspirin administration conferred no protection against cartilage degeneration.[10] In a prospective double-blind study[11] in which naproxen was compared with acetaminophen, a very high dropout rate precluded meaningful conclusions regarding the question of whether NSAIDs affect progression of OA in humans. No evidence of radiographic progression of OA was seen in either the experimental or the control group in a 2-year, placebo-controlled trial of diclofenac in patients with knee OA.[12]

Arguing that indomethacin, rather than exhibiting a DMOAD effect, may, in fact, accelerate joint damage in patients with knee OA, Rashad and associates[13] reported an increase in the rate of joint-space narrowing (implying loss of articular cartilage) in radiographs of patients with hip OA who were treated with that drug in comparison with those who received the weak cyclooxygenase (COX) inhibitor azapropazone, and patients in the indomethacin group came to arthroplasty sooner than those in the azapropazone group. However, that study had several limitations: Baseline pain scores were higher in the azapropazone group than the indomethacin group, and the timing of joint replacement surgery was not based on well-defined clinical criteria but was determined by a physician who was not blinded to the treatment group. Furthermore, even though the azapropazone patients had higher post-treatment pain scores, they were deemed to be surgical candidates later in their course of treatment than the indomethacin group, suggesting a bias to delay surgery.

In support of the contention that indomethacin is detrimental in OA, Huskisson and colleagues[14] concluded that its use accelerated joint breakdown in patients with knee OA. In a double-blind parallel study in which 376 patients with knee OA completed at least 1 year of treatment with indomethacin 75 mg/d, tiaprofenic acid 600 mg/d, or placebo, more than twice as many patients in the indomethacin group showed narrowing of the joint space in serial radiographs of the OA knee as those in the placebo group. However, a number of concerns exist relative to the design of that study, as enumerated by Doherty and Jones.[15] In summary, while the conclusion that indomethacin use leads to acceleration of joint breakdown in patients with OA may be correct, the supporting evidence is not wholly convincing.

Heparinoids

Glycosaminoglycan polysulfate (Arteparon), an aqueous extract of bovine tracheal and bronchial cartilage that contains synthetically oversulfated chondroitin-4-sulfate and chondroitin-6-sulfate and 3 mg/mL of peptides, stimulates cartilage matrix synthesis and is a

19

panprotease inhibitor.[2,4] Glycosaminoglycan peptide-complex (Rumalon), an aqueous extract of calf cartilage and bone marrow, when constituted in solution contains approximately 1.8 mg/mL glycosaminoglycans, which are principally chondroitin-4-sulfate and chondroitin-6-sulfate and 0.7 mg/mL peptide.[16] Evidence of a DMOAD effect has been observed with both of these agents in *in vivo* studies in animal models of OA.

Several clinical trials have reported efficacy of GAGPS in patients with OA. For example, Rejholec[17] studied the effects of GAGPS in patients with OA who also received NSAIDs and compared the outcomes to those in patients treated with NSAIDs alone or with GP-C plus NSAIDs. Although radiographic progression of OA was reported to be slower in both active treatment groups than in the controls, failure to include a placebo group or to control for NSAID use cast serious doubt on the significance of the findings. Furthermore, a recent 5-year controlled study failed to confirm that GP-C has a DMOAD effect in patients with knee OA.[18]

The fact that GAGPS and GP-C are derived from bovine tissues raised some concerns over possible transmission of bovine spongiform encephalopathy. In addition, their lack of demonstrated efficacy as DMOADs in adequately controlled human trials, bleeding complications related to the heparinoid structure of GAGPS, and cases of anaphylaxis related to the presence of antigenic protein components resulted in removal of both of these agents from clinical use.

In contrast to GAGPS and GP-C, the heparinoid sodium pentosan polysulfate (SP54), a polysaccharide sulfate ester prepared from beech hemicellulose, lacks antigenic protein constituents. Pentosan polysulfate has a mean molecular weight (MW) of 6000 d and is a potent inhibitor of MMPs, leukocyte elastase, and hyaluronidase.[19] Several studies have shown that treatment with PPS can preserve the PG concentration of articular cartilage and help maintain cartilage integrity in various animal models of OA.[4]

Calcium PPS, which has the advantage of being well absorbed after oral administration, has been shown to reduce loss of cartilage PGs in animal models. It remains to be demonstrated, however, that pentosans have a DMOAD effect in humans. The *in vitro* effects of pentosan and *in vivo* studies in animals and humans have recently been reviewed comprehensively by Ghosh.[20]

Intra-articular Corticosteroid Injection

As discussed in Chapter 16, *Intra-articular Injection of Corticosteroid*, Raynauld and associates[21] recently conducted a randomized double-blind clinical trial in which 68 patients with knee OA received intra-articular injections of triamcinolone acetonide or saline every 3 months for as long as 2 years. Results showed efficacy for the steroid injections with respect to improvement in pain and range of motion. However, the rate radiographic progression of joint space narrowing in the injected knee (a surrogate for thinning of articular cartilage) was comparable in the two treatment groups, ie, no "chondroprotective" effects of the steroid injections was demonstrated.

Intra-articular Hyaluronan Injection

Preclinical data are contradictory with respect to whether intra-articular (IA) injection of HA modifies progression of joint damage in OA and, if so, whether treatment is beneficial or detrimental. Numerous relevant methodologic differences exist among the animal studies that have examined this issue. In addition to the species used, the duration of treatment, source, and MW of the HA, timing of the intervention (prophylactic or therapeutic), and the outcome measures employed all may influence the results. Furthermore, as discussed below, one study in a canine model of OA and another in an ovine model raise a concern that rather than protecting against joint damage in OA, HA injection into the joint may, in fact, accelerate joint degeneration.

When dogs that had undergone anterior cruciate ligament transection were treated prophylactically with a series of IA injections of HA, no effect on morphologic changes of OA was apparent. However, a striking reduction in the PG concentration of the articular cartilage was seen in every dog 7 weeks after the last HA injection.[22] Although mechanical testing of the cartilage was not performed in the

19

above study, because the stiffness of articular cartilage is directly proportional to its PG concentration,[23] this finding raises a concern that HA treatment could accelerate joint damage in OA.

In support of this possibility, IA injection of HA in sheep that had undergone meniscectomy resulted in significantly more extensive osteophytosis and cartilage fibrillation and reduction in the net rate of PG synthesis by the OA cartilage in comparison with OA joints of sheep that had been injected with saline.[24,25] As indicated above, force-plate data indicate that the increase in severity of joint pathology after injection of the canine OA knee with HA was associated with an increase in loading of the arthritic knee, consistent with "analgesic arthropathy." Hurwitz and colleagues[26] have reported that the adductor moment at the knee in patients with medial compartment knee OA was greater while they were taking an NSAID than after withdrawal from the drug, when their knee pain was more severe, ie, pharmacologic amelioration of joint pain resulted in an increase in mechanical loading of the damaged joint.

Insufficient information is available to permit a conclusion concerning the effect of this treatment, if any, on the progression of OA in humans. In the single clinical trial that has examined this question, 36 patients with knee OA were treated conventionally or with weekly injections of Hyalgan for 3 consecutive weeks every 3 months (total of 12 injections). Based on arthroscopic observations at baseline and again 1 year later, Listrat and associates[27] concluded that HA treatment slowed the progression of chondropathy. However, that conclusion must be tempered by the relatively small number of patients in the study, by the fact that the HA group exhibited less severe chondropathy at baseline than those treated conventionally, and by the fact that the proportion of patients who required an NSAID during the study was twice as great in the control as in the HA group. Furthermore, although arthroscopy is useful for observation of damage to menisci, ligaments, and the articular surface, it is not a good tool with which to detect anatomic or biochemical changes in the OA joint, and it cannot be considered to have an accurate, sensitive, reproducible, and validated outcome measure for evaluation of chondropathy in OA. Cartilage thickness and the mechanical quality of the cartilage cannot be assessed unless a striking loss of cartilage has occurred. Probing the cartilage can provide some information about the resilience of the tissue, but the probe assesses change in only a small area and cannot simulate the effects of load bearing.

Tetracyclines

Based on prior observations that activities of MMPs (eg, collagenase, gelatinase, or stromelysin) are increased in OA articular cartilage and studies showing that tetracyclines inhibit metalloproteinases,[28,29] researchers have examined the effects of doxycycline on metalloproteinase activity *in vitro* and shown that doxycycline inhibited the activities of both gelatinase and collagenase in a concentration-dependent fashion.[30]

This observation led to studies in a canine model of OA, which showed that cartilage ulcerations on the medial femoral condyles could be prevented by prophylactic daily oral administration of doxycycline, 3.5 mg/kg (**Color Plate 23**).[31] In other dogs, only mild pitting of the articular cartilage or some partial thinning was observed. Reductions in levels of both total and active collagenase and total and active gelatinase in extracts of cartilage from the OA knee were seen in samples from the active treatment group.[31] Even when treatment was delayed until 4 weeks after cruciate ligament transection, a protective effect was seen.[32]

Studies of the mechanism(s) by which doxycycline inhibits metalloproteinase activity have suggested that it alters the conformation of procollagenase, rendering it more susceptible to breakdown in the tissue.[33] In addition, tetracyclines may interact with the zinc atom present at the catalytic site in MMPs or the calcium atoms that provide conformational stability to the enzyme, resulting in fragmentation of the proenzyme. However, doxycycline is not a particularly potent inhibitor of any of the MMPs that appear to be involved in cartilage destruction in OA and is unlikely to inhibit these enzymes *in vivo* at the tissue concentrations achieved after oral administration.[34] It is more likely that the remarkable protective effect which this drug demonstrates in animal models of OA involves control of the expression of MMP, through inhibition of transcription, as has been shown for MMP-3 in fibroblasts,[35] or inhibition of translation, as has been shown for type X collagen in chick chondrocytes.[36]

Recent studies suggest yet another possible mechanism by which doxycycline may protect against cartilage breakdown involving nitric oxide (NO). It has been shown that NO is spontaneously released from OA cartilage in quantities large enough to cause tissue damage.[37,38] A number of potentially detrimental effects of NO on articular cartilage have been elucidated; for example, NO may modulate the effects of interleukin-1 (IL-1) on cartilage matrix turnover. It suppresses extracellular matrix synthesis[39] and has been implicated in regulation of MMP production and activation of the latent proenzymes. In addition, it inhibits chondrocyte proliferation and induces chondrocyte death.[40-43] It was shown recently that tetracyclines block the RNA expression and translation of the enzyme nitric oxide synthase (NOS), although they have no significant effect on NOS activity.[44] Thus tetracyclines may protect articular cartilage from enzymatic degradation both by direct effects on MMPs and by a more proximal effect preventing synthesis of NOS. In support of this possibility, treatment with N-iminoethyl-L-lysine (L-NIL), a selective inhibitor of inducible NOS, reduced the severity of articular cartilage damage, synovial inflammation and osteophytosis, and the activities of collagenase and other metalloproteinases in cartilage and synovial fluid in a canine model of OA.[45]

Reports that the severity of cartilage damage in guinea pig[29] and rabbit[46] models of OA was reduced by oral administration of tetracycline support the above observations in the canine model of OA. These encouraging results have led to implementation of a placebo-controlled multicenter clinical trial in humans to ascertain whether treatment with doxycycline can prevent development of OA joint damage in knees at high risk for incident OA and/or slow the progression of OA in joints in which damage is already present.

Diacerhein

Diacerhein, which is derived from rhubarb, is the acetylated form of the anthraquinone, rhein. It has been shown to inhibit the expression of collagenase by chondrocytes exposed to IL-1 and to simulate synthesis of prostaglandin E_2 by chondrocytes in culture but has no effect on phospholipase A_2, cyclooxygenase, or 5-lipoxygenase.[47-52] Diacerhein has been reported to be effective in palliating symptoms of OA in humans, although beneficial effects are usually not seen with treatment periods shorter than 1 month.[53-55] In the canine cruciate–deficiency model of OA, chondropathy in the unstable knee, as assessed arthroscopically 16 weeks after transection of the anterior cruciate ligament and by direct observation 32 weeks after surgery, was significantly less severe in the diacerhein treatment group.[56]

In a recent 3-year placebo-controlled trial of diacerhein in humans with hip OA in which the dropout rate, unfortunately, was approximately 50% and approximately 7% per year underwent hip arthroplasty (mainly because of rapidly progressive OA), no DMOAD effect of diacerhein was apparent in those with rapid progression. However, among those who completed the study, diacerhein markedly decreased the rate of joint-space narrowing in the hip radiograph, mirroring results in the canine OA model and suggesting a DMOAD effect.[57]

Glucosamine Sulfate

Is glucosamine "chondroprotective"? Results of two recent, virtually identical randomized clinical trials,[58,59] both of which were supported by the manufacturer, have led to the suggestion that glucosamine not only improves joint pain in patients with knee OA but protects against articular cartilage damage, based upon analyses of changes in joint-space width in the standing anteroposterior knee radiograph. However, concern has been expressed about the interpretation of the results of these studies because of limitations of the radiographic methods employed.[60]

Narrowing of the medial tibiofemoral compartment joint space in paired standing knee radiographs, as used in these studies, may be due to differences in the position of the knee in the two examinations, in the severity of joint pain, in the distance between the knee and the cassette, or to other technical factors, as discussed in Chapter 8, *Radiography*. Indeed, unless rigorous attention is paid to such detail, the coefficient of variation for joint-space width on

19

repeated x-rays of the same knee taken within hours of each other may be as high as 25%.

It is difficult, furthermore, to reconcile the above positive results with the report of Setnikar and associates,[61] who were unable to detect radioactivity in deproteinized plasma after oral administration of radiolabeled glucosamine. On the other hand, radioactivity was detectable in serum proteins several hours after ingestion of the radionuclide, suggesting that the lack of free ^{14}C-D-glucosamine in deproteinized plasma was not due to failure to absorb the material but to first-pass clearance of glucosamine by the liver, where it was subsequently incorporated into plasma proteins (**Figure 19.1**).[62] These results suggest that it is unlikely that a significant quantity of glucosamine reaches the joints after oral administration.

An National Institutes of Health-supported multicenter study, the Glucosamine Chondroitin Arthritis Intervention Trial (GAIT) (currently in progress) is comparing glucosamine, chondroitin sulfate, the combination, and celecoxib with placebo in patients with knee OA. Although the primary outcome measure will be joint pain after 6 months of treatment, approximately 50% of the subjects will be maintained on treatment for 2 years and radiographs obtained at baseline will be compared with those obtained after 1 year and 2 years of treatment. As an alternative to the standing anteroposterior radiograph, a metatarsophalangeal view of the knee, which has been shown to possess excellent reproducibility in repeated examinations performed on the same day,[62] is being utilized in the GAIT study.

Finally, a caveat is required relative to DMOADs, in general. As indicated in Chapter 5, *Clinical Features*, the cross-sectional correlation between the severity of symptoms and the severity of structural damage in an OA joint is poor. A lack of correlation was apparent also in a longitudinal study of 145 patients with knee OA for whom radiographs and clinical data were available at baseline and 3 years later.[63] Although a strong correlation existed between the progression of individual radiographic features of OA (eg, joint-space narrowing, osteophytosis, subchondral sclerosis), *no* correlation was apparent between progression of joint pain and disability and progression of radiographic changes (**Table 19.1**). Therefore, even if a drug is shown

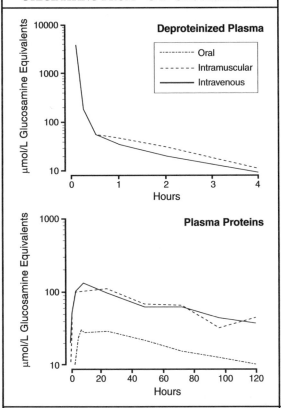

FIGURE 19.1 — RADIOACTIVITY ORIGINATING FROM ^{14}C-D-GLUCOSAMINE

Averages of two subjects each after intravenous, intramuscular, and oral administration. No radioactivity was detectable in deproteinized plasma after oral administration of the radiolabeled glucosamine.

Setnikar I, et al. *Arzneimittelforschung*. 1993;43:1109.

19

TABLE 19.1 — ASSOCIATION* BETWEEN RADIOGRAPHIC PROGRESSION OF KNEE OA (MEDIAL TIBIOFEMORAL COMPARTMENT) AND CHANGES IN OVERALL KNEE PAIN OVER 3 YEARS

Radiographic Feature	Radiographic Progression	Joint Pain	
		Worse	Better
Joint-space narrowing ($P = 0.677$)	Yes	1	7
	No	15	41
Osteophytes ($P = 0.663$)	Yes	1	7
	No	11	33
Sclerosis ($P = 0.566$)	Yes	0	3
	No	15	42

Abbreviation: OA, osteoarthritis.

* Fisher's exact test.

Dieppe PA, et al. *Osteoarthritis Cartilage*. 1997;5:87-97.

clearly to show the progression of joint damage in patients with OA, it should not be assumed *a priori* that it will have a beneficial effect on clinically important outcome measures, eg, joint pain, function, or quality of life.

REFERENCES

1. Lequesne M, Brandt K, Bellamy N, et al. Guidelines for testing slow acting drugs in osteoarthritis. *J Rheumatol*. 1994;41(suppl):65-73.

2. Burkhardt D, Ghosh P. Laboratory evaluation of anti-arthritic drugs as potential chondroprotective agents. *Semin Arthritis Rheum*. 1987; 17(suppl 1):3-34.

3. Lovejoy B, Cleasby A, Hassell AM, et al. Structural analysis of the catalytic domain of human fibroblast collagenase. *Ann NY Acad Sci*. 1994;732:375-378.

4. Altman RD, Howell DS. Disease-modifying osteoarthritis drugs. In: Brandt KB, Doherty M, Lohmander LS, eds. *Osteoarthritis*. Oxford, UK: Oxford University Press; 1998:417-428.

5. Di Pasquale G. Pharmacologic control of cartilage degeneration in osteoarthritis. In: Woessner JF, Howell DS, eds. *Joint Cartilage Degradation: Basic and Clinical Aspects*. New York, NY: Marcel Dekker; 1993:475-500.

6. Doherty M. 'Chondroprotection' by non-steroidal anti-inflammatory drugs. *Ann Rheum Dis*. 1989;48:619-621.

7. Brandt KD, Palmoski MJ. Effects of salicylates and other nonsteroidal anti-inflammatory drugs on articular cartilage. *Am J Med*. 1984;77: 65-69.

8. Palmoski MJ, Brandt KD. *In vivo* effect of aspirin on canine OA cartilage. *Arthritis Rheum*. 1983;26:994-1001.

9. Chrisman OD, Snook GA, Wilson TC. The protective effect of aspirin against degeneration of human articular cartilage. *Clin Orthop*. 1972;84:193-196.

10. Bentley G, Leslie IJ, Fischer D. Effect of aspirin treatment on chondromalacia patellae. *Ann Rheum Dis*. 1981;40:37-41.

11. Williams HJ. Comparison of naproxen and acetaminophen in the treatment of osteoarthritis of the knees. *Arthritis Rheum*. 1991;34:S84.

12. Dieppe P, Cushnaghan J, Jasani MK, McCrae F, Watts I. A two-year, placebo-controlled trial of non-steroidal anti-inflammatory therapy in osteoarthritis of the knee joint. *Br J Rheumatol*. 1993;32:595-600.

19

13. Rashad S, Revell P, Hemingway A, Low F, Rainsford K, Walker F. Effect of non-steroidal anti-inflammatory drugs on the course of osteoarthritis. *Lancet*. 1989;2:519-522.

14. Huskisson EC, Berry H, Gishen P, Jubb RW, Whitehead J. Effects of antiinflammatory drugs on the progression of osteoarthritis of the knee. LINK Study Group. Longitudinal Investigation of Nonsteroidal Anti-inflammatory Drugs in Knee Osteoarthritis. *J Rheumatol*. 1995;22: 1941-1946.

15. Doherty M, Jones A. Indomethacin hastens large joint osteoarthritis in humans—how strong is the evidence? *J Rheumatol*. 1995;22: 2013-2016.

16. Altman RD, Dean DD, Muniz OE, Howell DS. Prophylactic treatment of canine osteoarthritis with glycosaminoglycan polysulfuric acid ester. *Arthritis Rheum*. 1989;32:759-766.

17. Rejholec V. Long-term studies of antiosteoarthritic drugs: an assessment. *Semin Arthritis Rheum*. 1987;17(suppl 1):35-53.

18. Pavelka K, Gatterová J, Gollerová V, Urbanová Z, Sedlackova M, Altman RD. A 5-year randomized controlled, double blind study of glycosaminoglycan polysulphuric acid complex (Rumalon) as a structure modifying therapy in osteoarthritis of the hip and knee. *Osteoarthritis Cartilage*. 2000;8:335-342.

19. Klöcking HP, Hauptmann J, Richter M. Profibrinolytic and anticoagulant properties of the pentosan polysulphate derivative bego 0391. *Pharmazie*. 1991;46:543-544.

20. Ghosh P. The pathobiology of osteoarthritis and the rationale for the use of pentosan poylsulfate for its treatment. *Semin Arthritis Rheum*. 1999;28:211-267.

21. Raynauld JP, Buckland-Wright C, Ward R, et al. Safety and efficacy of long-term intraarticular steroid injections in osteoarthritis of the knee: a randomized, double-blind, placebo-controlled trial. *Arthritis Rheum*. 2003;48:370-377.

22. Smith GN Jr, Myers SL, Brandt KD, Mickler EA. Effect of intraarticular hyaluronan injection in experimental canine osteoarthritis. *Arthritis Rheum*. 1998;41:976-985.

23. Mow VC, Hung C. Mechanical properties of normal and osteoarthritic cartilage. In: Brandt KD, Doherty M, Lohmander LS, eds. *Osteoarthritis*. 2nd ed. Oxford, UK: Oxford University Press. In press.

24. Ghosh P, Read R, Armstrong S, Wilson D, Marshall R, McNair P. The effects of intraarticular administration of hyaluronan in a model of early osteoarthritis in sheep. I. Gait analysis and radiological and morphological studies. *Semin Arthritis Rheum*. 1993;22(suppl 1): 18-30.

25. Ghosh P, Read R, Numata Y, Smith S, Armstrong S, Wilson D. The effects of intraarticular administration of hyaluronan in a model of early osteoarthritis in sheep. II. Cartilage composition and proteoglycan metabolism. *Semin Arthritis Rheum.* 1993;22(suppl 1):31-42.

26. Hurwitz DE, Sharma L, Andriacchi TP. Effect of knee pain on joint loading in patients with osteoarthritis. *Curr Opin Rheumatol.* 1999;11: 422-426.

27. Listrat V, Ayral X, Patarnello F, et al. Arthroscopic evaluation of potential structure modifying activity of hyaluronan (Hyalgan) in osteoarthritis of the knee. *Osteoarthritis Cartilage.* 1997;5:153-160.

28. Greenwald RA, Simonson BG, Moak SA, et al. Inhibition of epiphyseal cartilage collagenase by tetracyclines in low phosphate rickets in rats. *J Orthop Res.* 1988;6:695-703.

29. Greenwald RA. Treatment of destructive arthritis disorders with MMP inhibitors. Potential role of tetracyclines. *Ann NY Acad Sci.* 1994;732: 181-198.

30. Yu LP Jr, Smith GN Jr, Hasty KA, Brandt KD. Doxycycline inhibits type XI collagenolytic activity of extracts from human osteoarthritic cartilage and of gelatinase. *J Rheumatol.* 1991;18:1450-1452.

31. Yu LP Jr, Smith GN Jr, Brandt KD, Myers SL, O'Connor BL, Brandt DA. Reduction of the severity of canine osteoarthritis by prophylactic treatment with oral doxycycline. *Arthritis Rheum.* 1992;35:1150-1159.

32. Yu LP Jr, Smith GN Jr, Brandt KD, O'Connor B, Myers SL. Therapeutic administration of doxycycline slows the progression of cartilage destruction in canine osteoarthritis. *Trans Orthop Res Soc.* 1993;18:724. Abstract.

33. Smith GN Jr, Brandt KD, Hasty KA. Procollagenase is reduced to inactive fragments upon activation in the presence of doxycycline. *Ann NY Acad Sci.*1994;732:436-438.

34. Smith GN Jr, Mickler EA, Hasty KA, Brandt KD. Specificity of inhibition of matrix metalloproteinase activity by doxycycline: relationship to structure of the enzyme. *Arthritis Rheum.* 1999;42:1140-1146.

35. Jonat C, Chung FZ, Baragi VM. Transcriptional downregulation of stromelysin by tetracycline. *J Cell Biochem.* 1996;60:341-347.

36. Davies SR, Cole AA, Schmid TM. Doxycycline inhibits type X collagen synthesis in avian hypertrophic chondrocyte cultures. *J Biol Chem.* 1996;271:25966-25970.

37. Stadler J, Stefanovic-Racic M, Billiar TR, et al. Articular chondrocytes synthesize nitric oxide in response to cytokines and lipopolysaccharide. *J Immunol.* 1991;147:3915-3920.

19

38. Palmer RM, Hickery MS, Charles IG, Moncada S, Bayliss MT. Induction of nitric oxide synthase in human chondrocytes. *Biochem Biophys Res Commun*. 1993;193:398-405.

39. Taskiran D, Stefanovic-Racic M, Georgescu H, Evans C. Nitric oxide mediates suppression of cartilage proteoglycan synthesis by interleukin-1. *Biochem Biophys Res Commun*. 1994;200:142-148.

40. Haüselmann HJ, Stefanovic-Racic M, Michel BA, Evans CH. Differences in nitric oxide production by superficial and deep human articular chondrocytes: implications for proteoglycan turnover in inflammatory joint diseases. *J Immunol*. 1998;160:1444-1448.

41. Tamura T, Nakanishi T, Kimura Y, Takahashi K, Inoue H, Takigawa M. Nitric oxide mediates interleukin-1-induced matrix degradation and basic fibroblast growth factor release in cultured rabbit articular chondrocytes: a possible mechanism of pathological neovascularization in arthritis. *Endocrinology*. 1996;137:3729-3737.

42. Sasaki K, Hattori T, Fujisawa T, et al. Nitric oxide mediates interleukin-1–induced gene expression of matrix metalloproteinases and basic fibroblast growth factor in cultured rabbit articular chondrocytes. *J Biochem*. 1998;123:431-439.

43. Lotz M. The role of nitric oxide in articular cartilage damage. In: Brandt KD, ed. *Osteoarthritis*. Philadelphia, Pa: WB Saunders Company; 1999;269-282.

44. Amin AR, Attur MG, Thakker GD, et al. A novel mechanism of action of tetracyclines: effects on nitric oxide synthases. *Proc Natl Acad Sci USA*. 1996;93:14014-14019.

45. Pelletier JP, Jovanovic D, Fernandes JC, et al. Reduced progression of experimental osteoarthritis *in vivo* by selective inhibition of inducible nitric oxide synthase. *Arthritis Rheum*. 1998;41:1275-1286.

46. Golub LM, Ramamurthy NS, McNamara TF, et al. Method to reduce connective tissue destruction. Kuraray Co, Ltd: Osaka, Japan; November 3, 1993. United States Patent 5,258,371.

47. Pomarelli P, Berti M, Gatti MT, Mosconi P. A nonsteroidal anti-inflammatory drug that stimulates prostaglandin release. *Farmaco*. 1980; 35:836-842.

48. Franchi-Micheli S, Lavacchi L, Friedmann CA, Zilletti L. The influence of rhein on the biosynthesis of prostaglandin-like substances in vitro. *J Pharm Pharmacol*. 1983;35:262-264.

49. La Villa G, Marra F, Laffi G, et al. Effects of rhein on renal arachidonic acid metabolism and renal function in patients with congestive heart failure. *Eur J Clin Pharmacol*. 1989;37:1-5.

50. Petrillo M, Montrone F, Ardizzone S, Caruso I, Blanchi Porro G. Endoscopic evaluation of diacerhein-induced gastric mucosal lesions. *Curr Ther Res*. 1991;49:10-15.

51. Pujol JP. Collagenolytic enzymes and interleukine I: their role in inflammation and cartilage degradation; the antagonistic effects of diacerhein on IL-1 action on cartilage matrix components. *Osteoarthritis Cartilage*. 1993;1:82. Abstract.

52. Cruz F, Tang J, Pronost S, Pujol JP. Mécanismes moléculaires impliqués dans l'inhibition de l'espression de la collagénase par la diacerhéine. *Rev Prat*. 1996;46:S15-S19.

53. Lingetti M, D'Ambrosio PL, Di Grezia F, Sorrentino P, Lingetti E. A controlled study in the treatment of osteoarthritis with diacerhein (Artrodar). *Curr Ther Res*. 1982;31:408-412.

54. Marcolongo R, Fioravanti A, Adami S, Tozzi E, Mian M, Zampieri A. Efficacy and tolerability of diacerhein in the treatment of osteoarthrosis. *Curr Ther Res*. 1988;43:878-887.

55. Nguyen M, Dougados M, Berdah L, Amor B. Diacerhein in the treatment of osteoarthritis of the hip. *Arthritis Rheum*. 1994;37:529-536.

56. Smith GN Jr, Myers SL, Brandt KD, Mickler EA, Albrecht ME. Diacerhein treatment reduces the severity of osteoarthritis in the canine cruciate-deficiency model of osteoarthritis. *Arthritis Rheum*. 1999;42:545-554.

57. Vignon E, Berdah L, Dougados M, Lequesne M, Mazieres B, Nguyen M. Evaluation of the structural effect of diacerhein: a three-year placebo-controlled trial. *Research and Therapeutics in Osteoarthritis, Interlukin-1 Inhibitors. 7th International Congress*. NEGMA Laboratoires; 2000:22. Abstract.

58. Reginster JY, Deroisy R, Rovati LC, et al. Long-term effects of glucosamine sulphate on osteoarthritis progression: a randomised, placebo-controlled clinical trial. *Lancet*. 2001;357:251-256.

59. Pavelka K, Gatterova J, Olejarova M, Machacek S, Giacovelli G, Rovati LC. Glucosamine sulfate use and delay of progression of knee osteoarthritis: a 3-year, randomized, placebo-controlled, double-blind study. *Arch Intern Med*. 2002;162:2113-2123.

60. Mazzuca SA, Brandt KD, Lane KA, Katz BP. Knee pain reduces joint space width in conventional standing anteroposterior radiographs of osteoarthritic knees. *Arthritis Rheum*. 2002;46:1223-1227.

61. Setnikar I, Palumbo R, Canali S, Zanolo G. Pharmacokinetics of glucosamine in man. *Arzneimittelforschung*. 1993;43:1109-1113.

19

62. Buckland-Wright JC, Wolfe F, Ward RJ, Flowers N, Hayne C. Substantial superiority of semiflexed (MTP) views in knee osteoarthritis: a comparative radiographic study, without fluoroscopy, of standing extended, semiflexed (MTP), and schuss views. *J Rheumatol*. 1999;26: 2664-2674.

63. Dieppe PA, Cushnaghan J, Shepstone L. The Bristol 'OA500' study: progression of osteoarthritis (OA) over 3 years and the relationship between clinical and radiographic changes at the knee joint. *Osteoarthritis Cartilage*. 1997;5:87-97.

20 Surgical Intervention

Joint Débridement and Lavage

For the subgroup of patients with knee osteoarthritis (OA) in whom loose bodies, flaps of cartilage, or disruption of the meniscus (eg, a bucket-handle tear) causes mechanical symptoms (eg, locking, giving way of the limb or catching), there is general agreement that arthroscopic surgery to remove the source of the mechanical problem can be helpful in alleviating knee pain and improving function.

However, arthroscopic lavage of the knee with débridement (eg, smoothing the surface of fibrillated articular cartilage or meniscus, trimming of osteophytes, and removal of inflamed synovium) is also widely employed in patients with symptomatic knee OA who do *not* have mechanical symptoms but who have not benefited from pharmacologic therapy. It is presumed that the lavage will remove fragments of cartilage or bone or soluble cartilage matrix macromolecules or crystals of calcium apatite or calcium pyrophosphate that may induce synovitis, thereby causing joint pain. Evidence is lacking, however, that removing or repairing nondisplaced meniscal tears or performing any of the other aspects of joint débridement mentioned above is of symptomatic benefit or alters the course of OA in patients who do not have mechanical symptoms. The magnitude of the problem is significant: approximately 12% of all people in this country over the age of 65 have frequent knee pain from OA, and more than 650,000 procedures involving arthroscopic lavage and/or débridement are performed annually at a cost of approximately $5,000 each.[1]

A recent study of this problem by Moseley and colleagues[2] is important insofar as it employed a control group of patients with knee OA who underwent sham arthroscopy. In this study, 180 patients with knee OA were randomly assigned to receive arthroscopic débridement, arthroscopic lavage, or placebo surgery, which involved skin incision and simulated débridement, but without insertion of the arthroscope. Patients and evaluators were blinded to treatment-group assignment and outcomes, which were assessed repeatedly over a 24-month period, including self-report of pain and function and objective tests of walking and stair climbing. One hundred and sixty-five patients completed the trial. At none of the evaluated time points did either intervention group report less pain or better function than the placebo group; no clinically meaningful differences between the three interventions were observed (**Figure 20.1**).

These results led to the conclusion that even if joint debris is associated with synovitis and clinical symptoms in patients with knee OA, removal of this debris has minimal effect on symptoms. Intra- and extra-articular factors, such as malalignment, periarticular muscle weakness, instability, and obesity—none of which is addressed by arthroscopic débridement or lavage—have greater effects on clinical outcomes than the trimming of cartilage surfaces and meniscus irregularities.[3] As suggested by Mosely and colleagues,[2] given that they are no more efficacious than placebo surgery, the approximately $3 billion spent annually on these procedures in this country might be used more effectively in management of OA if directed at other areas.

Arthroplasty

It is beyond the scope of this monograph to provide a comprehensive discussion of surgery for OA. It is important to recognize, however, that surgery plays an important role in the management of this disease. For patients in whom the comprehensive program of medicinal and nonmedicinal measures discussed earlier is ineffective, surgical intervention warrants consideration. Although a variety of surgical procedures, eg, soft tissue release, osteotomy, and arthrodesis, may be helpful in individual cases, overwhelmingly, surgical intervention for OA means total joint arthroplasty.

Total hip arthroplasty (THA) and total knee arthroplasty (TKA) are, in general, remarkably successful. As discussed below, pain relief is often striking and the complication rate low. Most subjects who undergo THA or TKA are able to return to essentially full function in activities of daily living. Furthermore, the benefits are typically long last-

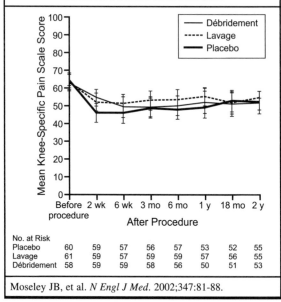

FIGURE 20.1 — COMPARISON OF KNEE PAIN SCORES OF PATIENTS WITH KNEE OA TREATED BY ARTHROSCOPIC DÉBRIDEMENT, ARTHROSCOPIC LAVAGE, OR A PLACEBO ARTHROSCOPIC PROCEDURE

No. at Risk	Before procedure	2 wk	6 wk	3 mo	6 mo	1 y	18 mo	2 y
Placebo	60	59	57	56	57	53	52	55
Lavage	61	59	57	59	59	57	56	55
Débridement	58	59	59	58	56	50	51	53

Moseley JB, et al. *N Engl J Med.* 2002;347:81-88.

ing, with the survival rate of the prosthesis now approximately 95% at 10 years and being nearly that high at 15 years. If cases of infection are excluded, the success rates for revision of the hip and knee arthroplasties that fail at these intervals approximate those for the primary surgery. Given that the patient with severe hip or knee OA is at risk of falling, it is worth noting that the surgical success rate for the fractured hip in this individual may be lower than that for total joint arthroplasty.

Physicians often regard orthopedic intervention for OA as "radical" and medical management as "conservative." However, for the patient with intractable joint discomfort, limited mobility, and a disease that profoundly affects quality of life, continuation of an ineffective medical regimen is, in fact, the radical approach and total joint arthroplasty, the more conservative. Furthermore, as shown by Fortin and associates,[4] excessive delay in total hip or knee replacement so that patients have poorer physical function and more pain preoperatively may result in poorer postoperative improvement, relative to that of patients with higher preoperative function.

More recently, Fortin and associates[5] have shown that the poorer functional recovery noted 6 months after total joint arthroplasty among subjects with greater pain and poor function at the time of surgery is still present 2 years after the procedure. Thus the data indicate that the timing of surgery is important; performance of surgery earlier in the course of functional decline may be associated with better outcomes.

Although OA is a disease whose severity increases with age, the risk of major surgery also increases with age. However, improvements in general medical care and anesthesia technique make arthroplasty a possibility even for the very elderly. With modern surgical techniques and hypotensive epidural anesthesia, the mortality of hip arthroplasty was reported only a few years ago to be as low as 0.1%.[6]

Reports of the risk of deep vein thrombosis after arthroplasty have ranged from 10% to 70%, with pulmonary embolism occurring in 1% to 4% of cases.[7] Prophylaxis with, eg, low molecular weight heparin, can reduce the incidence of pulmonary embolism to a negligible level, with few bleeding complications. Similarly excellent results (eg, 11% deep vein thrombosis and 1% pulmonary embolism) may be achieved with hypotensive epidural anesthesia and aspirin therapy.[6]

Late local complications of arthroplasty include deep infection, loosening, osteolysis, periprosthetic fractures, implant wear, and breakage.[7] Wear is unlikely to cause problems during the first 10 years after surgery but can result in instability and dislocation of the joint. Some 80% of all THA revisions are performed because of loosening, the risk of which is approximately 10% at 10 years and is greater in men and younger patients than in women and older patients.[8] The osteolysis triggered by wear particles can reduce the amount of bone stock needed for subsequent revision.

The overall infection rate after THA is <1%. Treatment of deep infection can occasionally succeed without removal of the implant. In patients with medical contraindications to surgery, antibiotics alone may slow down the destructive process. However, in most cases, deep infection is best treated by removal of the implant and other foreign material and debridement of the infected tissue, with prolonged antibiotic therapy based on the results of cultures.

Knutson has succinctly reviewed the local complications after TKA.[7] Based on an analysis of the Swedish knee arthroplasty registry, some 6% of revisions after TKA are performed for patellar problems, 7% for instability, and 15% for other mechanical reasons.[9] Loosening is the indication underlying approximately half of all revisions after TKA. However, the cumulative risk for revision 10 years after surgery is now as low as 3%. The risk is twice as great with unicondylar implants as with total knee implants. The cumulative risk of revision for deep infection of the knee is <1% at 10 years.

Several studies have confirmed that TKA reduces knee pain and improves function and quality of life in patients with knee OA.[10-15] It is the recommended treatment for patients with severe knee OA in whom medical therapy has been unsuccessful. On the other hand, controlled trials of TKA are scarce and no trials have been published that compare TKA with any other intervention. In most published studies, survival of the prosthesis is the primary (and often only) outcome measure, rather than patient-oriented outcomes. There are no evidence-based indications for TKA in patients with knee OA. The incidence rate for joint arthroplasty varies widely among countries and even among geographic regions within the same country.[16] For example, among individuals over the age of 65 years, approximately 0.5 to 0.7 TKAs are performed in the United Kingdom and Canada but >2/1000 in the United States.[16-18] It is widely considered that severe daily pain associated with loss of joint-space width on the knee radiograph are the chief indications for TKA, whereas comorbid conditions and technical difficulties are reasons for not performing the procedure.

Not only are the indications somewhat ambiguous, it is unclear which patients will benefit most from the procedure. It has been suggested that TKA is underutilized.[19,20] Dieppe and colleagues[21] have recently published a thoughtful analysis of why some individuals, but not others, with

20

knee OA seek medical attention and the factors that determine whether such individuals are referred to an orthopedic surgeon. **Table 20.1** contains a list of factors found by Dieppe and colleagues[21] to influence the decision of the primary care physician (ie, the "gatekeeper") to refer a patient with knee OA to an orthopedic surgeon for consideration of TKA.

TABLE 20.1 — FACTORS INFLUENCING THE "GATEKEEPER'S" DECISION TO REFER A PATIENT WITH KNEE OA TO AN ORTHOPEDIC SURGEON FOR CONSIDERATION OF TOTAL KNEE ARTHROPLASTY

- The gatekeeper's ability to make a correct diagnosis
- Experience of the gatekeeper
- Severity of the disease
- Ability of the gatekeeper to assess disease severity
- Attitude of the gatekeeper toward orthopedic surgery, in general, and total knee arthroplasty, in particular
- Relationship of the gatekeeper to local orthopedic surgeons
- Access to orthopedic surgery
- Access to alternatives, such as physical therapy
- Presence of referral guidelines
- Cost

Dieppe P, et al. *Rheumatology*. 1999;38:73-83.

In most health care delivery systems, access to orthopedic surgery for patients with knee OA depends upon referral to the surgeon by a primary care physician or rheumatologist. Little is known about the determinants of physician referral patterns. We found that family practice specialists and general internists in the United States are more likely to refer a hypothetical patient with hip OA for surgery than rheumatologists, presumably because rheumatologists are more knowledgeable about, or have greater belief in the value of, pharmacologic and nonpharmacologic treatment options of this disease[22] (**Table 20.2**).

Patients who are obese are often told that surgery cannot be performed until they lose weight (which they find difficult to accomplish). However, there is no evidence that obesity results in a poorer outcome.[23] A particular problem that warrants consideration is that people who attribute their symptoms to aging are more likely to consider that nothing can be done to help and less likely, therefore, to seek medical attention.[24,25] Indeed, joint pain in the elderly may be ignored because it is thought of as a normal consequence of aging.

Finally, it should be noted that a number of investigative surgical procedures, such as autologous chondrocyte transplantation,[26] use of mesenchymal stem cells,[27] and autologous osteochondral plugs (mosaicplasty),[28] are being evaluated for their utility in repair of isolated chondral defects, such as those as caused by traumatic injury. None of these procedures, however, is currently indicated for treatment of OA. Excellent reviews of the current status of research on regeneration of articular cartilage and articular cartilage transplantation have been published recently.[29,30]

REFERENCES

1. Owings MF, Kozak LJ. Ambulatory and inpatient procedures in the United States, 1996. Vital and health statistics. Series 13. No. 139. Hyattsville, Md.: National Center for Health Statistics, November 1998. DHHS publication no. (PHS) 99-1710.

2. Moseley JB, O'Malley K, Petersen NJ, et al. A controlled trial of arthroscopic surgery for osteoarthritis of the knee. *N Engl J Med.* 2002; 347:81-88.

3. Felson DT, Buckwalter J. Débridement and lavage for osteoarthritis of the knee. *N Engl J Med.* 2002;347:132-133.

4. Fortin PR, Clarke AE, Joseph L, et al. Outcomes of total hip and knee replacement: preoperative functional status predicts outcomes at six months after surgery. *Arthritis Rheum.* 1999;42:1722-1728.

5. Fortin PR, Penrod JR, Clarke AE, et al. Timing of total joint replacement affects clinical outcomes among patients with osteoarthritis of the hip or knee. *Arthritis Rheum.* 2002;46:3327-3330.

6. Sharrock NE, Cazan MG, Hargett MJ, Williams-Russo P, Wilson PD Jr. Changes in mortality after hip and knee arthroplasty over a ten-year period. *Anesth Analg.* 1995;80:242-248.

7. Knutson K. Arthroplasty and its complications. In: Brandt KD, Doherty M, Lohmander LS, eds. *Osteoarthritis.* Oxford, UK: Oxford University Press; 1998:388-402.

20

TABLE 20.2 — PHYSICAL FUNCTION AND PAIN 6 MONTHS AFTER TOTAL KNEE REPLACEMENT IN PATIENTS WHO HAD HIGH OR LOW FUNCTION AT BASELINE*

Outcome Measure	High Function at Baseline		Low Function at Baseline		Difference (high/low)	
	Mean = SD	95% CI	Mean ± SD	95% CI	Mean	95% CI
SF-36 physical function						
Baseline	37.3 ± 22.2	—	14.9 ± 12.2	—	22.4	15.5, 29.4
6 months	63.0 ± 25.0	—	47.0 ± 26.8	—	15.9	5.8, 26.0
Difference[†]	24.3	16.9, 31.8	31.6	23.6, 39.5	-7.2	-17.9, 3.5
WOMAC pain						
Baseline	7.8 ± 3.1	—	12.4 ± 2.7	—	-4.5	-5.7, -3.4
6 months	2.1 ± 2.5	—	5.9 ± 4.7	—	-3.8	-5.3, -2.3
Difference[†]	-5.6 ± 3.6	-6.6, -4.6	-6.8	-8.1, -5.4	1.1	-0.5, 2.8
WOMAC function						
Baseline	24.3 ± 8.2	—	44.2 ± 6.8	—	-19.9	-22.9, -17.0
6 months	9.5 ± 8.3	—	23.0 ± 16.6	—	-13.5	-18.7, -8.4
Difference[†]	-14.4	-16.9, -11.8	-21.8 ± 14.8	-26.0, -17.6	7.4	2.5, 12.2

Abbreviations: CI, confidence interval; SD, standard deviation; SF, short form; WOMAC, Western Ontario and McMaster Universities Osteoarthritis Index.

* The WOMAC subscale scores are a summation of the subscale itemized scores. A value of "0" was assigned if "none" was the answer reported, and a value of "4" if "extreme" was reported. Therefore, the range for WOMAC pain is 0-20 and for WOMAC function, 0-68. For the SF-36, a higher score represents better function; for WOMAC, a higher score represents worse limitation.

† From 6 months to baseline.

Fortin PR, et al. *Arthritis Rheum.* 1999;42:1722-1728.

20

8. Malchau H, Herberts P, Ahnfelt L. Prognosis of total hip replacement in Sweden. Follow-up of 92,675 operations performed 1978-1990. *Acta Orthop Scand*. 1993;64:497-506.

9. Knutson K, Lewold S, Robertsson O, Lidgren L. The Swedish knee arthroplasty register. A nation-wide study of 30,003 knees 1976-1992. *Acta Orthop Scand*. 1994;65:375-386.

10. Buckwalter JA, Lohmander S. Operative treatment of osteoarthritis. Current practice and future development. *J Bone Joint Surg*. 1994; 76:1405-1418.

11. Callahan CM, Drake BG, Heck DA, Dittus RS. Patient outcomes following tricompartmental total knee replacement. A meta-analysis. *JAMA*. 1994;271:1349-1357.

12. Rorabeck CH, Murray P. The cost benefit of total knee arthroplasty. *Orthopedics*. 1996;19:777-779.

13. Drewitt RF, Minns RJ, Sibley TF. Measuring outcome of total knee replacement using quality of life indices. *Ann R Coll Surg Engl*. 1992; 74:286-290.

14. Norman-Taylor FH, Palmer CR, Villar RN. Quality-of-life improvement compared after hip and knee replacement. *J Bone Joint Surg Br*. 1996;78:74-77.

15. Kirwan JR, Currey HL, Freeman MA, Snow S, Young PJ. Overall long-term impact of total hip and knee joint replacement surgery on patients with osteoarthritis and rheumatoid arthritis. *Br J Rheumatol*. 1994;33:357-360.

16. Wright JG, Coyte, P, Hawker G, et al. Variation in orthopedic surgeons' perceptions of the indications for and outcomes of knee replacement. *CMAJ*. 1995;152:687-697.

17. Coyte PC, Hawker G, Wright JG. Variations in knee replacement utilization rates and the supply of health professionals in Ontario, Canada. *J Rheumatol*. 1996;23:1214-1220.

18. Peterson MG, Hollenberg JP, Szatrowski TP, Johanson NA, Mancuso CA, Charlson ME. Geographic variations in the rates of elective total hip and knee arthroplasties among Medicare beneficiaries in the United States. *J Bone Joint Surg Am*. 1992;74:1530-1539.

19. Freund DA, Dittus RS. Assessing and improving outcomes: total knee replacement. Final report of the patient outcomes research team (PORT). Washington, AHCPR Pub. No. 97-N015, 1997.

20. Tennant A, Fear J, Pickering A, Hillman M, Cutts A, Chamberlain MA. Prevalence of knee problems in the population aged 55 years and over: identifying the need for knee arthroplasty. *BMJ*. 1995; 310:1291-1293.

21. Dieppe P, Basler HD, Chard J, et al. Knee replacement surgery for osteoarthritis: effectiveness, practice variations, indications and possible determinants of utilization. *Rheumatology.* 1999;38:73-83.

22. Mazzuca SA, Brandt KD, Katz BP, Li W, Stewart KD. Therapeutic strategies distinguish community based primary care physicians from rheumatologists in the management of osteoarthritis. *J Rheumatol.* 1993;20:80-86.

23. Stern SH, Insall JN. Total knee arthroplasty in obese patients. *J Bone Joint Surg Am.* 1990;72:1400-1404.

24. Prohaska TR, Keller ML, Leventhal EA, Leventhal H. Impact of symptoms and aging attribution on emotions and coping. *Health Psychol.* 1987;6:495-514.

25. Wolinsky FD, Johnson RJ. The use of health services by older adults. *J Gerontol.* 1991;46:S345-S357.

26. Brittberg M, Nilsson A, Lindahl A, Ohlsson C, Peterson L. Rabbit articular cartilage defects treated with autologous cultured chondrocytes. *Clin Orthop.* 1996;326:270-283.

27. Wakitani S, Goto T, Pineda SJ, et al. Mesenchymal cell-based repair of large, full-thickness defects of articular cartilage. *J Bone Joint Surg Am.* 1994;76:579-592.

28. Hangody L, Kish G, Karpati Z, Eberhart R. Osteochondral plugs: autogenous osteochondral mosaicplasty for the treatment of focal chondral and osteochondral articular defects. *Operative Tech Orthop.* 1997;7:312-322.

29. O'Driscoll SW. The healing and regeneration of articular cartilage. *J Bone Joint Surg Am.* 1998;80:1795-1812.

30. Buckwalter JA, Mankin HJ. Articular cartilage repair and transplantation. *Arthritis Rheum.* 1998;41:1331-1342.

20

INDEX

Note: OA stands for osteoarthritis. Page numbers in *italics* refer to figures.
Page numbers followed by t indicate tables. CP stands for color plates.

21

333

21

335

336

21

337

340

21

21